Integrative Pathways

Angele McGrady • Donald Moss

Integrative Pathways

Navigating Chronic Illness with a Mind-Body-Spirit Approach

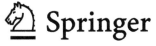 Springer

Angele McGrady, PhD
Department of Psychiatry
University of Toledo
Toledo, OH, USA

Donald Moss, PhD Dean
College of Integrative Medicine
and Health Sciences
Saybrook University
Oakland, CA, USA

ISBN 978-3-319-89311-2   ISBN 978-3-319-89313-6   (eBook)
https://doi.org/10.1007/978-3-319-89313-6

Library of Congress Control Number: 2018940264

Printed on acid-free paper

This Springer imprint is published by the registered company Springer International Publishing AG part of Springer Nature.
The registered company address is: Gewerbestrasse 11, 6330 Cham, Switzerland

"Research on mind/body health has exploded over the last several decades, documenting the profound interconnections between mental and physical health. Integrative models explaining these relationships, however, have been lacking. The Pathways Model addresses what clinical researchers in the field have been calling for, a research-based approach to health and wellness that clearly explains important concepts and provides an optimal foundation from which to approach health interventions."

—Patrick R. Steffen, PhD, BCB, *Professor of Psychology and Director of Clinical Training, Brigham Young University, President-elect, Association for Applied Psychophysiology and Biofeedback*

"The harsh reality is that the number of people who are currently suffering and who will be suffering the ravages of serious chronic illness is steadily increasing. In this exceptionally lucid and timely volume, the authors reach far, wide and deep into the clinical literature as well as their direct experiences of helping people. Together, they bring readers a sophisticated multi-level approach to a true integrative medicine that is inspiring. Their Pathways Model is rich in substance and flexible in approach, which all health care providers will appreciate. They thoughtfully acknowledge the power of the individual to make good health a priority and recovering from bad health a realistic and hopeful possibility."

—Michael D. Yapko, PhD, Author of *Depression is Contagious* and *Keys to Unlocking Depression*

"There is very little guidance for both treatment professionals and health and wellness coaches for how to work together, in an integrated manner, for the health and wellness of a person with some form of chronic illness. McGrady and Moss bridge this gap beautifully with their new book. As both a psychologist and coach who has trained thousands of health and wellness coaches, I am heartened to find such a contribution."

—Michael Arloski, PhD, PCC, CWP, NBW-HWC, *CEO and Founder, Real Balance Global Wellness Services, Inc.*, Author of *Wellness Coaching for Lasting Lifestyle Change (Whole Person Associates)*

Foreword

I have known Donald Moss and Angele McGrady for over 30 years and have always considered them to be among the most respected and skilled clinicians in our field. In this book, they have consolidated all of their valuable experience to construct a comprehensive model for treatment in Integrative and Integrated Care. Their insights into chronic illness, while relying heavily on sound scientific findings and principles, are firmly centered around compassion, mind-body science (psychophysiology), spirituality, and modern evidence-based psychotherapeutic approaches. This book should be invaluable for any clinicians willing to expand their horizons to multi-method approaches to difficult chronic illnesses.

The first chapter lays out the scope of the public issues created by chronic illness. It summarizes the underlying science relevant to the complex interactions between biology, neurophysiology, psychological phenomenon, and illness. It makes clear that narrow-minded approaches that rely only on medication, diet, or mind-body practices will not be sufficient to deal with the catastrophic consequences, both financially and in terms of human suffering of the mushrooming growth of chronic illness. A wonderful feature of the book is that case histories are scattered within the text to humanize the principles being discussed.

The Pathways Model is laid out in the second chapter. This is a model first published by the authors in 2013 and is expanded in great detail here. The Pathways consist of three levels that range from lifestyle changes to professional interventions. Factors broadly labeled as spiritual are always included. Case histories representing this approach are presented in the subsequent chapters that explore a number of disorders or presenting complaints.

Chapters 3–5 explore factors that are common to all of the pathways: coping, positive psychology, spirituality, and complementary/alternative medicine approaches. These chapters offer an informed, yet open-minded, approach to these sometimes controversial topics.

The remainder of the book is devoted to specific kinds of problems: pain, mood disorders, PTSD, anxiety, metabolic syndrome, cardiovascular disorders, lupus, cancer, traumatic brain injury, and substance abuse problems. In each chapter an overview of the disorder, existing evidence for etiology and treatment, and case histories that illustrate the pathways treatment are presented.

In conclusion, I am sure that anyone interested in approaches that are not simplistic or the latest fad will find this book of great value. It constantly forces the reader to think in compassionate ways about the patients with chronic disorders without blame or "silver bullets." It is the only book that I know of that includes a sophisticated approach to the place of biofeedback or applied psychophysiology within integrative healthcare. I can recommend it without reservation.

California School of Professional Psychology   Richard Gevirtz
Alliant International University
San Diego, CA, USA

Acknowledgments

As I finish this book, I remember the past, the legacy of scholarly work left by my parents, Drs. Fernand and Santina Vial, lifelong teachers and learners. In the present, I deeply appreciate my husband Patrick, son Kevin, and daughter-in-law Brandy for their love and encouragement as I conceptualized this book, researched it, wrote, and completed it. I wish success to my daughter Michele in her chosen career. I am most grateful to my "girlfriends" for their support and good humor and the time that we spend together. I appreciate my colleagues in the Department of Psychiatry for their insights as we discussed patients and the best educational approaches for medical trainees. Throughout my life, I have been blessed with personal and career mentors who guided me and believed in me. I thank my patients who shared their stories of suffering with me, trusted me, and showed incredible personal strength during our hours together. The cases used in this book are composites of many of those stories. Finally, as I look toward the future, I hope for happy and successful lives for Louwyn and Evelyn McGrady, who perhaps will carry on the legacy of love of learning from their parents, grandparents, and great grandparents.

Angele McGrady

I thank my wife Nancy for the example she has provided of living fully with chronic illness.

I am thankful for the assistance of our coauthor on Chap. 3, Jennifer Heintzman (Saybrook University).

I thank my research assistant, Shannon McLain, for her invaluable pursuit of relevant research. I thank my colleagues in integrative medicine, Angele McGrady, Fredric Shaffer, Eric Willmarth, Richard Gevirtz, Erik Peper, and Gabriel Sella, for their encouragement, example, and inspiration.

I thank my clients, who implemented so many of the lifestyle modifications described in this book, and shared their triumphs and setbacks with me. The case narratives are composites from their lives, modified for anonymity, but preserving, I hope, their passion for living and their determination to move toward *mindbodyspirit* well-being.

Donald Moss

Contents

About the Authors

Angele McGrady received her B.S. from Chestnut Hill College in Philadelphia, her Master's in Physiology from Michigan State University, and her Ph.D. in Biology from the University of Toledo. Later she completed her M.Ed. in Guidance and Counseling. She is a licensed Professional Clinical Counselor. She is certified by the Biofeedback Certification Institute of America and is also a certified sports counselor. Currently Dr. McGrady is a professor in the Department of Psychiatry at the University of Toledo. She has extensive experience teaching medical, graduate medical, and undergraduate students at the University of Toledo, and received the Dean's Award for Teaching Excellence from the medical school. Dr. McGrady is a Past President of the Association for Applied Psychophysiology and Biofeedback and is on the editorial board of the international journal *Applied Psychophysiology and Biofeedback*. In March 2000, she received the Distinguished Scientist Award from the Association for Applied Psychophysiology and Biofeedback. She lectures locally and nationally on topics related to stress, behavioral medicine, and biofeedback and conducts programs on wellness and building resiliency for healthcare professionals. Her curriculum vitae lists 83 publications and 22 book chapters. She has coedited one book, *Handbook of Mind-Body Medicine for Primary Care,* with Dr. Donald Moss and others and coauthored a book with Dr. Donald Moss: *Pathways to Illness, Pathways to Health,* published in 2013.

Donald Moss is Dean of the College of Integrative Medicine and Health Sciences at Saybrook University, Oakland, CA. There he has built training programs in biofeedback, clinical hypnosis, integrative mental health, wellness coaching, and integrative/functional nutrition. Dr. Moss is currently President of the Society for Clinical and Experimental Hypnosis and previously served as president of Division 30 (hypnosis) of the American Psychological Association and president of the Association for Applied Psychophysiology and Biofeedback (AAPB). He is also the ethics chair for the Biofeedback Certification International Alliance.

Moss is coeditor of *Foundations of Heart Rate Variability Biofeedback* (AAPB, 2016), coauthor of *Pathways to Illness, Pathways to Health* (Springer, 2013), and chief editor of *Handbook of Mind-Body Medicine for Primary Care* (Sage, 2003) and *Humanistic and Transpersonal Psychology* (Greenwood, 1998). He has a book in preparation for AAPB with coeditor Inna Khazan on *Mindfulness, Compassion, and Biofeedback Practice*. He has published over 60 articles and chapters on consciousness, psychophysiology, spirituality in health, and integrative medicine.

Chapter 1
Mind, Body, and Spirit in Chronic Illness

Abstract This chapter provides an introduction to chronic illness as conceptualized in the Pathways Model. Health care expenditures and the major conditions requiring costly medical care are discussed. The importance of environment, socioeconomic status, and developmental factors are highlighted. Several patient cases are utilized to demonstrate multiple risk factors, both biological and psychosocial, that increase the probability of developing a chronic illness. Patients describe in their own words the aspects of their background with which they have struggled. Adversity during the critical developmental period of childhood has ramifications for morbidity well into the adult years. Individuals who have experienced emotional, physical, or sexual abuse are at great risk for chronic illness, particularly pain conditions, depressive disorders, and cardiovascular disease. At similar risk are minimally educated, low-income patients who reside in a high stress neighborhood. The influence of lifestyle, particularly inactivity and high fat, high sugar diets is explored within the context of personal decisions and choices made by individuals. Isolated patients without social support who do not have a stable home suffer the effects of their environment both emotionally and physically. Chronic stress, due also to the illness itself, is associated with damaging effects mediated through the nervous system and the immune complex. First, the mind, body, and spiritual aspects of chronic illness are explored, and then they are correlated with the levels of intervention in the Pathways Model.

Keywords Chronic illness · Chronic stress · Lifestyle · Spirituality

Introduction: Health Care for Chronic Illness

Spending on health care in the United States has undergone a steady increase. Data from insurance claims, government spending, and facility surveys for the years 1996–2013 were analyzed in a comprehensive report of health care costs and the major conditions requiring these expenditures. From this information, trends in costs of care and spending on conditions separated by gender, age, and ethnicity were ascertained. Diabetes, ischemic heart disease, low back pain, and neck pain

© Springer International Publishing AG, part of Springer Nature 2018   1
A. McGrady, D. Moss, *Integrative Pathways*,
https://doi.org/10.1007/978-3-319-89313-6_1

were the conditions with the highest medical and surgical expenditures (Dieleman et al., 2016). From 1996 through 2013, $30.1 trillion dollars was expended on personal health care for physical and mental illness. Of the 143 conditions analyzed, spending on low back pain, neck pain, and diabetes increased the most over the 18 years' time span. It is noteworthy that the most expensive conditions are preventable at least in part and are linked to behavior and personal choices. The impact of pain, diabetes, and heart disease on the individual's functioning can be modified, and sometimes, significantly lessened by use of complementary therapies in conjunction with medical interventions. However, reimbursement for the former is generally low, despite increasing evidence for efficacy.

Behavioral Influences in Chronic Illness

The major behaviors associated with chronic illness are grouped under the heading of lifestyle and consist of nutrition, activity, and stress responses. Lifestyle medicine is informed by significant research indicating that these modifiable behaviors—especially physical inactivity, unhealthy eating, and hyper reactivity to stress—are the major drivers of mortality, disease, and health care costs in the United States. In addition, the global burden of disease from chronic illnesses related to behavior can be described as frightening; as the population ages, the burden is likely to increase (Global Burden of Disease Study 2013 Collaborators, 2015).

Being physically active decreases the risks for congestive heart failure, chronic obstructive pulmonary disease (COPD), and diabetes. Changing from inactivity, basically a sedentary lifestyle, to moderate activity confers a significant benefit to mental and physical health (Pearce, 2008). Interestingly, people with the most to gain from increasing physical activity are those classified as "inactive"; the group who has the most to gain from a weight loss program is the group that is most overweight; persons suffering from severe anxiety notice when their worry and nervousness has decreased by even a small amount and moderate improvement in anxiety is significant for many patients. Lifestyle factors overlap and interact. The patient who becomes more active experiences improved mood and is more motivated to walk more often or for longer distances. Patients who regularly relax their mind and body can focus more easily on preparing a healthy meal. The interaction among lifestyle factors is demonstrated by an interesting study of the benefits of a low-fat meal compared to consuming food high in saturated fat in two different stress conditions. (Kiecolt-Glaser et al., 2016) showed that a high saturated fat meal and a low saturated fat meal had the same effects on inflammatory markers and adhesion molecules *if* participants eating low fat also experienced recent distress.

Lifestyle medicine acknowledges the impact of peoples' behavior and choices in mental and physical health; the supporting database continues to grow and so does media and public interest (Rippe & Angelopoulos, 2011; Yeh & Kong, 2013). However, most Americans fail to meet recommendations for nutrition, with disparities evident by race/ethnicity, and socioeconomic status. High fat, low fiber, and low fruit and vegetable consumption are correlated with poorer health. Inactive people overloaded with calories generally feel unwell with a pervasive sense of malaise. It follows that the types of food that are consumed affect psychological state, particularly mood and cognition, the ability to concentrate and pay attention. Furthermore, people often make food choices depending on how they feel at the time and what they believe the positive effects of consumption of that food will be. Specific foods bring back memories that may be positive or negative. The smell of yeast rolls can elicit a pleasant memory of Mom's kitchen where there was safety and love or can bring back a painful image of walking past a bakery with no money to purchase bread.

Not feeling well does not bode well for motivation. For example, a patient with a painful back admitted that she had planned to cook a healthy meal but could not stand at the stove long enough; another patient similarly reported that he ran out of time to cook dinner for the family because he had to rest after work. Lack of motivation in general carries over into workplace performance. Eventually, persons who feel unwell or sluggish focus more and more on physical symptoms; they experience a decline in productivity, often resulting in criticism by their employer. The employee who cannot keep up with the demands of the job is often the one who will be the first to be laid off and will subsequently be faced with lower income, less buying power, and further decreases in self-esteem.

Changing behaviors related to choice of food and quantity of consumption has demonstrable positive effects short term and long term (Wang, Li, Chiuve, Hu, & Willett, 2015). When food choices were investigated over a 12-year period, improved nutritional quality was shown to correlate with fewer deaths. Dietary intervention studies show that in the examples of both cardiovascular disease and diabetes risk decreases quickly. Changes such as limiting saturated fat and increasing consumption of fruit, whole grains, and legumes help the individual to feel better and decreases risk for lifestyle-related chronic illnesses in the coming years.

Psychosocial Effects on Chronic Illness

Economic inequality is a major determinant of both lifestyle choices and prevalence of the major medical and psychiatric disorders. Poverty in childhood is associated with anxiety, depression, and behavior problems that persist into adulthood (Manseau, 2014). Household poverty is stressful. It is not only that children lack opportunity and suffer deprivation. But the type of stimulation to which they are exposed is in the form of loud noises, bright lights, traffic-congested streets, and violence, which is over-stimulation of the wrong kind, i.e., frightening stimulation instead of growth enhancing sound, light, and language (Todman & Holliday, 2015). Coping with food insecurity requires energy that those with reliable food resources can conserve for other activities. Hungry grade school children are thinking about food, not math problems or spelling words.

An obvious short-term repercussion of inactivity and unhealthy eating appears in body mass index (BMI), where disparities are evident along socioeconomic lines, specifically by gender, ethnicity, and economic status. To facilitate analysis of large data, simulation models were developed to identify environmental factors and behavioral patterns that affected lifestyle decision-making. The long-term goal was to find ways to reduce disparities in BMI between blacks and whites (Orr, Kaplan, & Galea, 2016), by first studying what social and economic factors influence the BMI. The distance from the supermarket in comparison to fast food locations or mini-marts, availability of safe open spaces for physical activity, and the quality of schools in the area were studied and found related to disparities in body mass index between blacks and white, with blacks being heavier.

For example, observing the retail food environment across neighborhoods illustrates that in predominantly African-American neighborhoods housing is closer to liquor stores or convenience stores than to supermarkets. Measured satisfaction with the location of the supermarket is not due exclusively to prices, but is related to the effort required to travel to shop and concentration of the minority population (Zenk et al., 2009). Yet, the assumption that the distance from a supermarket directly correlates with more unhealthy food choices is correct only to a point. Well-educated persons who believe that their choices are related to health outcomes will travel to stores where they can purchase healthy food, no matter the distance. Reducing *food deserts* (distance of greater than 2 miles between home and supermarket) is not the only factor in improving diet (Block & Subramanian, 2015).

Simulation also revealed an important effect of social norms. Increasing visibility of positive social behaviors related to healthy eating increased consumption by 7% in fruits and vegetables and lowered fast food consumption. Decisions about diet are partially influenced by whether people see others similar to themselves making choices of fruits and vegetables instead of foods with high fat and sugar density (Zhang, Giabbanelli, Arah, & Zimmerman, 2014).

Krueger and Reither (2015) summarized nine possible mechanisms, grouped into three categories: biological factors, health behaviors, and social environment to explain differences in obesity rates among ethnic groups. The differences are not trivial, with the highest rates in blacks (47%), followed by Hispanics, whites, and Asians (10.9%). Important conclusions emanating from this review highlighted the need to consider the context where the prevalence of obesity is greatest, such as low-income neighborhoods with less well-educated residents, the positive or negative influence of social connections, and the importance of early life experiences.

Expanding on this theme, education provides the gateway to obtain better employment and a higher wage. Without a high school education individuals earn minimum wage and therefore can only afford to live in low-income neighborhoods. The specific effect of home stability and neighborhood on lifestyle may be more dramatic in childhood but its effects continue into adulthood (Hudson, 2005). Years of education are correlated with life expectancy; those who do not finish high school have a much shorter life span than college graduates. Women with a high school education are predicted to live 74 years and men 68 years. In contrast, female college graduates have a life expectancy of 83 years and men 77 years. Efforts to dissect the factors that increase predicted life span have consistently emphasized education as the major factor. Between 1980 and 2000, the increases in life expectancy were far from uniform, favoring well-educated, high-income non-minority individuals (Meara, Richards, & Dutler, 2008; Todman & Diaz, 2014).

Over time, socioeconomic status may worsen, improve, or remain the same. If the individual seeks additional education, for example, the high school graduate attending a two-year college, that choice will improve the individual's ability to obtain more lucrative employment. In a study by Kiviruusu, Huure, Haukala, and Aro (2013) psychological or coping resources (the ability to problem solve and the degree of self-confidence) were studied over 10 years in people from different socioeconomic status levels; socioeconomic status (SES) was indexed only by years of education. Daily stress forced people to use energy for coping; psychological resources declined over time, and there was a stronger effect of SES on health. Worrying about food availability and living in noisy, poorly heated apartments produces wear and tear on the body, mind, and spirit. Adverse childhood events (ACE) become the foundation for delays in cognitive and emotional development. The child is forced to focus on adult themes instead of on academic learning and age appropriate social behavior. High risk behaviors often overlap and influence each other placing the individual with more than one high risk behavior at greater risk for chronic illness (Center for Disease Control, 2013). The memories of past adversity linger and may return during current stressful circumstances. In contrast, if the person can build psychological resources through therapy, support, and spirituality, then the effect of low SES is apparently less potent.

Multiple major life events in a year, whether positive or negative, increase the demand for adjustment and coping. Depression and anxiety simultaneously drain psychological resources and are the result of declining resources. Recalling the model of Cohen and Rodriguez (1995), affective disturbances that may be subclinical affect physical illness and illness behavior, which feedback to worsen mood and anxiety. Taxing the system over time creates allostatic load, which manifests in physical and emotional ways (Juster, McEwen, & Lupien, 2010). Chronic physical illness or emotional instability are major factors impacting allocation of personal and financial resources, as the person needs to make appointments, undergo testing, begins treatment, and commits to long-term care.

Coping with Chronic Illness

Receiving a diagnosis of a disorder sometimes provides relief as individuals have been experiencing bodily sensations or emotional reactions that they could not explain (Edwards, 2013). They have suffered but did not know why; perhaps they were blamed by family and friends. However, if the diagnosis has the adjective "chronic" attached to it, then the patients' relief is short lived. The patients realize that there will be times of better health and other times of declining health, but the uncertainty about prognosis may be the most draining (Johnson, Afari, & Zautra, 2009; Johnson, Zautra, & Davis, 2006). Patients may realize much later that some of the control over the illness belongs to them, but initially, they often feel overwhelmed and identify more with dependence than with feeling powerful. Again, conflicting emotional reactions, such as hope, anger, and sadness, may accompany the realization that their illness will be in them for months and years. Individuals who tend to be more perfectionistic may blame themselves and attribute the illness to their own fault; they "should have known;" they "ought to have kept their weight down."

Naming the illness can bring additional stress. A diagnosis of congestive heart failure may emphasize *failure* as in personal failure. Patients want to follow a treatment plan, but each day that they do not follow it to the letter is further evidence of personal failure. Stoeber and Janssen (2011) differentiate between perfectionistic concerns and positive striving for better outcomes. The patient with Type 2 diabetes must accept that there is no perfect control of blood glucose and some variations will not be explainable. Resentment easily builds in patients with the perfectionistic mindset who believe: "no matter what I do, I will need insulin injections within five years." In contrast to heart failure, the diagnosis of *heart attack* connotes a different psychological response, often aggression. A person can fight back after a heart *attack* but can one fight a *failing* heart? (Yu, 2008).

Anger is frequently observed in persons with chronic illness. Frustration emerges after months of vague diagnoses, unsympathetic friends or family, and growing financial burdens due to missed work. The clinician must address anger issues if this emotion is the major reaction to a diagnosis or a treatment plan (Brennan, 2011). Patients are not necessarily aware of why they feel angry or why they are behaving badly toward the people who are taking care of them. Rapid, almost reflex-like reactions can occur outside of conscious awareness, including words, facial expression, and body language. Adults who grew up in households frequently filled with angry voices or physical aggression may demonstrate the same reactions to the health care team after diagnosis and during treatment. They have not learned to express emotions in healthier, less confrontational ways, so when they are frightened or unsure, they react defensively.

Repeated exposure to criticism from others is damaging to the self-esteem of the person with chronic illness. One harsh statement or misunderstanding is hurtful, but frequent negative interactions with health care workers and their perceived disapproval of the patient slowly create a reservoir of rage. As described in several of the case examples in this volume, patients with chronic illness referred for mental health treatment often arrive with resentment and anger, in addition to depression and anxiety, which have complicated their medical illness and interfered with the course of treatment to that point. Most distressing are the belief that one has done everything to maintain health and the experience of the person who was completely healthy at the last checkup. For example, an illness with a genetic component not expected to emerge until older age is diagnosed in middle adulthood. When information about genetic susceptibility is presented to the patient for the purposes of clarification, it may instead have the opposite effect—the patient becomes angrier and feels more helpless. "This couldn't happen to me." "I take care of myself".

Case of Nadine

Nadine was a 57-year-old white woman who came to the clinic with complaints of depression and pain from fibromyalgia. She had applied for disability from social security but her application was rejected. She reported symptoms of tearfulness and sadness and loss of motivation and occasional difficulties concentrating. She had resigned from her job because her functioning became impaired due to pain; she was afraid of being written-up and decided to resign before she was fired.

At the second session, Nadine said that she was aware of the risk factors for chronic illness, including the fact that she had been the victim of physical abuse during her childhood. Nadine was the youngest of three children. She was an unwanted child born 10 years later than her brother and was made to suffer for it, experiencing physical punishment for even minor transgressions. Her parents fought often and sometimes their fights became violent. When she began to get ill in her early 50s Nadine researched fibromyalgia and the frequently comorbid depression. She said: "I know that I have most of the risk factors for chronic illness, so it seems that I was destined to get this. It's hard to think that my childhood had such a great effect on my life as I am living it now. We are financially stable because my husband has a good job, but I can't work anymore. My husband tries to understand but becomes frustrated when we have to cancel plans because I have so much pain. My father died a few years ago, my mother is alive and in fairly good health at age 85, but I speak to her rarely. I am still so angry with both of them. My parents' abuse of me sealed my fate."

Risk Factors for Chronic Illness

Most chronic illnesses have an identifiable genetic component, which contributes in varying degrees to the emergence of that illness. Epigenetics is the science of interacting genetics and environment when experience, learning, and social interactions modify the genetic template without altering the basic DNA sequence. Most chronic illnesses emerge as epigenetic phenomena. The identifiable hereditary factors predict only a small portion of the prevalence with multiple genes involved in a single illness. Heredity factors will not be covered here, so the reader is referred to the chapter on genetics in McGrady and Moss (2013).

Some of what individuals experience during the early years of life is forgotten and no longer resides in the conscious or unconscious mind. But some memories, both positive and negative, are retained. Fear during the original event makes memories more permanent because of the emotion tied to the memory and the repeated re-experiencing of the event. Synapses strengthen due to strong stimulation, information coming into the brain from multiple sources (sight, smell, sound), and the value attached to the stimulus reinforce the memory (Purves et al., 2012).

In addition, fear responses are linked to threats to survival and are therefore reinforced further. What the person perceives as important is repeated in the mind, thereby providing a strengthening message to those synapses (Gardner, 2008). In this context, one can understand why unrelated numbers are the hardest to recall, words linked to emotion are easier to remember than neutral phrases and negative experiences consolidate more completely than pleasant memories. Fear and negative events that occur during childhood have documented effects on physical and emotional health in the short term and increase the risk of chronic illness (Heim, Shugart, Graighead, & Nemeroff, 2010). The mechanisms responsible for these effects are detailed further in later sections.

Environmental Effects on Chronic Illness

An exploration of the effects of environment on human behavior during illness leads us to delve into basic biology textbooks. Non-human mammals must constantly adapt to changes in their surroundings to survive. Exposure to harsh environments in nature forces animals to adapt or perish. The chameleon changes colors to blend in with bushes and other vegetation. Birds living in the rain forest grow strong, longer beaks. When winter comes to the northern hemisphere, days are shorter and colder and animals store food and grow thicker coats. When the snow and the ice come to the land, the bears go into a common den, where they will be close to others and not alone to face the harsh conditions (Blix, 2016). The heat and broiling sun come to the dessert, but still plants grow and flower. There is hardly any water, but the gecko has prepared for this and thrives. In the high mountains, the air is thin and the soil is barren. Grass is sparse and there are only rocks. Still, some plants emerge and adapted animals live and bear young (Michigan State University, 2001).

All living creatures including people are faced with harsh, hostile environments at some time in their lives. What can be learned and applied to human survival from the animals in the arctic or desert? Consciously or unconsciously, people change in response to their personal environment, house or apartment, and of course, weather conditions in their area in addition to interactions with family and friends. People become attached to their "place" meaning the familiar brick or shingles of their residence, and the people with whom they feel connected (Knez, 2005). If exposed to multiple moves, children no longer feel relevant to a home, neighborhood, or school. Coupled with instability within the home, minimal attachment to place intensifies the experience of being disconnected, not fitting in, or searching for people with similar tendencies, whether those are positive or negative influences. When survival is threatened, animals will stay close to the pack leader, rarely venturing out on their own. In nature, isolation is death.

The Case of Celine

Celine was a 19-year-old college student who was referred for panic disorder. She was attending college full time and working part time at a local bakery. Celine was the daughter of a US Navy captain and a stay-at-home mom; she had two younger sisters. Her father had been promoted up the ranks in the Navy, which necessitated nine moves before Celine finished high school. When the team conducted the Pathways evaluation of Celine and asked her about her concept of home, she laughed at us:

What do you mean by home? I moved nine times against my will between kindergarten and 12th grade. Each move except for two was extremely difficult. The reason that the two were less traumatic [that was her word choice] was that I was already so miserable in those places that I didn't think it could get any worse. I'm pretty outgoing and do make friends pretty easily, but when you ask me about home I'm stumped for an answer. My college apartment is filled with my roommates' junk. I like them as people but they're messy and unorganized. In a year, I will graduate and then what? When I think about the future, my anxiety overwhelms me. I don't know where to go or what I want to do. My parents have moved again during the time that I have been in college. In a way, my roommates' junk makes me feel secure because it reminds me of their presence—I believe they are coming back "home".

Home is a concept with universal meaning; it is cross cultural and multigenerational. When home connotes stability and happiness, the person is drawn to it and craves the return to home. Turning a corner of the neighborhood street and seeing a lighted window magnetizes the pull toward home (Museum of Modern Art, 2015). People anticipating "home" experience an increase in heart rate and breathing even as they imagine and anticipate the physical safety of home and the people waiting for them. In contrast, if the image of "home" contains violent scenes, pain, or deprivation, the person's physiological response may be the same (rapid heart rate and breathing), but safety does not ensue when they open the door. Instead, the system goes on high alert mentally and physically. Furthermore, leaving "home" is contextually different depending on whether the individuals are fleeing "home," being moved against their will to a nursing facility, or whether the person is leaving for college, marriage, or job opportunity because of their own choice.

Life changes require adaptation and drain energy, whether these changes are positive or negative. Coping resources are taxed due to an accumulation of negative events, but an overload of positive situations can also exhaust the system. The listing of "life events" in the Social Readjustment Scale totals positive and negative events during the past year, and the total is correlated with risk for mental or physical illness (Hobson et al., 1998; Holmes & Rahe, 1967). The more coping energy required in daily life, the greater the stress on the mind-body-spirit. Early adversity in the form of low socioeconomic status has enduring effects, partially because of repeated stress on the mind-body-spirit, requiring adaptation and adjustment during the same time that the brain is developing. Certain circumstances, as in the case of Darnell described below, may elicit memories of past difficulties which were overcome but remain just below the surface.

The Case of Darnell

Darnell was a 30-year-old black man who was referred to us by his girlfriend who threatened to leave him if he didn't get help. Darnell was laid off from his job at the local auto factory where he had worked for 8 years. He was proud of his work record. During the past year, he had experienced headaches and back pain, which had steadily increased in frequency. He had not sought any medical attention for the pain because he was worried that the doctor would want him to take time off, and he did not want to lose the pay. Now, after the layoff, he continued to have pain but not as often. There was no specific call back date from his employer so he spent his days playing video games and hanging out with other laid off co-workers. His girlfriend became more and more frustrated and angry with him.

Darnell grew up as one of two children of a single mother who worked full time. The family struggled to keep afloat because mom's job was minimum wage. Mom worked and as a baby, Darnell was left with neighbors or relatives. Darnell was 2 years older than his sister and from the age of eight he was given responsibility for her. On one occasion, Darnell's sister hurt herself and bled profusely. Darnell and his sister were terrified that she was dying so they ran into the hallway of their apartment screaming. A neighbor came out and took the children to the local emergency room. Mom was called at her job to come to the hospital; she arrived furious that they had not been able to take care of themselves. For Darnell, now under the stress of job loss and financial insecurity, the anger, frustration, and hopelessness of those years returned in full force. Darnell felt helpless again and frightened that his girlfriend would leave him. He sought the distractions of video gaming and used more alcohol to blunt some of the fear. Mentally, he was back in the low-income neighborhood of his childhood. He felt paralyzed to make a change and at the same time felt terrified at the consequences of not making a change. He feared losing all that he had worked for and everything important to him.

Darnell was fortunate because he had a girlfriend who cared about him and forced him into coming to a therapist for an evaluation. Isolation worsens the effects of stress in people, they become more vulnerable without support. After trauma, feeling disconnected from family and friends leads to higher risk for emotional illness. The severity of trauma, the proximity to traumatic stimuli, and the person's coping ability are important factors, but are not the sum-total of influence on risk. The person's sense of connectedness with others, and the perceived availability of social support and community resources are also highly relevant (Dorahy et al., 2009). Darnell had pulled himself out of the deprivation of his childhood, but a "triggering" event—the layoff—challenged his sense of self-efficacy; in his mind, he was a child again. Unfortunately, the effects of low SES and the resulting health disparities are often transmitted from generation to generation unless a positive "signal" event occurs or the person develops mastery coping skills and better self-esteem (Thoits, 2010).

Personal Choices About Health-Related Behaviors

It is important to return to basic principles to begin to understand the choices people with chronic illness make and the actions that they take. An important driver of behavior is fear. If the world is experienced as a dangerous place, then the person may be extremely reluctant to compromise safety in any regard whether this is physical safety in sport, or emotional safety in fear of mental abuse (Bourne, 1998). Similarly, if the medical world (hospital, clinic, medication) is thought to be harmful or threatening or the health care providers seem not to act in the patient's best interest, the patient will resist. Fear can also lead to the patient hiding their own wishes, becoming subservient to the predominant social group (doctors), and acquiescence to the ideas and wishes of the medical system. Disclosure of one's own needs or one's own beliefs may be perceived as very hazardous for the person who is dominated by a core fear because the person expects criticism or disdain from others. The fear of rejection of one's body as diseased and imperfect may play out in psychological self-criticism (negative statements about the self), in behavioral self-criticism (cutting or harming the self), or in a combination of the two (starvation in anorexia). Often, a turning point in therapy is reached by accepting the patient's refusal of a treatment or lifestyle suggestion; instead of the patient continuing to verbalize intractable opposition, acceptance of the patient's decision softens the resistance and opens the door for productive dialogue.

People also make decisions based on their beliefs about the situation and their assessment of their abilities to act in their own behalf. Robert, a 36-year-old man just diagnosed with Type 2 diabetes expressed the following thoughts: "If I act in this way, I expect this consequence. If I control my blood glucose with diet, I may not need insulin." Mental calculation of the anticipated effort and the cost in time and dollars balance against the expected outcome of making that change. Prior research has shown that outcome expectancies are related to self-care behaviors in individuals with Type 2 diabetes mellitus. However, individuals with Type 2 diabetes generally have low outcome expectancies regarding the effect of exercise on blood glucose (Gibson et al., 2012). Having to make a decision quickly increases the role of instinct over rational thought. In chronic illness, pain, high blood glucose, and decreased perfusion to the brain create difficulties in concentration and cloud decision-making abilities. Fast, less well thought-out decisions, based mostly on primitive instincts, are not in most patients' best interest and should be deflected by the health care provider. Unfortunately, in a busy medical practice, quick decisions about care are often encouraged instead of discouraged.

Perceived behavioral control is comprised of self-efficacy—the person's ability to perform a difficult behavior, its controllability, and the extent to which the actual action depends on the person and not others. An intended behavior may be limited by problems in execution. If people are realistic when they decide to change a behavior, perceived behavioral control is close to actual control. The theory of planned behavior (Ajzen, 2002) is guided by beliefs about the normative expectations of other people, factors that encourage or prevent performance of the behavior, and beliefs about the consequences of the behavior. Social groupings (family, neighborhood, school, and work) will affect both the person's perceptions and the probability of positive or negative outcomes. These factors are particularly relevant to lifestyle choices, which are strongly influenced by the social context and beliefs about personal efficacy.

Spirituality in Chronic Illness: The Case of Jeremy

Jeremy was a 19-year-old male who grew up as the son of a church pastor. He was an only child in a stable home in a small-sized Midwestern city. Four years ago, Jeremy was diagnosed with Type 1 diabetes mellitus, after only a few weeks of symptoms. His parents were both frightened and devastated. They had been overprotective during Jeremy's youth, watching his diet closely and making sure he got enough sleep so they couldn't understand why this had happened to their son. After high school, many teens left the area for college or employment, anxious to leave the small city and explore larger worlds. Jeremy's parents often talked about temptation increasing proportionally with the distance from home. After the diagnosis, Jeremy's father told him that the illness was a sign from God that he should not leave for college but stay in town. As Jeremy recalled his father's words, he became visibly anxious, talking more rapidly.

> I will be tempted, will fall into the hands of the devil. I will turn away from my faith. I will not be able to take care of my diabetes. What if I give into the temptation to use alcohol? My friends have had a beer or two—nothing drastic, but it is against our faith. My parents are older than those of most of my friends and growing up the only child of a pastor has not always been easy. But I do have friends. Most of them are going away to college and I want to go too. Now I am afraid. What if my parents are right and I can't take care of myself or I fall away from the church? I was taught that God is good and takes care of us. I don't understand why God won't take care of me in another city. Our bodies are sacred, temples of God, which need to be respected and considered holy. What is diabetes doing to my body? Is it still sacred? People believe that diabetes results from overeating, drinking too much, and not caring about health—that wasn't me at all. Why did God give me this illness?

A basic tenet of spirituality is that the body is sacred and that the body, mind, and spirit are one entity. This viewpoint has been correlated with pro-health behaviors. If the body is sacred, then the corollary belief is that it should not be mistreated by alcohol overuse, unhealthy food, or self-harm (Grossoehme, VanDyke, & Seid, 2008). Higher religiosity can be comforting and enhance a sense of well-being. For example, in one study older individuals who engaged in religious practices reported lower anxiety about their appearance as they aged (Homan & Boyatzis, 2010). Integration of the religious or spiritual parts of life with one's own self gives the person a sense of connection with the greater good. Motivation in a spiritual context can be normative and/or even transcendent. People can overcome difficulties and can cope with chronic illness if they believe that life has meaning and purpose, whether they are healthy or not; sometimes, the illness is perceived as conferring a particular meaning to existence and expanding appreciation for life (Martos, Kezdy, & Horvath-Szabo, 2011).

Maintaining a sense of the sacred is connected with meaning in life and personal strivings. How much is invested in a particular effortful endeavor is related to the extent of intersection with the spiritual realm. Personal strivings possess qualities that can be described as holy or spiritual. People invest time, thought, and energy in the most sanctified strivings. The more they believe that the strivings reflect the spiritual realm, the more positive emotions and sense of meaning will result from pursuit of the strivings (Mahoney et al., 2005). In Jeremy's case, the onset of diabetes challenged his most basic beliefs. His parents' spiritual interpretation of the illness fed into their already present fears that their son would leave home and not return. Jeremy felt very safe at home, in contrast to the earlier described case of Celine who laughed at the idea of home. But he felt very stuck at home under the conditions of his illness and his parents' expressed worries and catastrophic statements and what would happen if he left.

In the story of the prodigal son, one son leaves home for adventure; the other son stays to work with his father. Nouwen (2009) explored the rationale and emotions of both sons. The son who stayed behind may have lost an opportunity to explore and to test himself away from the security of home. He felt unappreciated because he was loyal to his father and continued to work on the family farm. Does the prodigal son undergo greater spiritual growth because he fell into sin, wasted his years, and couldn't make it in the world away from home? The question arises in a spiritual context: Does one have to fail before one can be successful—that is, must one experience falling-down before knowing what it feels like to get up? Do people without chronic illness still experience the learning and growth opportunity that comes with the effort to regain balance and health in the chronically ill? Jeremy seems to be struggling with decisions similar to those of both sons in the parable of the prodigal son.

Psychosocial Risk Factors Get Under the Skin

There are a myriad of factors that could be discussed in this section, but only a few were selected due to space considerations. The reader is referred to McGrady and Moss (2013), specifically to the chapters on *Psychosocial Etiology of Illness* and *Psychophysiological Etiology of Illness,* for a more in-depth analysis of the mechanisms by which external factors can "get under the skin" and impact the biological and molecular domains.

The primary pathways linking psychological and social factors with the emergence of chronic illness have been identified as the hypothalamic-pituitary-adrenal axis (HPA) and neuro-immune connections. Anxiety, panic, anger, and sadness connect to physical disorders and illness behavior through multiple pathways, including biological routes mediated by the HPA axis and neuro-immune modulation. It is not necessary for the negative emotions to meet criteria for psychiatric illness (generalized anxiety *disorder*, panic *disorder*, or major depressive *disorder*) to disrupt physical health. Further, the feelings of being unwell (subthreshold for diagnosis) and acting sick feedback to the emotions and cognitions (Cohen & Rodriguez, 1995). Behavioral connections between psychosocial factors and illness comprise the lifestyle habits described previously, but also include the important influence of sleep. Insomnia, non-restorative sleep, and nightmares increase the risk for diabetes, lower the threshold for pain, and interfere with extinction of the fear network to specific stimuli, in addition to facilitating the emergence of anxiety and depression (Smith, Edwards, McCann, & Haythornthwaite, 2007). Withdrawal during illness is adaptive short term as it allows the person to rest, regain strength, stay away from other people, and facilitate the replenishment of resources and mind-body-spirit healing (Segerstrom, 2010). However, long-term isolation is detrimental to a healthy emotional life as well as harmful to the physical body.

Cortisol is a major stress hormone, particularly adapted for short-term stress reactions. Its levels vary as part of the ancient fight-flight-freeze response, which remains our basic behavioral repertoire for reacting to stress. Aggression and withdrawal have been extensively studied as short-term reactions to stress, while freezing less so, although it has as long of a history as the more commonly recognized flight-or-fight reactions. Freezing is a state of attentive mobility that helps individuals prevent detection by the perceived harmful source of the fear (in animals—predators; in humans—threats of many types). In humans, the periaqueductal gray matter in the brain, in concert with inhibition of the motor system, is suggested to underlie the freeze response (Hermans, Henckens, Roelofs, & Fernandez, 2013). Part of the freeze response involves a heightened focus on the perceived current or anticipated threat, highly adaptive during the actual stress experience.

When a stressful situation is of short duration, the presence of cortisol helps the individual focus on that stressor and the necessary adaptation. Cortisol reduces the retrieval of aversive memories, interrupts the vicious cycle of spontaneous retrieving, re-experiencing, and re-consolidating traumatic memories while enhancing fear extinction, facilitating storage of corrective experience. Higher cortisol acutely facilitates reductions in threat appraisal, allowing the person to handle the situation and then recover (de Quervain, Aerni, Schelling, & Roozendaal, 2009). In the MIDUS study, individuals between the ages of 25 and 74 were contacted in 1994–1995 and again in 2004–2005; assessments include cortisol and psychological testing. The group that had lost spouses during this time had smaller awakening responses of cortisol and lower levels in the early part of the day, demonstrating a pattern shift which has ramifications for the chronicity of the stress response and for reactivity to current stress (Morozink, Friedman, Coe, & Ryff, 2010). Normally, cortisol is high in the early morning, preparing the individual for activity; its levels decrease during the day with the lowest levels occurring in the evening, as the person winds down and prepares for bed. The imbalance in cortisol levels implies a reduction in the ability of the individual to cope with stimuli while the levels are abnormally low and increased arousal when levels are high at the wrong time.

Unfortunately, chronically stressful situations or re-experienced traumatic experiences are handled physiologically as if they were immediate and short term. Patients with anxiety disorders demonstrate increased vigilance and hyperarousal in contrast to those who are not highly anxious. These response systems vary depending on whether the threat is perceived to be avoidable or not (Low, Weymar, & Hamm, 2015). There is no certainty about how long a stressor has to last before it is labeled chronic or how serious a stressor has to be before it results in sustained effects on the brain. In a fascinating series of studies on persons who were in a minor motor vehicle accident, Wang et al. (2016) showed that there are changes 2 weeks after a minor accident and after 3 months, specifically reductions in volume of the prefrontal cortex. In some victims of auto accidents, fear stimuli (fearful faces) elicited more reactivity, hyperarousal (autonomic nervous system and cortisol), and abnormal emotional processing compared to others involved in similar accidents.

Cumulative stressful life events were also shown to correlate with decreases in gray matter volume in the hippocampus and anterior cingulate after 3 months. Individuals without a psychiatric diagnosis demonstrated these changes compared to baseline. Importantly, those areas of the brain mentioned above are implicated in post-traumatic stress disorder (Papagni et al., 2011). Cognitive labeling of an experience as adverse or negative begins the cascade of physiological reactions. If common, neutral stimuli are perceived repeatedly as having an emotional component or being potentially threatening, frequent mobilization of the system designed for acute responses occurs. In time, the brain changes and the brain changes feed back to emotion and behavior. A pattern of seeing only the negative about the self, the future, and the present is the hallmark of major depressive disorder (Phillips, Drevets, Rauch, & Lane, 2003).

Effects of Stress on the Gastrointestinal System

There are many possible physiological targets for the effects of stress, including the cardiovascular, respiratory, gastrointestinal, and pain systems. The gastrointestinal system will be discussed below since there is not a specific chapter devoted to this topic. The reader is encouraged to consult the chapters on pain conditions, heart disease, and the metabolic syndrome in this volume and the chapter on digestive disorders in McGrady and Moss (2013).

At every stage of the digestive process, the autonomic nervous system controls motility, digestion, and absorption (Sowder, Gevirtz, Shapiro, & Ebert, 2010).

Signals from the brain have an influence on the motor, sensory, and secretory functions of the gut and the signaling is bidirectional (Dinan, Stilling, Stanton, & Cryan, 2015). Gut microbes are part of the system affecting the brain and behavior. By the time the child is two and a half years old, the microbiota (bacterial environment) resembles that of an adult and is fairly stable, containing bacteroidetes and firmicutes. Genetically engineered germ-free mice, obviously without normal intestinal bacteria have lower brain-derived neurotrophic factor (BDNF), are less social, do less self-grooming, and exhibit stronger responses to mild stress. Transplantation of microbiota modifies the internal environment in a positive way, decreasing over-anxious reactions to stress. Efforts to "clean the gut" and replace unhealthy bacteria with healthy combinations may be seen as extreme to some readers. However, it is generally agreed that feeling sick to the stomach contributes to general malaise. Unhealthy food choices, for example, excessive consumption of high fat foods, often create GI distress short term, and long term by changing the bacterial environment (Junger, 2013).

The effects of stress on digestion and absorption result in either rapid passage of food throughout the tract and frequent bowel movements or pain from low motility and constipation. Irritable bowel syndrome, peptic ulcer disease, and GERD (gastro-esophageal reflux disease) are almost synonymous with psychological distress (Konturek, Brzozowski, & Konturek, 2011). Patients with irritable bowel syndrome over react to minimal symptoms, catastrophize possible consequences, and perceive their coping abilities to be inadequate (Lackner, Quigley, & Blanchard, 2004). Mood and anxiety disorders are frequently comorbid with GI disorders, but it is not usually clear whether the psychological factors preceded the GI problems or vice versa (Roy-Byrne, Davidson, Kessler, Asmundson, & Goodwin, 2008). Suffering with chronic digestive problems and abdominal pain leads the individual, fearing embarrassment to become isolated, and stay away from social groups. These behaviors along with worry and sadness may evolve into social anxiety disorder and major depression (Suarez, Mayer, Ehlert, & Nater, 2010).

The Immune System in Chronic Illness

Inflammation may be the final common pathway linking psychological and social adversity to chronic illness. Social adversity, even prenatally, was shown to intensify inflammatory processes and increase C-reactive protein levels (CRP), a marker of inflammation (Slopen et al., 2015). A harsher family climate, such as growing up in a low-income, noisy, violent neighborhood is associated with multiple demands for coping. Stress is an everyday occurrence, drains the coping resources of the individual and the family and decreases the ability and perhaps the desire for self-control. Deprivation creates the mindset of entitlement and focuses on what is available right now. Adversity depletes self-control and lays the foundation for ill health (Hostinar, Ross, Chen, & Miller, 2015). In summary, the HPA axis is engaged many times a day to cope with the constant stress. Low SES persons demonstrate higher C-reactive protein and interleukin-6 (IL-6). HPA stimulates production of proinflammatory cytokines, which in turn cascade into stimulating CRP, necessary in reactions to acute stress, but damaging with repeated and prolonged stress.

Neurotransmitters associated with the autonomic nervous system (norepinephrine and serotonin) affect inflammation differently. NE affects proinflammatory cytokines; so drugs that block NE shift balance toward humoral immunity; serotonin inhibits the production of interleukin; drugs that affect serotonin shift balance toward cellular immunity (Uher et al., 2014).

The psychosocial factors discussed earlier are relevant to this discussion of the effects of stress on the immune system. For example, the sense of psychological well-being as demonstrated by a sense of mastery, positive affect, and personal autonomy related with lower IL-6. People with relatively few years of education, but a solid sense of well-being will not demonstrate the same imbalance in function of the immune system as those individuals who are neither well educated nor perceive themselves as psychologically healthy. Further, higher education combined with the sense of well-being correlated with lower levels of IL-6. Fewer years of education and low sense of well-being also correlated with higher interleukin-6 (IL-6) (Morozink et al., 2010). The HPA axis and the neuro-immune system operate within complex feedback loops, sharing information, and reacting to each change.

Learning to React

One of the ways children learn is by observation and copying behaviors of others with whom they have frequent contact. From a behavioral perspective, children mimic the behaviors and the emotional reactions that they see and place value on those behaviors depending on the superiority of the person. The recognition of faces and their expression provides models for emotional and behavioral reactions. Early in development, babies can distinguish human and monkey faces equally well, but the human faces are reinforced and the ability to distinguish monkey faces disappears (Sacks, 2010). The adults' smile or the angry face directed toward the child both have physiological and neural consequences. Facial musculature coupled with hearing angry or loving voices permits the detection of the emotion and in time, the child learns the consequences of different facial expressions (Parr, Waller, & Fugate, 2005). Observing the display of positive and negative emotions has different effects on the cortical structures involved in attaching meaning to those displays (Rahko et al., 2010). Specifically, the amygdala plays an important role in processing of threat conveyed by facial expression; this observation is supported by evidence that damage to the amygdala results in impaired perception of emotions, particularly fear (Mattavelli et al., 2014).

Mirror neurons in several areas of the brain translate sensory perceptual activity, body language, and eventually words, allowing the observer to understand and attempt to forecast the thoughts and feelings of the observed person (Izzard, 2009). Fabbi-Destro and Rizzolatti (2008) postulates that areas in the insula that are responsible for sensation contain two populations of neurons: one for experiencing the sensation and another for observing people experiencing the sensation. Some believe that the neural basis for emotion is contained in an "as-if loop" in the insula by which a person is sensitive to another's emotion as if it is happening to them.

The size of the brain area used in emotional and sensory perception (neocortex) is related to the evolution of primates to group-dwelling species and allows for finer communication between members of the group. The terminal neurons that produce facial expressions receive upper level neural input from the layers of the neocortex involved in emotional processing (Purves et al., 2012). Yuen et al. (2010) found that corticosterone released in highly stressed states enhances the activity of mirror neurons as well as long-term potentiation via NMDA and AMPA receptors in the limbic region. Humans are more likely to copy other people, whether or not they are competent in that regard, because of the effect of cortisol. The stress response affects the speed of learning and the consistency of the retention of the memory; one trial learning occurs after a strong negative stimulus whose memory will be retained for a long time.

Engaging in Positive Change: The Pathways Model

The Pathways Model proposes a multi-level intervention paradigm with emphasis on self-awareness, personal choices, and patient-provider active collaboration (McGrady & Moss, 2013). A team approach to care allows providers of different disciplines to be more or less involved depending on the results of the initial evaluation. The astute clinician recalls that each illness has its own time course, waxing and waning in severity; current symptoms are not identical with the most frequent effects of the disorder. Translation of the patient's experience into clinical terms requires attention and compassion from the provider. For example, "I need to sleep 12 hours a day" is different from "I want to sleep all the time." "I can't remember anything" could be a problem with cognitive functioning, attention clouded by brain fog in a patient with fibromyalgia, lack of motivation from depression, or intrusive pain. Unmasking psychological factors from a portrayal of physical symptoms can be a daunting task, even for an experienced mental health provider (Schildkrout, 2011). The mental health clinician must remember that she was neither present at the beginning of symptom development nor at the time of diagnosis of the physical disease.

Level One in the Pathways Model seems simple at first, but serves the important function of re-establishing normal rhythms, critically important to facilitate Levels Two and Three. A patient with disrupted or compromised breathing, sleeping, and eating behaviors will have difficulty focusing on building skills or engaging in complex treatments. Disease burden must be lifted, sometimes with very active participation from the provider; at other times, the patient can be guided at first, and then can proceed in the health coaching model. Stability of physiological systems gives patients a greater sense of control and improves mental stability.

Skill building occurs in Level Two. Basic relaxation strategies are taught and patients are encouraged to incorporate those skills into their daily lives. The Level Two skills listed are not all inclusive so related skill sets can be utilized such as the problem-solving approach of D'Zurilla and Nezu (2007). Techniques of managing stress-related problems in a step-by-step approach can be learned and applied successfully to the demands of chronic illness. Patients can set goals in each of the levels of the Pathways Model or can set overall goals for improvement in physical or mental state, using process goals in each level. What is most important is that patients base their goals on what is important to them and that the goal setting process is done collaboratively between patient and providers (Reuben & Tinetti, 2012).

Based on the skills acquired in Level Two, potentially stressful situations can be anticipated and prepared for, using relaxation, basic imagery, and cognitive restructuring. Recalling the lessons learned from the animal adaptation literature is often helpful to patients since it momentarily directs their thoughts away from themselves. During times of high stress, which may occur during a flare up or exacerbation of the illness itself, patients are distracted from managing the demands of the chronic illness. If the stressor is outside of the illness, focus on the stressor is adaptive, but inattention to monitoring blood glucose, peak flow (in asthma), and neglecting activity very soon has damaging effects. When stress is prolonged, the Pathways approach suggests to patients that their own self-care remains important and that giving up on activity, nutrition, or the activities that give life meaning is counterproductive.

In Level Three, interventions increase in intensity and require a licensed mental health provider or physician. During psychotherapy, psychophysiological therapy, and medical interventions, the patient is encouraged to maintain a growth mindset. For example, a fixed mindset assumes that our character and abilities are static and are not changeable by experience. A growth mindset thrives on challenge. Struggles and failure are not evidence of weakness or stupidity, but should be considered a means for personal growth Dweck (2006). Even when illness flares or worsens, the attitude that "nothing can improve; my condition can only get worse" is discouraged, in contrast to "I can grow spiritually and emotionally, despite my physical handicaps."

Balance is an important part of the Level Three interventions. Achieving balance between attention to the illness, family responsibilities, and work or school necessitates understanding of the concept of an energy budget. The person begins a task with a certain amount of energy, which depends on both physical and mental factors. Physical factors include the hours that the person slept and whether the sleep was restful, food eaten, and the quality of food. Mental factors are the ability to focus, remain calm, and being mindful. Once engaged in the task, energy can be burnt up with mental anxiety or physical tension. Or the energy budget can be managed appropriately, so that the person addresses the task and continues until it is complete. Recovery is as important as how much energy is expended because without recovery, re-engagement in the next task is more difficult (Loehr & Schwartz, 2003). Maintaining balance means that goals remain in place, despite setbacks, but the person may have to devote more energy to the stressor. At the conclusion of the stressful period, the person rebuilds resources, resets both emotionally and physically, fosters their sense of control, and returns to a positive mood state. Hope, expectation of better days, improved health and mood engenders success for future tasks (Lyubomirsky, King, & Diener, 2005).

References

Ajzen, I. (2002). Perceived behavioral control, self-efficacy, locus of control, and the theory of planned behavior. *Journal of Applied Social Psychology, 32*(4), 665–683.

Blix, A. S. (2016). Adaptations to polar life in mammals and birds. *Journal of Experimental Biology, 219*, 1093–1105.

Block, J. P., & Subramanian, S. V. (2015). Moving beyond "food deserts:" Reorienting United States policies to reduce disparities in diet quality. *PLoS Medicine, 12*(12), e1001914.

Bourne, E. (1998). *Healing fear: New approaches to overcoming anxiety.* Oakland, CA: New Harbinger.

Brennan, I. (2011). *Anger antidotes.* New York, NY: W.W. Norton.

Center for Disease Control. (2013). *Adverse childhood experiences study pyramid.* Atlanta, GA: Centers for Disease Control and Prevention. Retrieved January 18, 2013, from https://www.cdc.gov/violenceprevention/acestudy/about.html

Cohen, S., & Rodriguez, M. S. (1995). Pathways linking affective disturbances and physical disorders. *Health Psychology, 14*(5), 374–380.

D'Zurilla, T. J., & Nezu, A. M. (2007). *Problem-solving therapy: A positive approach to clinical intervention* (3rd ed.). New York, NY: Springer.

de Quervain, D. J., Aerni, A., Schelling, G., & Roozendaal, B. (2009). Glucocorticoids and the regulation of memory in health and disease. *Frontiers in Neuroendocrinolology, 30*, 358–370.

Dieleman, J. L., Baral, R., Birger, M., Bui, A. L., Bulchis, A., Chapin, A., & Murray, C. J. (2016). U.S. spending on personal health care and public health, 1996-2013. *Journal of the American Medical Association, 316*(24), 2627-2646.

Dinan, T. G., Stilling, R. M., Stanton, C., & Cryan, J. F. (2015). Collective unconscious: How gut microbes shape human behavior. *Journal of Psychiatric Research, 63*, 1–9.

Dorahy, M. J., Corry, M., Shannon, M., MacSherry, A., Hamilton, G., McRobert, G., et al. (2009). Complex PTSD, interpersonal trauma, and relational consequences: Findings from a treatment-receiving Northern Irish sample. *Journal of Affective Disorders, 112*, 71–80.

Dweck, C. S. (2006). *Mindset: The new psychology of success.* New York, NY: Random House.

Edwards, L. (2013). *A social history of chronic illness in America: In the kingdom of the sick.* New York, NY: Walker Publishing Company, Inc.

Endless house: Intersections of art and architecture (Exhibit). (2015). New York, NY: Museum of Modern Art.

Fabbi-Destro, M., & Rizzolatti, G. (2008). Mirror neurons and mirror systems in monkeys and humans. *Physiology, 23*, 171–179.

Gardner, D. (2008). *The science of fear: Why we fear the things we shouldn't—And put ourselves in greater danger* (1st ed.). Strand, London, UK: Penguin Books Ltd..

Gibson, B., Marcus, R. L., Staggers, N., Jones, J., Samore, M., & Weir, C. (2012). Efficacy of a computerized simulation in promoting walking in individuals with diabetes. *Journal of Medical Internet Research, 14*(3), e71.

Global Burden of Disease Study 2013 Collaborators. (2015). Global, regional, and national incidence, prevalence, and years lived with disability for 301 acute and chronic diseases and injuries in 188 countries, 1990-2013: A systematic analysis for the Global Burden of Disease Study 2013. *Lancet, 386*, 743–800.

Grossoehme, D. H., VanDyke, R., & Seid, M. (2008). Spirituality's role in chronic disease self-management: Sanctification of the body in families dealing with cystic fibrosis. *Journal of Health Care Chaplaincy, 15*(2), 149–158.

Heim, C., Shugart, M., Graighead, W. E., & Nemeroff, C. B. (2010). Neurobiological and psychiatric consequences of child abuse and neglect. *Developmental Psychobiology, 52*, 671–690.

Hermans, E. J., Henckens, M. J., Roelofs, K., & Fernandez, G. (2013). Fear bradycardia and activation of the human periaqueductal grey. *Neuroimage, 66*, 278–287.

Hobson, C. J., Kamen, J., Szostek, J., Nethercut, C. M., Tiedman, J. W., & Wojnarowicz, S. (1998). Stressful life events: A revision and update of the social readjustment rating scale. *International Journal of Stress Management, 5*(1), 1–23.

Holmes, T., & Rahe, R. (1967). The social readjustment rating scale. *Journal of Psychosomatic Research, 11*, 213–218.

Homan, K. J., & Boyatzis, C. J. (2010). Religiosity, sense of meaning, and health behavior in older adults. *International Journal for the Psychology of Religion, 20*(3), 173–186.

Hostinar, C. E., Ross, K. M., Chen, E., & Miller, G. E. (2015). Modeling the association between lifecourse socioeconomic disadvantage and systemic inflammation in healthy adults: The role of self-control. *Health Psychology, 34*(6), 580–590.

Hudson, C. (2005). Socioeconomic status and mental illness: Tests of the social causation and selection hypotheses. *American Journal of Orthopsychiatry, 75*(1), 3–18.

Izzard, C. E. (2009). Emotion theory and research: Highlights, unanswered questions and emerging issues. *Annual Review of Psychology, 60*, 1–25.

Johnson, L., Afari, N., & Zautra, A. (2009). The illness uncertainty concept: A review. *Current Pain and Headache Reports, 13*(2), 133–138.

Johnson, L. M., Zautra, A. J., & Davis, M. C. (2006). The role of illness uncertainty on coping with fibromyalgia symptoms. *Health Psychology, 25*(6), 696–703. https://doi.org/10.1037/0278-6133.25.6.696

Junger, A. (2013). *Clean gut*. New York, NY: Harper One.

Juster, R. P., McEwen, B. S., & Lupien, S. J. (2010). Allostatic load biomarkers of chronic stress and impact on health and cognition. *Neuroscience and Biobehavioral Reviews, 35*, 2–16.

Kiecolt-Glaser, J. K., Fagundes, C. P., Andridge, R., Peng, J., Malarkey, W. B., Habash, D., & Belury, M. A. (2016). Depression, daily stressors, and inflammatory responses to high-fat meals: When stress overrides healthier food choices. *Molecular Psychiatry, 22*(3), 476–482. https://doi.org/10.1038/mp.2016.149

Kiviruusu, O., Huure, T., Haukala, A., & Aro, H. (2013). Changes in psychological resources moderate the effect of socioeconomic status on distress symptoms: A 10-year follow-up among young adults. *Health Psychology, 32*(5), 627–636.

Knez, I. (2005). Attachment and identity as related to a place and its perceived climate. *Journal of Environmental Psychology, 25*(2), 207–218.

Konturek, P. C., Brzozowski, T., & Konturek, S. J. (2011). Stress and the gut: Pathophysiology, clinical consequences, diagnostic approach and treatment options. *Journal of Physiology and Pharmacology, 62*(6), 591–599.

Krueger, P. M., & Reither, E. M. (2015). Mind the gap: Race/ethnic and socioeconomic disparities in obesity. *Current Diabetes Reports, 15*(11), 95.

Lackner, J. M., Quigley, B. M., & Blanchard, E. B. (2004). Depression and abdominal pain in IBS patients: The mediating role of catastrophizing. *Psychosomatic Medicine, 66*, 435–441.

Loehr, J., & Schwartz, T. (2003). *The power of full engagement*. New York, NY: Free Press.

Low, A., Weymar, M., & Hamm, A. O. (2015). When threat is near, get out of here: Dynamics of defensive behavior during freezing and active avoidance. *Psychological Science, 26*(11), 1706–1716.

Lyubomirsky, S., King, L., & Diener, E. (2005). The benefits of frequent positive affect: Does happiness lead to success? *Psychological Bulletin, 131*(6), 803–855.

Mahoney, A., Pargament, K. I., Cole, B., Jewell, T., Magyar, G. M., Tarakeshwar, N., et al. (2005). A higher purpose: The sanctification of strivings in a community sample. *International Journal for the Psychology of Religion, 15*(3), 239–262. https://doi.org/10.1207/s15327582ijpr1503_4

Manseau, M. W. (2014). Economic inequality and poverty as social determinants of mental health. *Psychiatric Annals, 44*(1), 32–37.

Martos, T., Kezdy, A., & Horvath-Szabo, K. (2011). Religious motivations for everyday goals: Their religious context and potential consequences. *Motivation and Emotion, 35*, 75–88.

Mattavelli, G., Sormaz, M., Flack, T., Asghar, A. U., Fan, S., Manssuer, L., et al. (2014). Neutral responses to facial expressions support the role of the amygdala in processing threat. *Social Cognitive and Affective Neuroscience, 9*(11), 1684–1689. https://doi.org/10.1093/scan/nst162. Epub 2013 Oct 4.

McGrady, A., & Moss, D. (2013). *Pathways to illness, pathways to health*. New York, NY: Springer.

Meara, E. R., Richards, S., & Dutler, D. M. (2008). The gap gets bigger: Changes in mortality and life expectancy, by education, 1981-2000. *Health Affairs, 27*(2), 350–360.

Michigan State University. (2001). *Michigan forests forever teachers' guide*. Michigan State University Extension. Retrieved from http://mff.dsisd.net/Environment/WinterAnimals.htm

Morozink, J. A., Friedman, E. M., Coe, C. L., & Ryff, C. D. (2010). Socioeconomic and psychosocial predictors of interleukin-6 in the MIDUS national sample. *Health Psychology, 29*(6), 626–635.

Nouwen, H. (2009). *Home tonight: Further reflections on the parable of the prodigal son*. New York, NY: Doubleday.

Orr, M. G., Kaplan, G. A., & Galea, S. (2016). Neighbourhood food, physical activity, and educational environments and black/white disparities in obesity: A complex systems simulation analysis. *Journal of Epidemiology and Community Health, 70*, 862–867.

Papagni, S. A., Benetti, S., Arulanantham, S., McCrory, E., McGuire, P., & Mechelli, A. (2011). Effects of stressful life events on human brain structure: A longitudinal voxel-based morphometry study. *Stress, 14*(2), 227–232.

Parr, L. A., Waller, B. M., & Fugate, J. (2005). Emotional communication in primates: Implications for neurobiology. *Current Opinion in Neurobiology, 15*, 716–720.

Pearce, P. Z. (2008). Exercise is medicine™. *Current Sports Medicine Reports, 7*(3), 171–175.

Phillips, M. L., Drevets, W. C., Rauch, S. L., & Lane, R. (2003). Neurobiology of emotion perception II: Implications for major psychiatric disorders. *Biological Psychiatry, 54*, 515–528.

Purves, D., Augustine, G. V., Fitzpatrick, D., Hall, W. C., LaMantia, A. S., White, L. E., & McNamara, J. O. (2012). *Neurosciences* (5th ed.). Sunderland, MA: Sinauer Associates.

Rahko, J., Paakki, J. J., Starck, T., Nikkinen, J., Remes, J., Hurtig, T., & Kiviniemi, V. (2010). Functional mapping of dynamic happy and fearful facial expression processing in adolescents. *Brain Imaging and Behavior, 4*(2), 164–176.

Reuben, D. B., & Tinetti, M. E. (2012). Goal-oriented patient care—An alternative health outcomes paradigm. *The New England Journal of Medicine, 366*(9), 777–779.

Rippe, J. M., & Angelopoulos, T. J. (2011). Lifestyle medicine: Continuing to grow and mature. *American Journal of Lifestyle Medicine, 5*(1), 4–6.

Roy-Byrne, P. P., Davidson, K. W., Kessler, R. C., Asmundson, G. J. G., & Goodwin, R. D. (2008). Anxiety disorders and comorbid medical illness. *Focus, 6*, 467–485.

Sacks, O. (2010). *The mind's eye*. New York, NY: Alfred A. Knopf.

Schildkrout, B. (2011). *Unmasking psychological symptoms*. New York, NY: Wiley.

Segerstrom, S. (2010). Resources, stress, and immunity: An ecological perspective on human psychoneuroimmunology. *Annals of Behavioral Medicine, 40*, 114–125.

Slopen, N., Loucks, E. B., Appleton, A. A., Kawachi, I., Kubzansky, L. D., Non, A. L., et al. (2015). Early origins of inflammation: An examination of prenatal and childhood social adversity in a prospective cohort study. *Psychneuroendocrinology, 51*, 403–413.

Smith, M. T., Edwards, R. R., McCann, U. D., & Haythornthwaite, J. A. (2007). The effects of sleep deprivation on pain inhibition and spontaneous pain in women. *Sleep, 30*(4), 494–505.

Sowder, E., Gevirtz, R., Shapiro, W., & Ebert, C. (2010). Restoration of vagal tone: A possible mechanism for functional abdominal pain. *Applied Psychophysiology and Biofeedback, 35*(3), 199–206.

Stoeber, J., & Janssen, D. (2011). Perfectionism and coping with daily failures: Positive reframing helps achieve satisfaction at the end of the day. *Anxiety, Stress, & Coping, 24*(5), 477–497.

Suarez, K., Mayer, C., Ehlert, U., & Nater, U. M. (2010). Psychological stress and self-reported functional gastrointestinal disorders. *The Journal of Nervous and Mental Disease, 198*(3), 226–229.

Thoits, P. A. (2010). Stress and health: Major findings and policy implications. *Journal of Health and Social Behavior, 51*(S), 541–553.

Todman, L. C., & Diaz, A. (2014). A public health approach to narrowing mental health disparities. *Psychiatric Annals, 44*, 27–31.

Todman, L. C., & Holliday, C. S. (2015). Adverse features of the built environment. In M. T. Compton & R. S. Shim (Eds.), *The social determinants of mental health* (pp. 193–212). Arlington, VA: American Psychiatric Association.

Uher, R., Tansey, K. E., Dew, T., Maier, W., Mors, O., Hauser, J., & McGuffin, P. (2014). An inflammatory biomarker as a differential predictor of outcome of depression treatment with escitalopram and nortriptyline. *American Journal of Psychiatry, 171*, 1278–1286.

Wang, X., Xie, H., Cotton, A. S., Duval, E. R., Tamburrino, M. B., Brickman, K. R., et al. (2016). Preliminary study of acute changes in emotion processing in trauma survivors with PTSD symptoms. *PLoS One, 11*(7), e0159065. https://doi.org/10.1371/journal.pone.0159065

Wang, D. D., Li, Y., Chiuve, S. E., Hu, F. B., & Willett, W. C. (2015). Improvements in US diet helped reduce disease burden and lower premature deaths, 1999-2012; overall diet remains poor. *Health Affairs, 34*(11), 1916–1922. https://doi.org/10.1377/hlthaff.2015.0640

Yeh, B. I., & Kong, I. D. (2013). The advent of lifestyle medicine. *Journal of Lifestyle Medicine, 3*(1), 1–8.

Yu, D. S. F. (2008). Heart failure: The manifestations and impact of negative emotions. In L. Sher (Ed.), *Psychological factors and cardiovascular disorders: The role of psychiatric pathology and maladaptive personality features* (pp. 135–151). New York, NY: Nova Biomedical Books.

Yuen, E. Y., Liu, W., Karatsoreos, I. N., Ren, Y., Feng, J., McEwen, B. S., & Yan, Z. (2010). Mechanisms for acute stress-induced enhancement of glutamatergic transmission and working memory. *Molecular Psychiatry, 16*(2), 156–170.

Zenk, S. N., Schulz, A. J., Lachance, L. L., Mentz, G., Kannan, S., Ridella, W., & Galea, S. (2009). Multilevel correlates of satisfaction with neighborhood availability of fresh fruits and vegetables. *Annals of Behavioral Medicine, 38*, 48–59.

Zhang, D., Giabbanelli, P. J., Arah, O. A., & Zimmerman, F. J. (2014). Impact of different policies on unhealthy dietary behaviors in an urban adult population: An agent-based simulation model. *American Journal of Public Health, 104*(7), 1217–1222.

Chapter 2
The Pathways Model for Improved Health and Wellness

Abstract The Pathways Model was developed by Angele McGrady and Donald Moss (Pathways to illness, pathways to health, Springer, New York, NY, 2013), as an integrative model for improving health and remediating illness. The Pathways Model utilizes a coaching-based approach to assess the individual's readiness for health-supportive changes and articulates a three-level plan for enhancing health and wellness. The Pathways Model begins with the formation of an "alliance for health" with each prospective patient. The Pathways self-care plan is a personally forged and committed program for self-directed changes, in coordination with professional support.

The Pathways Level One plan includes self-directed lifestyle changes and behavioral change to restore the body's biological rhythms. Level One activities are simple and practical, reflecting the individual's life experience and choices. The Level Two plan involves acquiring specific skills for improved coping and self-regulation. Level Two activities can be supported by educational resources and community programs, such as a relaxation training CD, community-based mindfulness or meditation classes, or instruction at a yoga or wellness center. The Pathways Level Three plan consists of interventions delivered by a trained health care professional, including health psychologists, psychotherapists, physicians, physical therapists, nutritionists, herbalists, naturopaths, acupuncturists, and others.

This chapter promotes the inclusion of religious and spiritual practices at each Level in the Pathways Model, and advocates for including complementary therapies in the Pathways Model.

Keywords Pathways Model · Lifestyle medicine · Coaching · Complementary therapies · Spirituality

Portions of this chapter are adapted with permission from D. Moss (2015), integration of mindfulness training into a comprehensive "Pathways Model" treatment program: The case of Jorge, *Biofeedback, 43*(3), 137–141.

The Need for an Integrative Model to Support Comprehensive Health-Supportive Change

The changing face of illness. The face of illness has changed, and human beings are eager for new approaches to pursue health and wellness. The illnesses that brought patients into medical clinics 100 years ago, including infectious diseases, bacterial parasites, and unhealed physical trauma, have been conquered to a large extent. Instead, today's patients present with diseases of lifestyle, stress-related conditions, and chronic illnesses (Moss, McGrady, Davies, & Wickramasekera, 2003). Hypertension, depression, anxiety, diabetes, fibromyalgia, chronic fatigue, and chronic pain are more typical problems today. Many of the complaints presented by patients in the clinic are strongly influenced by life stress, relationship strain, sedentary lifestyle, and poor dietary choices. The conditions may involve biomedical or genetic elements, but the decisions made by patients in their everyday lives often cause the medical conditions to worsen or improve.

Conventional medicine is best prepared to treat conditions that can be documented by laboratory tests, imaging, and objective evidence. Many of today's health problems worsen for no measurable reason. In turn, physicians are best prepared to provide medication or surgical intervention. For today's most common disorders, prescribed medicines often provide symptomatic relief at best, and surgery sometimes compounds lifestyle-based problems. Increasing numbers of people seek out advice for health problems at the health food store, or visit Reiki energy healers, massage therapists, naturopaths, and other non-mainstream medicine practitioners, instead of conventional medical care.

Complementary and integrative health For over two decades, the field of health care has referred to non-mainstream approaches as complementary and alternative medicine (CAM). From 1998 through 2014, the division of the National Institutes of Health dealing with non-mainstream therapies was known as the National Center for Complementary and Alternative Medicine (NCCAM). The *Complementary Medicine* label indicated non-mainstream approaches that are used in combination with mainstream medical interventions, whereas the *Alternative Medicine* label indicated non-mainstream therapy approaches that are used in place of mainstream medicine. In late 2014, NCCAM was renamed as the National Center for Complementary and Integrative Health, showing a greater emphasis on bringing complementary and mainstream approaches together in a coordinated way (NCCIH, 2016).

> "The most effective approach for many of the stress-related and chronic conditions troubling patients today is one of lifestyle change, self-care, and illness 'self-management.'"

In many cases, patients are reluctant to share their use of non-mainstream health remedies with their allopathic physicians, and there is little coordination between so called complementary and alternative medicine (CAM) practitioners and the primary care physician. One recent Dutch study found that 92% of patients sampled preferred a physician who would accept and refer them for CAM practices, yet only 30% informed their physician about CAM use (Miek, van de Vijver, Busch, Fritsma, & Seldenrijk, 2012). A 2004 review found similar patterns in North American patients over the previous decade with as many as 77% of patients not disclosing CAM use to physicians (Robinson & McGrail, 2004).

Throughout this book, we will utilize the term "complementary therapy" and emphasize the integration of complementary therapies, behavioral interventions, and mainstream medicine into one seamless health care program. Communication among mainstream and complementary practitioners is imperative to overcome the all too common fractionation of care. We will return to a discussion of complementary and integrative health care later in this chapter.

Lifestyle medicine The most effective approach for many of the stress-related and chronic conditions troubling patients today is one of lifestyle change, self-care, and illness "self-management." George and Thomas (2010), for example, have estimated that patients must provide 90% of their own care for diabetes. Unfortunately, less than half of medical patients follow through consistently with medical recommendations for self-care practices and lifestyle changes. The number of research publications on patient "compliance" and "adherence" with physician recommendations suggests the size of the problem.

For over two decades, experts in health and wellness promotion have identified a core group of behavioral and lifestyle changes that can greatly diminish illness and enhance wellness. Smoking cessation, regular sleep habits, aerobic activity, moderation in alcohol use, positive nutritional choices, and stress management form a core of wellness recommendations that would greatly lessen the incidence of hypertension, diabetes, cardiovascular illness, and a variety of other medical and mental health problems.

Dean Ornish has shown by a series of credible research studies that his program of whole foods, plant-based (vegetarian) diet, smoking cessation, physical exercise, stress management, yoga, and meditation produce measurable and clinically significant improvements in patients with cardiovascular illness. These changes include reductions in triglycerides, cholesterol, and blood pressure, and increase myocardial perfusion (Ornish, 1996; Ornish et al., 1998; Silberman et al., 2010). The Ornish team also showed in another large-scale study that following participation in the Ornish program, cardiac patients with depressive illness also showed significant improvements in mood (Pischke, Frenda, Ornish, & Weidner, 2010).

Ornish and colleagues have advocated for "Lifestyle Medicine," a branch of evidence-based medicine dedicated to research, prevention, diagnosis, and treatment of conditions and illnesses caused by maladaptive lifestyle and unhealthy environments (Sagner et al., 2014).[1] Lifestyle medicine has broader applications than the original Ornish research, offering promise for the chronic non-communicable diseases, cardiovascular diseases, cancer and diabetes, which threaten world health (Sagner et al.,

---

[1] Sagner et al. (2014) used the term "morbidogenic environments," indicating that the environment can be conducive to illness.

2014). The same group of authors has proposed a model of lifestyle medicine for implementation in primary care (Egger, Katz, Sagner, & Stevens, 2014).

> "The Pathways Model utilizes health and wellness coaching to assist the individual in gaining a sense of self-efficacy, an inner conviction that 'I can make changes in my behavior and they will make a difference in my health.'"

Nevertheless, the general population is losing ground on many of these variables. Sedentary lifestyles, avoidance of physical activity, poor nutritional choices, and weight gain are epidemic, with two-thirds of the US population qualifying as overweight and one-third as obese (Thorpe, Florence, Howard, & Joski, 2004). A more recent study by Christopher Murray of Institute for Health Metrics and Evaluation at the University of Washington found that although in the United States mean longevity continues to increase, the United States is not keeping pace with other developed countries in population health.[2] When Murray et al. (2015) examined their data in terms of years of life lost (YLL) to premature mortality and especially years lived with disability (YLD), the rankings for the United States compared to other developed nations worsened in each category examined. The leading risk factors degrading US population health were tobacco smoking, high body mass index, high blood pressure, high fasting plasma glucose, physical inactivity, excessive alcohol use, and preferences for high fat, low fruit, and low vegetable diet.

The Pathways Model: An Overview

The Pathways Model was developed by Angele McGrady and Donald Moss (2013) to promote the development of an integrative model for modifying lifestyle, improving health and remediating illness. The Pathways Model is one approach within the broader emerging field of Lifestyle Medicine (Sagner et al. 2014). The Pathways Model utilizes a coaching-based approach to assess the individual's readiness for health-supportive changes and articulates a three-level plan for enhancing health and wellness. Rather than seek external strategies to increase the patient's compliance with a physician dictated health plan, the Pathways Model begins by offering the patient an alliance for health, a jointly formulated program for personally chosen changes and strategies.

The Pathways Model presented in this book provides a comprehensive approach to integrating lifestyle changes, behavioral changes, self-care, and self-regulation skills into the care for chronic conditions. The Pathways Model conceives of illness as a pathway emanating from genetic predisposition, through diet and level of

---

[2] Of great concern, a report from the National Center for Health Statistics in December 2016 reported the first reduction in US population life expectancy in many years. Life expectancy in 2015 was 78.8, a decrease of 0.1 since 2014 (National Center for Health Statistics, 2016).

"Human beings who can clearly see and understand their own role in illness creation, through past choices and lifestyle habits, can better dedicate themselves to new pathways, to wellness and health."

exercise, through a series of lifestyle choices, through the impact of life and work stress, culminating in medical conditions that are largely avoidable, and that in some cases are reversible. Human beings who can clearly see and understand their own role in illness creation, through past choices and lifestyle habits, can better dedicate themselves to new pathways to wellness and health.

The Pathways Model addresses the continuum of health and disease, and the role of both health risk-behaviors and well-behaviors in shaping the individual's overall health. The process begins with a Pathways Assessment that explores the onset of the individual's illness or health problems and identifies negative behaviors and lifestyle factors that may have contributed to the onset or continuance of health problems. In addition, the Pathways Assessment explores the individual's current readiness for change (Prochaska & Norcross, 2001; Prochaska & Velicer, 1997). When human beings do not believe that change is possible, and doubt that any action will make a difference in their current health problems, then the best designed wellness plan will have no effect because they will take no action.

The Coaching Approach to Enhanced Human Being and Well-Being

The Pathways Model utilizes health and wellness coaching to assist the individual in gaining a sense of self-efficacy, an inner conviction that "I can make changes in my behavior and they will make a difference in my health." Albert Bandura has promoted the importance of self-efficacy for health and with colleagues has conducted a number of studies on disease self-management programs, self-efficacy, and health improvements (Bandura, 2004). In one study, a 7-week disease self-management education program produced a reduction in health care utilization over 2 years of follow-up, and the magnitude of that use was negatively correlated with self-efficacy (Lorig et al., 2001). The more self-efficacy a subject displayed, the less he or she utilized health care.

The Pathways Model adopts the coaching model and advocates a step-wise approach to lifestyle change, beginning with small self-directed changes, and proceeding to more demanding changes only when the individual has experienced some initial successes with small steps.

Appropriate conceptual models of the human functioning that support this Pathways coaching approach include humanistic psychology, positive psychology, and self-determination theory. Traditional dynamic psychotherapy and psychology, following Freud, emphasized a model emphasizing deficiencies and weaknesses in the human being and his or her development, and interventions to compensate for deficiencies. Interventions explored early traumatic experiences and psychodynamic psychotherapy was an exhaustive and exhausting multi-year process.

Abraham Maslow, the founder of humanistic psychology, suggested shifting the focus of research to the human being's potential and capacity for growth (Maslow, 1968). He pointed out that in spite of inner weaknesses, there is something in human nature that continues to press toward actualization (Moss, 1999). Maslow proposed that studying well-functioning, "self-actualized" human beings might provide a better roadmap for helping human beings move toward health.

Positive psychology, as articulated by Martin Seligman, Steen, Park, and Peterson (2005) and Mihaly Csikszentimihalyi (1999), has, in many ways, fulfilled Maslow's vision for a more positive model of human experiencing and unleashed a torrent of empirical research on human happiness and positive functioning. Positive psychology asks how and under what conditions humans can best develop their functional capacity and well-being.

Self-determination theory is a model of human motivation and personality; it emerged from social psychology, and places the emphasis on basic needs such as autonomy, competency, and relatedness which are necessary for healthy functioning and well-being (Ryan & Deci, 2002; Pearson, 2011; Spence & Oades, 2011). Self-determination theory has explored empirically the motivators that facilitate healthy self-regulation (Brown & Ryan, 2004). Phelps (2014), drawing on self-determination theory, observed that the more autonomous a behavior is, the more personal commitment the individual will show for the behavior. Chapter 3 will present an expanded overview of positive psychology, self-determination theory, and the concepts of resilience, thriving, and post-traumatic growth as conceptual frameworks for intervention with chronic illness.

The field of coaching, including both life coaching and health coaching, has evolved with an emphasis on developing short-term strategies for facilitating personal change. This facilitation of change comes through inviting human beings to become self-aware of personal values and motivations and to make appropriate choices to pursue their goals. Wolever et al. (2010) conducted a study of 56 diabetic patients, who were randomized to receive either treatment as usual or a telephone-based regimen of health coaching. The patients in the coaching condition were guided to create a personalized vision of positive health and to choose goals aligned with their personal values. Only those patients in the coaching group showed improvements in self-reported medication adherence, exercise frequency, coping with stress, and perceived health status. In addition, patients in the coaching group who had an elevated HgA1C at baseline significantly reduced their levels. The Pathways Model embraces the concepts and values of positive psychology and self-determination theory, and the objective of coaching human beings toward positive self-directed changes in health behaviors and lifestyle.

The Three Levels in the Pathways Model

The Pathways Model promotes a three-level, step-wise framework for facilitating personal changes in health-related lifestyle:

Level One focuses on changes in everyday behaviors that are designed to re-establish normal body rhythms. Changes at Level One are self-directed and simple. The individual may commit to improve the use of simple sleep hygiene principles to enhance the quality and quantity of sleep. She or he might commit to walk to a nearby park or to utilize calming music for self-soothing at the end of the day's work. The everyday life interventions in Level One are developed through an initial Pathways evaluation, including comprehensive self-assessment and professional assessment (McGrady & Moss, 2013, pp. 63–73).

Level Two focuses on the individual learning self-regulation skills and utilizing community resources and educational materials to support learning and lifestyle changes. The individual may use an educational CD to learn mindfulness meditation or attend a yoga class at the local YMCA. Progressive relaxation, autogenic training, and guided imagery are all basic self-regulation skills that can be learned with the use of written handouts, educational CDs or DVDs, and community-based classes.

"The Pathways Model promotes a three-level, step-wise framework for facilitating personal changes in health-related lifestyle."

Level Three involves professional interventions, the utilization of services provided by a health practitioner, such as hypnosis, energy therapy, psychotherapy, acupuncture, or medication management. The authors have found that patients benefit much more from professional services, when a well-organized program of lifestyle changes and self-care practices is already underway. The patient participates more actively in the interventions planned by the professional, and the process of change is more sustainable.

This book extends the Pathways Model to chronic illness, with practical guidelines for both self-care and professional intervention. *Pathways to Illness, Pathways to Health* (2013) focused primarily on human beings with conditions from which they could recover. Some chronic conditions were included, such as addictive disorders, diabetes, and fibromyalgia. However, the majority of the case narratives highlighted patients who were able to reverse much or all of their symptoms; in many ways, they *recovered!* In this volume, we highlight human beings with a variety of chronic and irreversible medical and emotional disorders, such as chronic pain, bipolar disorder, lupus erythematosus, and cancer, and show how they have utilized the Pathways Model to manage their conditions, moderate their systems, and enhance their quality of life. For the most part, they do not expect to *recover* from their illness, but they can *thrive* in their lives. Chapter 3 will present a model, based on positive psychology, self-determination theory, and the new model of post-traumatic growth, for thriving with one's chronic condition.

The Pathways Model treatment documented in the case narratives in this book were variously carried out with the collaboration of counselors, health and clinical psychologists, health coaches, and nurse practitioners. Licensed medical and mental health professionals complete the initial evaluation; these individuals assess physical and emotional health, lifestyle, and health-related behaviors. Diagnoses are established and overall treatment goals are developed. Optimally, the primary care physician and/or specialty physicians such as oncologists and cardiologists are included in the Pathways team. This is an *interprofessional* model of collaborative care across disciplines.

> "When human beings face illness, disability, and the possibility of death, they often struggle with existential and spiritual questions."

Regardless of discipline, whether psychologist, counselor, nurse, or coach, the Pathways interventions making up Level One and Level Two are largely coaching interventions. The Pathways team invites the patient into a collaborative "alliance for health," and engages in motivation interviewing to mobilize patient's active involvement in the Pathways health plan. The old model of a professional prescribing and the patient complying is overturned. The patient actively sets goals and selects specific lifestyle changes, behavioral steps, and interventions, in dialogue with the Pathways team.

Expanding the Pathways Model: I. Religion and Spiritual Practices

This volume also emphasizes two areas of health and behavior that were not highlighted in *Pathways to Illness, Pathways to Health* (2013). First is the area of religion, spiritual practices, and health. Spirituality, illness, and health are intermingled in a multitude of ways. When human beings face illness, disability, and the possibility of death, they often struggle with existential and spiritual questions.

The authors (McGrady and Moss) considered adding a Level Four to the Pathways Model, suggesting that human beings can transform their lives and their illnesses through spiritual transcendence at another new and higher level in their Pathways programs. However, on second thought, we recognized that religion and spirituality are not separate from the other three levels. Rather, they deserve a place at each level. Human beings can make small self-directed changes in their spiritual practices, can benefit from educational materials and community resources for pursuing spiritual renewal, and can turn to ministers, pastoral educators, parish nurses, and other spiritual counselors for professional guidance in applying religion and spiritual practices to their health. Chapter 4 will explore religion, religious practices, and spiritual disciplines as factors in managing and enhancing health.

Expanding the Pathways Model: II. Complementary Therapies

The second area deserving more attention within the Pathways Model is the benefit available from complementary or non-mainstream therapies. An increasing number of North Americans utilize a wide variety of non-mainstream therapies. As discussed earlier, complementary and alternative medicine (CAM) has served as an umbrella label for all therapies outside of the mainstream of conventional Western medicine. The term Complementary Medicine was applied to those non-mainstream therapies that are used in combination with conventional medical interventions to *complement* conventional care (NCCIH, 2016). Complementary therapies can sometimes be conceptualized in ways compatible with the Western biomedical model, which highlights physiology, biochemistry, and identifiable disease mechanisms. Mind-body approaches such as biofeedback and hypnosis are somewhat outside of the mainstream of medical practice, yet each operates in ways that "make sense" to science, and each addresses well-recognized disease mechanisms. For example, patients using biofeedback enhance their awareness of their physiology and learn to modify physiological processes related to the target condition (Shaffer & Moss, 2006). Similarly, neuro-imaging during hypnosis shows that hypnosis modifies activity in brain pain centers in specific ways related to the language and suggestions in the hypnosis induction. Hypnotic suggestions to reduce the unpleasantness of pain influence brain activity in the anterior cingulate cortex, while hypnotic suggestions to reduce the magnitude or intensity of pain sensations primarily influence the somatosensory cortex (Hofbauer, Rainville, Duncan, & Bushnell, 2001; Jensen & Patterson, 2014; Rainville, Duncan, Price, Carrier, & Bushnell, 1997).

The term Alternative Medicine, in contrast, was applied to those therapies that were seen as replacing conventional medical treatments; serving as an alternative to mainstream medical care (NCCIH, 2016). With the increasing dialogue between medical researchers and CAM researchers, however, there are fewer and fewer truly alternative therapies. Therapies, such as Reiki energy healing, that were once believed to be entirely separate from conventional care, are now frequently delivered in hospital and clinical settings, especially those providing cancer care, palliative care, and end-of-life care. In addition, a study by Astin (1998) showed that only 4.4% of patients used alternative therapies in isolation. Thus, the vast majority of patients utilize these one-time "alternative therapies" as complements to conventional care and appreciate them for their beneficial effects in moderating stress, soothing pain, and reducing discomfort generally.

Some alternative therapies have been conceptualized in terms incompatible with Western scientific models. Energy medicine, for example, is often claimed to enhance the flow of Chi and circulate Chi around the body. Chi is a kind of energy or life force, and energy therapies aim to restore an energetic balance to the body. Or energy therapies may be seen as restoring balance to the Chakras, energy centers according to the Ayurvedic medicine system of India. Both Chi and the Chakras seem to be incompatible conceptually with a biomedical model that emphasizes variables measured by blood work or imaged with a PET scan or functional MRI. Nevertheless, Western science is attempting to come to terms with these alternative models, conducting research first to assess whether the interventions based on the hypothetical energy have measurable health effects, and secondarily to measure whether the hypothesized fluctuations of energy during energy medicine sessions correlate with measurable Western physiological processes or mechanisms.

Health effects of energy-based interventions Many studies show therapeutic benefit for Qi Gong, Reiki, and other energy therapies. Jahnke, Larkey, Rogers, Etnier, and Lin (2010) did a comprehensive review of 77 methodologically adequate research studies and concluded that research consistently showed the therapeutic effects of Qi Gong and Tai Chi, including improved bone density, cardiopulmonary condition, physical function, reduced falls, self-efficacy, and immune function.

Western scientific investigation of non-mainstream therapy mechanisms The National Center for Complementary and Integrative Health (formerly the National Center for Complementary and Alternative Medicine) has provided grant funding since at least 2002 for basic, mechanistic, and pre-clinical research in all domains of non-mainstream medicine in order to provide a stronger foundation for ongoing and planned clinical studies (NCCAM, 2002). The research has specifically targeted a number of areas including changes in immune pathways induced by non-mainstream therapies, animal research, and imaging studies on the mechanisms involved in therapeutic massage, investigations of the therapeutic pathways being impacted by manual therapies such as spinal manipulation, and many other areas (NCCAM, 2002; NIH, 2015).

Philosophical and paradigmatic values of complementary and integrative medicine In addition, there are many values associated with complementary and integrative medicine that seem to appeal to the health consumer. Many complementary and integrative approaches emphasize:

1. A holistic view of body, mind, and spirit
2. Regard for the patient as a unique human being
3. A personal supportive relationship between healer and patient
4. An active role for the patient in the healing process
5. The use of lifestyle and habit changes to optimize health
6. Interventions to elicit the body's inner resources for healing
7. An aversion to invasive and harsh treatments that crush the disease but harm the patient
8. An openness to prayer, meditation, and spiritual practices as tools for healing
9. An integration of physical, psychological, and spiritual practices
10. An acceptance of unconventional interventions and models that appear to demonstrate efficacy (Adapted from Moss et al., 2003, p. 13)

"The authors of the present volume advocate that these complementary and integrative medicine values are much needed for the average medical patient today, often suffering with diseases of lifestyle, stress-related conditions, and chronic illnesses."

The authors of the present volume advocate that these complementary and integrative medicine values are much needed by the average medical patient today, often suffering with diseases of lifestyle, stress-related conditions, and chronic illnesses. It is our belief that these features belong in primary care, and not just in some separate complementary medicine clinic. Chapter 6 will present the vision of a true partnership between complementary therapies and mainstream medicine within a broader integrative health care.

Summary

In closing, illness in the twenty-first century presents a new face, and the best answer to that new face is often lifestyle change, self-care, and illness "self-management." The Pathways Model provides an integrative model for delivering this new approach to health care. It offers a model of multi-level interventions: beginning with Level One, including simple self-directed behavior change, continuing with Level Two, emphasizing the acquisition of self-regulation skills and the use of educational materials and community resources for wellness, and culminating in Level Three, the delivery of evidence-based professional therapies.

The Pathways Model includes the use of health and wellness coaching strategies to enlist the patient in an alliance for health, fostering personal involvement and self-efficacy for a program of behavioral and lifestyle change. The Pathways Model also promotes the application of positive, health enhancing religious and spiritual practices, and evidence-based complementary therapies for the cultivation of wellness and the management of illness.

References

Astin, J. (1998). Why patients use alternative medicine: Results of a national survey. *Journal of the American Medical Association, 279*(19), 1548–1553.

Bandura, A. (2004). Health promotion by social cognitive means. *Health Education and Behavior, 31*(2), 143–164.

Brown, K. W., & Ryan, R. M. (2004). Fostering healthy self-regulation from within and without: A self-determination theory perspective. In P. A. Linley & S. Joseph (Eds.), *Positive psychology in practice* (pp. 105–124). Hoboken, NJ: Wiley.

Csikszentimihalyi, M. (1999). If we are so rich, why aren't we happy? *American Psychologist, 54*(10), 821–827.

Egger, G., Katz, D., Sagner, M., & Stevens, J. (2014). The art and science of chronic disease management come together in a lifestyle-focused approach to primary care. *International Journal of Clinical Practice, 68*(12), 1406–1409. https://doi.org/10.1111/ijcp.12500

George, S. R., & Thomas, S. P. (2010). Lived experience of diabetes among older, rural people. *Journal of Advanced Nursing, 66*(5), 1092–1100. https://doi.org/10.1111/j.13652648.2010.05278.x

Hofbauer, R. K., Rainville, P., Duncan, G. H., & Bushnell, M. C. (2001). Cortical representation of the sensory dimension of pain. *Journal of Neurophysiology, 86*(1), 402–411.

Jahnke, R., Larkey, L., Rogers, C., Etnier, J., & Lin, F. (2010). A comprehensive review of health benefits of Qigong and Tai Chi. *American Journal of Health Promotion, 24*(6), e1–e25. https://doi.org/10.4278/ajhp.081013-LIT-248

Jensen, M. P., & Patterson, D. R. (2014). Hypnotic approaches for chronic pain management. *American Psychologist, 69*(2), 167–177. https://doi.org/10.1037/a0035644

Lorig, K. R., Ritter, P., Stewart, A. L., Sobel, D. S., Brown, B. W., Bandura, A., et al. (2001). Chronic disease self-management program: 2-Year health status and health care utilization outcomes. *Medical Care, 39*(11), 1217–1223.

Maslow, A. H. (1968). *Toward a psychology of being* (3rd ed.). New York, NY: Wiley.

McGrady, A., & Moss, D. (2013). *Pathways to illness, pathways to health*. New York, NY: Springer. https://doi.org/10.1007/978-1-4419-1379-1.

Miek, J., van de Vijver, L., Busch, M., Fritsma, J., & Seldenrijk, R. (2012). Integration of complementary and alternative medicine in primary care: What do patients want? *Patient Education and Counseling, 89*(3), 417–422.

Moss, D. (Ed.). (1999). *Humanistic and transpersonal psychology: A historical and biographical sourcebook*. Westport, CT: Greenwood.

Moss, D. (2015). Integration of mindfulness training into a comprehensive "Pathways Model" treatment program: The case of Jorge. *Biofeedback, 43*(3), 137–141.

Moss, D., McGrady, A., Davies, T., & Wickramasekera, I. (Eds.). (2003). *Handbook of mind-body medicine in primary care*. Thousand Oaks, CA: Sage.

Murray, C., Atkinson, C., Bhalla, K., Birbeck, G., Burstein, R., Chou, D., et al. (2015). The state of US health, 1990–2010: Burden of diseases, injuries, and risk factors. *Journal of the American Medical Association, 310*(6), 591–608. https://doi.org/10.1001/jama.2013.13805

National Center for Complementary and Alternative Medicine. (2002). *Basic and preclinical research on complementary and alternative medicine*. Program Announcement Number PA-02-124. Retrieved from http://grants.nih.gov/grants/guide/pa-files/PA-02-124.html

National Center for Complementary and Integrative Health. (2016). *Complementary alternative or integrative health. What's in a name?* Retrieved from https://nccih.nih.gov/health/integrative-health

National Center for Health Statistics. (2016). *Mortality in the US, 2015*. NCHS Data Brief No. 267. Retrieved from https://www.cdc.gov/nchs/products/databriefs/db267.htm

National Institutes of Health. (2015). *Basic and preclinical research on complementary and alternative medicine (CAM) (R15)*. Program Announcement Number PA-06-064. Retrieved from http://archives.nih.gov/asites/grants/09-17-2015/grants/guide/pa-files/PA-06-064.html

Ornish, D. (1996). *Dr. Dean Ornish's program for reversing heart disease*. New York, NY: Ivy Books/Ballantine Books.

Ornish, D., Scherwitz, L., Billings, J., Brown, S. E., Gould, K. L., Merritt, T. A., & Brand, R. J. (1998). Intensive lifestyle changes for reversal of coronary heart disease. Five-year follow-up of the Lifestyle Heart Trial. *Journal of the American Medical Association, 280*, 2001–2007.

Pearson, E. S. (2011). The 'how to' of health behavior change brought to life: A theoretical analysis of the co-active coaching model and its underpinnings in self-determination theory. *Coaching: An International Journal of Theory, Research, and Practice, 4*(2), 89–103.

Phelps, C. (2014). *The lived experience of individuals with Type 2 diabetes who have sustained successful lifestyle change and achieved long-term positive health outcomes: A detailed look at the female experience* (Doctoral dissertation). Retrieved from the ProQuest dissertation database (UMI No. 3642969).

Pischke, C. R., Frenda, S., Ornish, D., & Weidner, G. (2010). Lifestyle changes are related to reductions in depression in persons with elevated coronary risk factors. *Psychological Health, 25*(9), 1077–1100.

Prochaska, J. O., & Norcross, J. C. (2001). Stages of change. *Psychotherapy, 38*(4), 443–448.

Prochaska, J. O., & Velicer, W. F. (1997). The transtheoretical model of health behavior change. *American Journal of Health Promotion, 12*, 38–48.

Rainville, P., Duncan, G. H., Price, D. D., Carrier, B., & Bushnell, M. C. (1997). Pain affect encoded in human anterior cingulate but not somatosensory cortex. *Science, 277*(5328), 968–971.

Robinson, A., & McGrail, M. R. (2004). Disclosure of CAM use to medical practitioners: A review of qualitative and quantitative studies. *Complementary Therapies in Medicine, 12*(2–3), 90–98.

Ryan, R. M., & Deci, E. L. (2002). An overview of self-determination theory: An organismic-dialectical perspective. In E. L. Deci & R. M. Ryan (Eds.), *Handbook of self-determination research* (pp. 3–36). Rochester, NY: The University of Rochester Press.

Sagner, M., Katz, D., Egger, G., Lianov, L., Schulz, K. H., Braman, M., et al. (2014). Lifestyle medicine potential for reversing a world of chronic disease epidemics: From cell to community. *International Journal of Clinical Practice, 68*(11), 1289–1292. https://doi.org/10.1111/ijcp.12509

Seligman, M. E. P., Steen, T. A., Park, N., & Peterson, C. (2005). Positive psychology progress: Empirical validation of interventions. *American Psychologist, 60*(5), 410–421.

Shaffer, F., & Moss, D. (2006). Biofeedback. In C.-S. Yuan, E. J. Bieber, & B. A. Bauer (Eds.), *Textbook of complementary and alternative medicine* (2nd ed., pp. 291–312). Abingdon, Oxfordshire, UK: Informa Healthcare.

Silberman, A., Banthia, R., Estay, I. S., Kemp, C., Studley, J., Hareras, D., & Ornish, D. (2010). The effectiveness and efficacy of an intensive cardiac rehabilitation program in 24 sites. *American Journal of Health Promotion, 24*(4), 260–266.

Spence, G. B., & Oades, L. B. (2011). Coaching with self-determination in mind: Using theory to advance evidence-based coaching practice. *International Journal of Evidence Based Coaching and Mentoring, 9*(2), 37–55.

Thorpe, K., Florence, C., Howard, D., & Joski, P. (2004). The impact of obesity in rising health spending. *Health Affairs,* Suppl Web Exclusives, W4-480-6.

Wolever, R. Q., Dreusicke, M., Fikkan, J., Hawkins, T. V., Yeung, S., Rakefield, J., et al. (2010). Integrative health coaching for patients with Type 2 diabetes: A randomized clinical trial. *The Diabetes Educator, 36*(4), 629–639. https://doi.org/10.1177/0145721710371523

Chapter 3
Chronic Illness, Global Burden, and the Pathways Approach

Abstract This chapter proposes that the major challenge for human health in the twenty-first century is chronic diseases and chronic conditions. This is a global problem, burdening health care systems and economies worldwide. WHO statistics show that almost 70% of deaths annually are caused by chronic diseases, especially cardiovascular disease, cancer, chronic respiratory diseases, and diabetes. Factors contributing to the increase in chronic illnesses worldwide are aging populations, rapid urbanization, and the globalization of unhealthy lifestyles. This global burden of chronic disease is felt most strongly in minority and low-income populations and in developing countries. The first order of interventions includes community-based public health interventions, for example, initiatives to ban tobacco and alcohol advertising, replace trans fats with polyunsaturated fats, and increase breastfeeding. The chapter also introduces functional medicine and the Pathways approach to chronic conditions, two perspectives integrating a holistic evolutionary systems-based approach, with attention to lifestyle variables, affective regulation, early trauma, and environmental influences. The example of obesity is utilized to illustrate the influence of lifestyle, nutrition, stress, trauma, and the human biome on chronic conditions.

Keywords Chronic illness · Global burden · Functional medicine · Obesity · The human biome · Stress · Emotional dysregulation · Adverse childhood experiences

Introduction

This chapter introduces emerging community health perspectives on chronic illness, which frame it as the major challenge to health in the twenty-first century. The chapter reviews the evidence that chronic illness has become an increasing burden to the

This chapter was written with the assistance of co-author, Jennifer Heintzman, Ph.D., College of Integrative Medicine and Health Sciences, Saybrook University, Oakland, CA.

developing world, as well as the developed world, now contributing substantially to deaths and to health care costs worldwide. The primary factors contributing to this global problem are lifestyle based, and call for community-based interventions targeting lifestyle change.

Individual health education and treatment also remain a priority, and this chapter introduces both functional medicine and the Pathways approach to chronic illness, supporting lifestyle modification, behavioral change, and quality of life on an individual basis. This approach is relevant across the spectrum of income groups and nations, as lifestyle-based chronic conditions afflict increasing numbers worldwide. Concepts drawn from functional medicine, lifestyle medicine, stress theory, affective regulation, and research on the effects of trauma on health is explored to emphasize the challenges presented by chronic illness today.

The Global Problem of Chronic Disease

Concepts of Chronic Disease

Chronic diseases are defined by the World Health Organization (WHO, 2015) as those health conditions that are not transmittable from person to person, are slow to progress, and are long-lasting. In its current literature, WHO refers to chronic disease as non-communicable diseases (NCDs). NCDs comprise one of three categories of disease and injury identified by the World Health Organization (2016a, 2016b) in order to track statistical information related to global incidences of mortality and morbidity. The other two categories include: (1) communicable, maternal, perinatal, and nutritional conditions; and (2) injuries. Neither the term chronic disease nor the term non-communicable disease is ideal, since in fact, some chronic conditions, such as cervical cancer, do have an infectious origin, and some communicable diseases, such as HIV/AIDS, are chronic (Adeyl, Smith, & Robles, 2007).

According to WHO (2015, 2016b) statistics, NCDs are responsible for 38 million deaths globally each year, or almost 70% of all reported deaths. The majority of these deaths (82%) were caused by cardiovascular disease (heart attacks and strokes), cancer, chronic respiratory diseases (asthma and chronic obstructive pulmonary disease), and diabetes.

The Australian Institute of Health and Welfare provided a definition that was both straightforward and comprehensive, emphasizing the global impact of chronic illness on the human being:

> The term **chronic disease** applies to a group of diseases that tend to be long-lasting and have persistent effects. Chronic diseases have a range of potential impacts on a person's individual circumstances, including quality of life and broader social and economic effects. (Australian Institute of Health and Welfare, 2015)

Global burden of chronic disease The global burden of chronic disease is rising rapidly according to WHO statistics set out in the *Global Action Plan for the*

Prevention and Control of NCDs 2013–2030 (WHO, 2013). The WHO report predicts that global deaths due to NCDs will increase by 15% between 2010 and 2020. This rise is anticipated due to the significant driving forces identified as contributing to the development of chronic diseases, which include aging populations, rapid urbanization, and the globalization of unhealthy lifestyles (Randall & Ford, 2011). Unhealthy lifestyles have been linked to increased blood pressure, elevated glucose levels and cholesterol, and ultimately to obesity, which is a significant chronic condition worldwide (WHO, 2003, 2011).

World Health Organization (2015) statistics indicate that all age groups, including children, adults, and the elderly, are susceptible to NCDs. Of the total number of global deaths due to chronic disease that occur each year, 16 million, or nearly half of them, are premature deaths, which means they have occurred to individuals who are below the age of 70 years. The reason all age groups are susceptible to developing NCDs is that people in all age groups are vulnerable to the primary risk factors for developing chronic diseases. These risk factors, as identified by WHO, include exposure to tobacco or alcohol, an unhealthy diet, and a lack of physical activity.

"Nearly three-quarters of the 38 million chronic disease related deaths that occur annually around the world, or 28 million, occur in developing countries (low- and middle-income nations)."

Until recently, NCDs, or chronic diseases, have been regarded as conditions largely affecting people in the developed, high-income countries. The pattern in the global burden of chronic disease has now shifted in the direction of developing nations. Nearly three-quarters of the 38 million chronic disease-related deaths that occur annually around the world, or 28 million, occur in developing countries (low- and middle-income nations). Statistics indicate that NCDs are closely related to poverty (WHO, 2013). Not only are the majority of global chronic disease-related deaths occurring in developing nations, but also 82% of premature deaths due to chronic disease are occurring in low- to middle-income countries (WHO, 2016b). In developing nations, the vulnerable and the socially disadvantaged get sicker and die sooner than people living in developed nations. The vulnerable and disadvantaged in low- and middle-income countries are at a greater risk to: be exposed to harmful substances such as tobacco and alcohol, eat poorer quality of food, experience greater stress, and have limited access to health care services (WHO, 2011). Of course, the drinking of alcohol and the consumption of a poor diet occurs in both low- and high-income countries worldwide. However, individuals in high-income countries have greater access to health services that buffer them from the risks of developing chronic diseases (Randall & Ford, 2011). Although chronic diseases remain the major cause of death and disability in developed countries, the global burden of such chronic diseases is felt most strongly in minority and low-income populations.

World Health Organization (WHO) Approach to Chronic Disease Management

In 2011, the WHO policy response to the global NCD burden was endorsed by the 66th World Health Assembly and subsequently 190 countries agreed with the policy. One aspect of the policy response was the creation of the *Global Action Plan for the Prevention and Control of NCDs 2013–2030* (WHO, 2013, 2015). The plan established nine voluntary global health targets, one of which was to reduce the number of premature deaths due to NCDs worldwide by 25% by 2025. The majority (90%) of premature deaths due to NCDs in the world occur in low- and middle-income countries (WHO, 2011). The majority of these premature deaths could be prevented given the fact that most premature deaths are linked to common risk factors such as alcohol and tobacco use, inactivity, and poor diet (Hamilton, Healy, Dunstan, Zderic, & Owen, 2008; Pratt, Norris, Lobelo, Roux, & Wang, 2012).

The WHO *Global Action Plan for the Prevention and Control of NCDs 2013–2030* (2013) encourages a comprehensive approach to the management of NCDs, which focuses strategies on the detection, screening, and treatment of NCDs. The plan lays out a three-pronged approach to chronic disease management aimed at: (1) reducing the risks associated with developing NCDs, (2) promoting interventions that prevent and control NCDs, and (3) mapping the epidemic of NCDs and their risk factors worldwide in order to monitor national progress in reaching the voluntary global targets agreed to by member nations by 2025. In 2015, nations began setting national targets and measuring their progress (WHO, 2015).

In order to prevent the majority of premature deaths and disability due to chronic disease worldwide, the WHO *Global Action Plan* (2013) outlines a selection of the most cost-effective and impactful interventions focused on reducing the risk factors associated with NCDs, as well as promoting interventions designed to prevent and control chronic disease. Countries that agreed to the *Global Action Plan* have been able to choose to implement interventions that align with their national needs and their financial resources. Suggested interventions include: the banning of harmful tobacco and alcohol advertising, replacing trans fats with polyunsaturated fats, promoting breastfeeding of infants, and implementing simple screening measures to detect and prevent diseases such as cervical cancer (WHO, 2015).

In addition to promoting and implementing chronic disease prevention and control strategies, the WHO *Global Action Plan* (2013) makes clear that the greatest impact in NCD management will be achieved by re-orienting national health systems to address the needs and manage the care of individuals with NCDs, including offering palliative care (WHO, 2015).

The ability of countries to adopt implementation strategies to prevent and control NCDs and to structure their public health systems to care for and treat individuals with NCDs is related to their national wealth. It is problematic that low- and middle-income countries that have the greatest need to intervene and manage chronic disease (compared to high-income countries) have the least financial ability to do so (WHO, 2015). High-income countries are four times as likely as low-income countries to cover NCD-related health care services through health insurance. Countries with inadequate health insurance coverage are unlikely to provide universal access to essential NCD interventions.

The World Bank (Adeyl et al., 2007) supports the WHO policy response to non-communicable diseases. Like WHO, the World Bank has identified public health interventions and improved medical care for individuals with NCDs as essential strategies for impacting the massive global chronic disease burden. The World Bank emphasizes that NCDs place a significant economic burden on countries, particularly as significant numbers of individual's age, leave the paid labor force, and are more likely to develop NCDs. The economic burden will be felt by multiple entities, including individuals, households, communities, employers, health care systems, and governments. This burden will affect mostly the poor, and hence, the rich-poor gap in health outcomes must be addressed. This economic burden strengthens the World Bank's emphasis on the need for a cost-effective analysis of interventions for the control, prevention, treatment, and management of NCDs. According to the World Bank, the most cost-effective interventions for the prevention of NCDs include tobacco taxes.

The World Bank (Adeyl et al., 2007) also addresses the issue of service delivery issues as being central to achieving better NCD outcomes. Given that a key component of management of chronic diseases is the need for long-term care, the World Bank report highlights the importance of community engagement to improve access to health care services and to promote patient self-care. Community engagement is defined by the World Health Organization as "a process by which people are enabled to become actively and genuinely involved in defining the issues of concern to them, in making decisions about factors that affect their lives, in formulating and implementing policies, in planning, developing, and delivering services and in taking action to achieve change" (1992).

Evolving Understandings of Chronic Diseases

In recent years, the World Health Organization (2011, 2013) and the World Bank (Adeyl et al., 2007) have identified an upward trend in mortality and morbidity related to chronic or non-communicable diseases worldwide. Both WHO reports and World Bank reports project that the burden of chronic disease will increase rapidly in the years to come. Deaths due to NCDs are projected to increase by 15% between 2010 and 2020, with the greatest increase occurring in Africa, Eastern Mediterranean, and South East Asia, where they will increase by more than 20% (WHO, 2011, 2013). Currently, NCDs are the major cause of death in middle- and high-income countries, but according to the World Bank (2007) NCDs are projected to be the major cause of death in low-income countries by 2015 as well. In low-income countries, communicable diseases, death related to childbirth, and nutrition-related deaths have historically dominated mortality statistics. These are the issues that, until recently, have constituted the global health priorities.

"This shift in the global pattern of disease in the direction of chronic diseases being the leading cause of mortality and morbidity worldwide is taking place at an accelerated rate, and the shift is occurring at a faster rate in developing countries than it did in developed, high income countries a half-century ago."

Shifts in public health care priorities In the past, public health policy has been dominated by an emphasis on communicable or infectious diseases, while chronic and non-communicable diseases were understood to be largely limited to the developed regions of the world. However, newer statistical research (Adeyl et al., 2007; WHO 2003, 2011, 2013) indicates that developing countries are suffering increasingly high levels of public health problems related to chronic diseases. Currently, chronic diseases dominate mortality statistics in five out of six regions identified by the World Health Organization (2011). In 23 selected low-and middle-income countries, accounting for 80% of the total burden of chronic disease mortality in developing nations, chronic diseases are responsible for 50% of the total disease burden. Age-standardized death rates are more than 50% higher in 15 of these 23 countries than in high-income countries (Abegunde, Mathers, Adam, Ortegon, & Strong, 2007; WHO, 2011).

This shift in the global pattern of disease in the direction of chronic diseases being the leading cause of mortality and morbidity worldwide is taking place at an accelerated rate, and the shift is occurring at a faster rate in developing countries than it did in developed, high-income countries a half-century ago (Abegunde et al., 2007). The issue is complicated by the fact that some developing nations are experiencing a double burden of disease: They are being challenged by significant and simultaneous burdens of communicable and non-communicable diseases. In countries such as India, projections indicate that communicable diseases will still occupy a critically important position in the health policy agenda in that country until at least 2020 (Abegunde et al., 2007).

The shift in the global pattern of disease identified by the World Health Organization and the World Bank has also been acknowledged by the United States Department of State (n.d.). The US Department of State has explained that historically chronic diseases have been found primarily in high-income countries, while low-income, developing nations were occupied primarily with combating infectious diseases. Now, however, developing nations are also experiencing chronic diseases such as heart disease, lung disease, cancer, diabetes, and respiratory disease, as the major cause of death and disability. By 2020, chronic non-communicable diseases will account for seven out of ten deaths worldwide, as they already do in the United States.

Chronic Illness in the United States

The 1998 Medical Expenditure Panel Survey (MEPS) compiled health data by interviewing a nationally representative sample of more than 24,000 Americans (Anderson & Horvath, 2004). This research showed that 45% of working-age Americans and 85% of seniors have at least one chronic condition. Findings from the study also determined that health care costs related to chronic conditions account for 78% of all health care spending in the United States annually. The researchers who conducted the study warned that the MEPS did not include American adults living in institutions such as nursing homes, and as a result, the number of individuals reported living with chronic conditions in the United States and the cost of their care is likely even higher than indicated by the study findings. In 2012, the Center for Disease Control and Prevention (CDC) determined that about 50% of all adults, 117 million individuals in the United States, has been diagnosed with a chronic condition, and about 25% of adults are diagnosed with two or more chronic conditions (CDC, 2016a).

Chronic Illness, Death, and Disability

" ... health care costs related to chronic conditions account for 78% of all health care spending in the United States annually."

According to the Centers for Disease Control and Prevention, chronic diseases are the leading cause of death and disability in the United States (CDC, 2016a). Chronic diseases are responsible for seven out of ten deaths in the United States, and two conditions, cardiovascular disease (CVD)[1] and cancer, are responsible for nearly half (48%) of all deaths (CDC, 2016a).

The Centers for Disease Control National Health Report (CDC, 2014) evaluated the findings from 17 CDC surveys and three non-CDC sources to determine national health trends in the United States between 2005 and 2013. The national health report concluded that the leading causes of death for that period remained primarily the same, with the exception that the rank order of prevalence for the top ten causes of death changed minimally. (The top 10 causes of death in the United States are: heart disease, cancer, respiratory disease, stroke, unintentional injury, Alzheimer's disease, diabetes mellitus, pneumonia and influenza, kidney disease, and intentional self-harm).

---

[1]CVD here includes primarily coronary heart disease and stroke, high blood pressure, and heart failure.

The report also concluded that the age-adjusted mortality rates for the majority of the leading causes of death are on the decline. However, a closer look at the numbers indicates that in some areas the actual number of deaths per annum is on the rise. The authors of the report suggest that the reason for this increase may be related to the increase in the US population size, as well as to decreased engagement in protective behaviors such as physical activity among adults, and increased engagement in risky behaviors such as alcohol consumption and tobacco exposure. Overall, the national health report is clear that much of the health burden related to the ten leading causes of death in the United States, including the massive burden due to chronic disease, could be reduced or avoided altogether through improved nutrition, increased physical activity, improved vaccination rates, the avoidance of tobacco use, and other behavioral interventions.

In an effort to reduce the prevalence of chronic disease in the United States, and to help individuals manage their chronic illnesses better, or prevent them altogether, the Centers for Disease Control and Prevention (CDC, 2016b) has focused its efforts on promoting strategies designed to reduce the risk factors associated with chronic disease. The CDC has implemented prevention strategies aimed at government policy changes and initiatives that:

- Lead to more smoke-free environments in workplaces and public spaces
- Ensure access to healthy foods, particularly in underserved communities
- Tax unhealthy food, tobacco, and alcohol products
- Ban trans fatty acids in food items
- Encourage healthier restaurant menus
- Increase the number of fluoridated community water systems in the United States
- Promote cancer screening, as well as heart and stroke prevention
- Lead to better designed communities built to encourage physical exercise
- Enable safe walking and biking
- Lead to better or increased access to physical education programs in schools and childcare environments

These strategies are largely in alignment with the Pathways Model (McGrady & Moss, 2013), although the Centers for Disease Control did not address the role of stress in chronic disease, and neglected the power of stress management in enhancing wellness. Where these recommendations were implemented, they have supported individuals in making healthier lifestyle choices.

The Individual Problem of Chronic Disease

The public health perspective outlined above and the corresponding community-based initiatives address only part of the problem regarding the prevalence of chronic disease in the United States. Individual human beings afflicted with chronic illness also need strategies to manage their chronic conditions and to restore quality of life. At this point, we will supplement the public health perspective on chronic illness, by introducing the functional medicine point of view, and highlighting the role of chronic stress, emotional dysregulation, adverse childhood experiences, and psychological trauma.

Chronic Disease from a Functional Medicine Perspective

The concept of functional medicine was developed in 1989 (or 1990) by Jeffrey Bland, a biochemist with training and experience in the fields of nutritional medicine and systems biology (Bland, 2015). Functional medicine emerged in parallel with sharp increases in the number of individuals suffering from complex chronic illnesses in the United States. At the same time, the traditional acute care medical approach to illness demonstrably failed to prevent and treat these chronic diseases. The development of functional medicine was supported by growing interest nationwide in complementary and alternative medicine and by a related movement away from simplistic pharmaceutical drug therapy to treat symptoms of illness.

The traditional medical model has been effective in responding to infectious diseases and acute traumas, but ineffective in responding to the epidemic of chronic diseases. The functional medicine approach was designed in a way that moves beyond the management of acute symptoms of disease and addresses the underlying causes of chronic disease. It applies scientific research findings and a systems-biology orientation to better understand the antecedents of disease, as well as the triggers and the mediators of chronic disease. It seeks to develop a picture—not just of *what* is wrong with a chronically ill individual—but of *why* an individual is experiencing complex health issues.

"In other words, lifestyle choices and environmental factors can turn on or off certain genes, which can lead to the development of chronic disease."

The functional medicine systems-oriented approach is focused on three complementary and interrelated goals. It seeks to: (1) address the underlying causes of chronic illness, instead of simply treating the symptoms; (2) support unwell individuals on a path to optimal quality of life and mental-emotional-spiritual well-being, in spite of chronic illness; and (3) guide all individuals to embrace practices that will prevent illness altogether. In order to develop a complete understanding of the client, the functional medicine clinician considers the genetic predisposition of the individual to develop chronic illness, the individual's personal lifestyle, and the environmental factors influencing the individual's health.

The functional medicine approach operates with an understanding that genetics plays a role in the development of chronic illnesses, but genetic predisposition to disease is only part of the story. Research has shown that "humans are not genetically hardwired for most diseases; instead, gene expression is altered by myriad influences, including environment, lifestyle, diet, activity patterns, psycho-social-spiritual factors, and stress" (Jones & Quinn, 2016, p. 3). In other words, lifestyle choices and environmental factors can turn on or off certain genes, which can lead to the development of chronic disease. So, from a functional medicine perspective, chronic disease is driven by food, lifestyle, and environment, in an interaction with genetics (Jones & Quinn, 2016, p. 2). In order to respond to complex chronic illnesses that are impacted by food, daily activities of living, and environmental factors, health practitioners have to address the *pathways to disease*, which include poor nutrition, inactive lifestyles, chronic stress, toxic environments, a lack of social and emotional support (relatedness), and problems in spirituality, purpose, and meaning in the lives of many Americans.

An Example: Obesity from a Functional Medicine Perspective and a Holistic, Pathways Perspective

Obesity as a Chronic Illness

Obesity is among the most prevalent and the most preventable chronic diseases affecting Americans and is a major contributor to other chronic illnesses, especially cardiovascular diseases and diabetes. The problem will be addressed here through North American and European research, but we nevertheless emphasize that globalization of American and Western lifestyles is rendering obesity, like other chronic conditions, a global problem (WHO, 2017). The World Health Organization has reported that in 2014 there were 1.9 billion overweight adults worldwide and 600 million obese individuals (WHO, 2016c).

Obesity in the United States

"High obesity rates place millions of Americans at heightened risk for developing chronic illnesses such as diabetes, heart disease, high blood pressure, nonalcoholic fatty liver disease, osteoarthritis, some forms of cancer, and stroke …"

Obesity has been identified as a serious health concern in the United States, with statistics indicating that more than one-third of American adults, or 78.6 million people, are obese (CDC, 2014). Nearly 69% of American adults are overweight or obese, and 1 in 20 are extremely obese. One in five children and adolescents in the United States currently are obese. According to research reported in *The State of Obesity* (Levi, Segal, Rayburn, & Martin, 2015), which analyzed health survey interview data gathered from more than 400,000 adults annually, obesity rates have more than doubled in the past 35 years and as a result, obesity has reached epidemic proportions. High obesity rates place millions of Americans at heightened risk for developing chronic illnesses such as diabetes, heart disease, high blood pressure, nonalcoholic fatty liver disease, osteoarthritis, some forms of cancer, and stroke (United States Department of Health and Human Services, 2012).

Evolutionary perspective In attempting to understand *why a*n individual develops a chronic illness such as obesity, the functional medicine perspective considers biological evolution. From an evolutionary perspective, obesity can be explained in three ways (Speakman, 2013). First, it may be viewed as a positive genetic adaptation. For instance, obesity might be seen as an adaptation in areas of the world where food supplies are erratic. Unfortunately, research that has looked at cultural variations in nutritional stability does not support this explanation (Benyshek & Watson, 2006; Nesse & Stearns, 2008). Second, the development of obesity may be viewed as non-adaptive, and therefore, genetically selected only due to its association with another positive trait. However, no clear associated and adaptive trait has been identified for obesity. Third, obesity may be perceived as the expression of a random genetic mutation. This is based on an understanding that most mutations in genes are neutral and do not result in the development of disease. Gene mutations only get "turned on" in some individuals under certain circumstances (Speakman, 2013), such as in chemically toxic environments. This suggests that the development of chronic diseases in these circumstances is preventable.

Factors that contribute to the expression of altered genes and the subsequent development of obesity include poor nutrition, a sedentary lifestyle, chronic stress, and exposure to environmental toxins (Hyman, 2010). According to *Dietary Guidelines for Americans, 2015–2020* (United States Department of Health and Human Services & United States Department of Agriculture, 2015), the typical diet consumed by most Americans is low in fruits, vegetables, and healthy fats, and high in grains. Overall, Americans are not choosing nutrient dense foods, but instead are getting more than half their calories from added sugars, refined starches, and unhealthy vegetable oils. Additionally, many Americans do not have access to healthy, affordable food choices. In fact, more than 48 million Americans live in households that experience food insecurity (United States Department of Health and Human Services & United States Department of Agriculture, 2015).

Functional Medicine Assessment and Obesity

Functional medicine is an approach to health and well-being that guides the practitioner to expand her or his options for helping clients by addressing the lifestyle issues underlying their illnesses and supporting them to make changes. According to *The Institute for Functional Medicine*, the functional medicine assessment begins with an explanation for the client about the difference between conventional and functional medicine, highlighting the fact that functional medicine focuses on understanding and treating the origins of disease in the individual, as opposed to treating the symptoms of disease. The functional medicine practitioner begins by taking a functional medicine history. The practitioner gathers extensive information about the client's health history going back prior to conception, i.e., the health status of the client's mother during the pregnancy. Details about the client's medical symptoms are elicited, and a full nutritional assessment is done. The practitioner conducts a thorough physical exam. In addition, he or she incorporates into the assessment the results from all necessary medical tests conducted to identify clinical imbalances in various organ systems of the client's, such as cardiovascular, digestive, endocrine, exocrine, lymphatic, muscular-skeletal, nervous system, and urological. Along with this information, the functional medicine clinician considers the mental, emotional, and spiritual factors, as well as life experiences, and the client's attitudes and beliefs, and exposure to toxins that may be contributing factors to the client's disease.

The practitioner then has the task of organizing all of the information gathered about the client in order to identify cause-and-effect relationships between the antecedents, triggers, and mediators of the client's illness, which become clear as a thorough personal, family, social, and medical history across the life span reveals connections. The functional medicine clinician can then pinpoint the modifiable lifestyle factors that could be altered in the client's life, in order to support him or her on the path back to health. These include sleep and relaxation, exercise and movement, nutrition and hydration, stress and resilience, relationships and networks of support, trauma, microorganisms, and environmental toxins. With a complete picture of the client's health story, the practitioner and client work together to prioritize the next steps to be taken to return the client to health. These may include further assessment and interventions such as referrals to nutrition professionals, lifestyle behavior coaches or educators, or other health care providers and specialists including to other forms of therapy. The client's progress is tracked and, using additional assessments, an evaluation of the effectiveness of various therapies is made. Additions and adjustments to the treatment plan are made as needed at each clinical visit until the client is functioning well and is in full health. The functional medicine approach to assessment has been adopted by medical practitioners across the United States and has been incorporated into various training programs for clinicians as well (Grisanti & Weatherby, 2008; Hughes, 2014; Jones & Quinn, 2016).

Obesity does not develop from one unique cause and is not an isolated condition (Grundy, 1998; Valavanis, Mougiakakou, Grimaldi, & Nikita, 2010). Instead, it is a complex disease that occurs as a result of a combination of environmental and lifestyle factors in conjunction with a genetic predisposition for the development of the disease. The typical twenty-first-century North American's lifestyle is marked by a diet replete with refined foods that are high in simple carbohydrates and nutrient poor, chronic stress, insomnia, a lack of exercise and movement, chronic infections, and environmental toxins that contribute to hormone imbalances, poor gastrointestinal or "gut" health, persistent low-grade inflammation, and weight gain.

Dietary and lifestyle solutions can help the client trying to recover from obesity by improving the client's nutritional intake through the addition of high quality, nutrient dense foods; by adding movement to the client's daily life; by lessening his or her stress levels; and improving her or his sleep habits. However, as researchers (Cox, West, & Cripps, 2015; DiBaise et al., 2008; Ley, 2009) develop a growing understanding of the biological basis of obesity, it is evident that gastrointestinal or "gut" health plays a complex role. When healthy gut bacteria become overrun by unhealthy gut bacteria in the gastrointestinal system, the intestinal tract, which is supposed to funnel all toxins through the body to the point of elimination, becomes permeable. It "leaks" toxins into its surroundings and this in turn leads to low-grade persistent inflammation, which is often associated with obesity. The chronic low-grade inflammatory state causes a continuous triggering of the immune system. This in turn contributes to additional dysfunction including leptin resistance, impaired fat and glucose metabolism, insulin resistance, and beta-cell destruction.

While re-establishing healthy bacteria in the intestines is an important goal in recovery from obesity, research (Monteiro & Azevedo, 2010) indicates that acid levels in the stomach must be addressed as well, if efforts are to be successful. A low-acid level in the stomach prevents the stomach from being able to extract the necessary nutrients from foods, and the typical high carbohydrate, high sugar North American diet contributes to a low-acid environment in the stomach. In addition, while a low-acid environment prohibits the absorption of necessary proteins, fat, vitamins and minerals, it enables the extraction of more calories from food. These calories are then stored as fat, which is not the case in individuals with a healthy gut who eat the same amount of food (DiBaise et al., 2008). The stomach functions at an optimal pH level of 1.0–2.0. This low pH level is more acidic than car battery acid, and it is this high acid level that keeps the stomach free from microbes. If acid levels in the stomach start to fall and pH levels rise, the stomach's ability to destroy pathogens becomes compromised. Thus, the restoration of proper acid levels in the stomach and re-establishing the gut microbiota to a healthy state are necessary steps in improving the biological conditions that contribute to obesity.

Overwork, Sedentary Lifestyle, and Stress

Americans are working long hours each week. According to a Gallup, Inc. (2014) survey, the average American work week is 47 hours, and most jobs in the United States involve little physical movement. In addition, Americans are spending over 10 hours each day watching or engaged in media programming (Neilsen, 2016). Overall, 83 million Americans 6 years of age and older are leading sedentary lives involving minimal or no physical exertion (Physical Activity Council, 2016). Stress levels among Americans have reached an all-time record high. According to the 2015 Stress in American Survey (American Psychological Association, 2015), the average stress level reported by adults increased in 2015 over 2014 levels, and a greater number of Americans reported experiencing stress levels above what they believed was healthy. Twenty-four percent of Americans reported experiencing extreme stress levels. The top sources of stress for Americans are money, work, family responsibilities, personal health problems or health problems affecting a family member, and the economy.

Emotional Dysregulation, Autonomic Dysregulation, and Eating Behavior

Emotional dysregulation is a chronic condition for some individuals and is an accompaniment of stressful situations for others. Emotional dysregulation is both an affective and an autonomic nervous system phenomenon; it involves the individual's inability to modulate and manage negative affective states and mood lability, and an accompanying imbalance between sympathetic and parasympathetic nervous activation (Wooley et al., 2004). Excessive sympathetic activation is a marker for many stress-related disorders, ranging from hypertension to anxiety disorder to compulsive overeating (Everly & Lating, 2013; Martínez-Martínez, Mora, Vargas, Fuentes-Iniestra, & Martínez-Lavín, 2014). In addition, disturbed sympathetic nervous system regulation plays a direct role in cardiovascular illness, metabolic abnormalities, and insulin resistance (Lambert, Straznicky, Dixon, & Lambert, 2015).

Current research shows that emotional dysregulation is a contributor to emotional eating, eating in the absence of hunger, and to some extent food addiction (Baldofski et al., 2016). Gowey et al.'s study of obese adolescent and young adult females found strong associations between psychological dysregulation (cognitive, emotional, and behavioral dysregulation) and greater body mass index, problematic eating patterns and behaviors, and body dissatisfaction (Gowey et al., 2016). There are also direct associations among emotional dysregulation, depressive symptoms, and disturbed eating (bulimia) reported among diabetic youth (Young-Hyman et al., 2016). This extensive body of research suggests that interventions should not only address external lifestyle variables such as activity level and dietary choices, but also internal variables such as stress management and emotional/autonomic regulation skills.

> "Maternal emotional dysregulation impacts both the infant's early eating behaviors and infant weight."

Maternal emotional dysregulation impacts both the infant's early eating behaviors and infant weight. One study showed that mothers' emotional regulation during pregnancy predicts infant body mass index at 3 years of age (de Campora, Larciprete, Delogu, Meldolesi, & Giromini, 2016). In addition, in a study of overweight Italian mothers, de Campora, Giromini, Larciprete, Li Volsi, and Zavattini (2014) found high levels of emotional dysregulation and disturbed feeding interactions (including interactional conflicts, infant food refusal, and the affective state of the dyad during feeding) with the infants at 7 months. Early infant and mother-child dyadic intervention should also be included in efforts to address the obesity epidemic.

In addition, emotional dysregulation and functional medicine perspectives are interlinked. For example, Foster, Rineman, and Cryan (2017) have gathered evidence showing that: (1) gut microbiota influence stress-related behavior, and (2) deficiencies in gut flora produce exaggerated hypothalamic-pituitary axis stress response in animals and humans, and (3) gut microbiota can influence depression-like behavior.

Psychological Trauma, Chronic Illness, and Obesity

An abundance of research has documented the link between early experiences of trauma and later diagnosis with chronic illness and chronic conditions. One early study of almost 10,000 adults evaluated at a San Diego clinic found a strong correlation between the number of adverse/traumatic childhood events an individual had experienced and the later development of a variety of health and mental health problems. The number of adverse childhood events strongly predicted the presence of adult diseases including ischemic heart disease, cancer, lung disease, skeletal fractures, and liver disease (Felitti et al., 1998). Early exposure to trauma increases the release of an overabundance of stress hormones, disposing the individual to adult illness. The more exposure to trauma, the greater the number of adult illnesses. Williamson et al. (2002) used the same database to show that early trauma and abuse also strongly increased the risk for adult obesity. The higher the number and severity of each type of abuse and trauma, the higher the rates of obesity. More recent population-based studies have confirmed a strong link between early trauma, disordered eating, and obesity (D'Argenio et al., 2009; Fuemmeler, Dedert, McClernon, & Beckham, 2009). The D'Argenio et al. study in particular showed that a variety of early life stressors, not only abuse, increased the risk for adult era obesity. Importantly, they showed that psychiatric disorders did not account for this effect.

The number of North Americans who have experienced childhood abuse, life stress, and trauma is extremely high. The types of adverse experiences include early sexual abuse, physical abuse, parental divorce, financial dislocations, and domestic violence, and all of these early events produce abnormal levels of stress hormones, emotional dysregulation, and poor adaptive coping, raising the risk for disordered eating and obesity.

Environmental Toxins, Chronic Illness, and Obesity

Over extended periods of time, daily limited exposure to environmental toxins can have a cumulative effect, which may be detrimental. Perhaps not surprisingly, exposure to environmental contaminants among Americans is on the rise. This includes exposure to organic pollutants and heavy metals, which have been shown to alter the functioning of the neuro-endocrine-immune system and the mitochondrial system of individuals, and contribute to the development of obesity and other chronic diseases, as well as mental health disorders such as attention deficit disorder, autism spectrum disorder, depression, and dementia (Hyman, 2007). A complete assessment must be conducted with the obese individual in order to evaluate and treat the total physiological burden on the individual's mind and body. Toxins and contaminants contribute to the total burden and their presence and impact must be assessed as well. In the case of the development of obesity, toxins can influence metabolism by altering immune system functioning, mitochondrial functioning, and hormone regulation, as well as the functioning of other systems. For example, consider the herbicide ATZ (Atrazine), which has been used widely in the United States since the beginning of the obesity epidemic in the 1960s. Exposure to ATZ has been correlated with the development of insulin resistance and obesity (Hughes, 2014).

Conclusions

Obesity is a multi-factorial illness requiring the integrative, health care approach set forth in the Pathways Model (McGrady & Moss, 2013). It is a disease that is characterized by alterations in genetic expression; physiological imbalances in the endocrine system and the immune system; and imbalances in the daily life and the environment of the individual. As a complex and chronic illness, its treatment often requires that several factors be addressed. Dietary interventions, lifestyle changes, and the elimination of environmental hazards should be considered. Some examples include: Eliminating nutrient poor and inflammatory foods, increasing access to nutrient dense foods, ensuring optimal hydration, increasing daily opportunities for movement and exercise, improving sleep, increasing leisure and restful experiences, reducing work and family stress. In addition, building resilience, addressing trauma issues, improving relational support, enhancing meaning and purpose in an individual's life may all be incorporated in an effort to address the imbalances in the person's life and to impact positively the health and well-being of that individual.

Obesity is a chronic socio-psycho-biological problem; weight management treatment must be multifaceted and long term. The obese individual must be re-educated for basic affective regulation and life coping, and supported physiologically, behaviorally, socially, emotionally, and spiritually, if disordered eating patterns are to be overcome. Physiological support can include psychophysiological interventions such as heart rate variability biofeedback and stress management skills training to reduce autonomic dysregulation. McGrady (2010) has documented the benefit of biofeedback-assisted relaxation for diabetes and hypertension.

A comprehensive assessment is necessary to individualize the treatment program to address those factors most dominant for a specific individual, in order to impact positively the overall health and well-being of the individual. Medical management is also critical, since obesity is typically one component within the metabolic syndrome, with high risk for hypertension, abnormal blood glucose, hyperlipidemia, and cardiovascular disease (Ahima, 2016; Han & Lean, 2016; McGrady & Moss, 2013).

References

Abegunde, D., Mathers, C., Adam, T., Ortegon, M., & Strong, K. (2007). The burden and costs of chronic diseases in low-income and middle-income countries. *The Lancet, 370*(9603), 1929–1938. https://doi.org/10.1016/s0140-6736(07)61696-1

Adeyl, O., Smith, O., & Robles, S. (2007). *Public policy and the challenge of chronic noncommunicable diseases.* Washington, DC: The World Bank Publications. Retrieved from http://siteresources.worldbank.org/INTPH/Resources/PublicPolicyandNCDsWorldBank2007FullReport.pdf

Ahima, R. S. (Ed.). (2016). *The metabolic syndrome: A textbook.* Cham, Switzerland: Springer.

American Psychological Association. (2015). *2015 Stress in America.* Retrieved from http://www.apa.org/news/press/releases/stress/2015/snapshot.aspx

Anderson, G., & Horvath, J. (2004). The growing burden of chronic disease in America. *Public Health Reports, 119*(3), 263–270. https://doi.org/10.1016/j.phr.2004.04.005

Australian Institute of Health and Welfare. (2015). *Chronic diseases.* Retrieved from http://www.aihw.gov.au/chronic-diseases/

Baldofski, S., Rudolph, A., Tigges, W., Herbig, B., Jurowich, C., Kaiser, S., et al. (2016). Weight bias internalization, emotion dysregulation, and non-normative eating behaviors in pre-bariatric patients. *International Journal of Eating Disorders, 49*(2), 180–185. https://doi.org/10.1002/eat.22484

Benyshek, D. C., & Watson, J. T. (2006). Exploring the thrifty genotype's food-shortage assumptions: A cross-cultural comparison of ethnographic accounts of food security among foraging and agricultural societies. *American Journal of Physical Anthropology, 131*, 120–126.

Bland, J. (2015). Functional medicine: An operating system for integrative medicine. *Integrative Medicine, 14*(5), 18–20.

Centers for Disease Control and Prevention. (2014). *CDC national health report: Leading causes of morbidity and mortality and associated behavior risk and protective factors—United States, 2005–2013.* Retrieved from https://www.cdc.gov/mmwr/preview/mmwrhtml/su6304a2.htm

Centers for Disease Control and Prevention. (2016a). *Chronic disease overview.* Retrieved from https://www.cdc.gov/chronicdisease/overview/

Centers for Disease Control and Prevention. (2016b). *The four domains of chronic disease prevention: Working toward health people in healthy communities.* Retrieved from https://www.cdc.gov/chronicdisease/pdf/four-domains-factsheet-2015.pdf

Cox, A., West, N., & Cripps, A. (2015). Obesity, inflammation, and the gut microbiota. *The Lancet, Diabetes and Endocrinology, 3*(3), 209–215. https://doi.org/10.1016/S2213-8587(14)70134-2

D'Argenio, A., Mazzi, C., Pecchioli, L., Di Lorenzo, G., Siracusano, A., & Troisi, A. (2009). Early trauma and adult obesity: Is psychological dysfunction the mediating mechanism? *Physiology and Behavior, 98*(5), 543–546. https://doi.org/10.1016/j.physbeh.2009.08.010

de Campora, G., Giromini, L., Larciprete, G., Li Volsi, V., & Zavattini, G. C. (2014). The impact of maternal overweight and emotion regulation on early eating behaviors. *Eating Behavior, 15*(3), 403–409. https://doi.org/10.1016/j.eatbeh.2014.04.013

de Campora, G., Larciprete, G., Delogu, A. M., Meldolesi, C., & Giromini, L. (2016). A longitudinal study on emotional dysregulation and obesity risk: From pregnancy to 3 years of age of the baby. *Appetite, 96*, 95–101. https://doi.org/10.1016/j.appet.2015.09.012

DiBaise, J., Zhang, H., Crowell, M., Krajmalnik-Brown, R., Decker, G., & Rittmann, B. (2008). Gut microbiota and its possible relationship with obesity. *Mayo Clinic Proceedings, 83*(4), 460–469. https://doi.org/10.4065/83.4.460

Everly, G. S., & Lating, J. M. (2013). *A clinical guide to the treatment of the human stress response.* New York, NY: Springer.

Felitti, V. J., Anda, R. F., Nordenberg, D., Williamson, D. F., Apitz, A. M., Edwards, V., et al. (1998). Relationship of childhood abuse and household dysfunction to many of the leading causes of death in adults: The Adverse Childhood Experiences (ACE) study. *American Journal of Preventative Medicine, 14*(4), 245–258.

Foster, J. A., Rineman, L., & Cryan, J. F. (2017). Stress and the gut-brain axis: Regulation by the microbiome. *Neurobiology of Stress, 7*, 124–136. https://doi.org/10.1016/j.ynstr.2017.03.001. Retrieved from http://ac.els-cdn.com/S2352289516300509/1-s2.0-S2352289516300509-main.pdf?_tid=d9f07b0e-6a62-11e7-91de-00000aacb35e&acdnat=1500236025_c38207bff-794182cb2a6ae0e474f6e30

Fuemmeler, B. F., Dedert, E., McClernon, F. J., & Beckham, J. C. (2009). Adverse childhood events are associated with obesity and disordered eating: Results from a U.S. population-based survey of young adults. *Journal of Traumatic Stress, 22*(4), 329–333. https://doi.org/10.1002/jts.20421

Gallup Inc. (2014). *The "40-hour" workweek is actually longer—By seven hours.* Gallup.com. Retrieved from http://www.gallup.com/poll/175286/hour-workweek-actually-longer-seven-hours.aspx

Gowey, M. A., Reiter-Purtill, J., Becnel, J., Peugh, J., Mitchell, J. E., Zeller, M. H., et al. (2016). Weight-related correlates of psychological dysregulation in adolescent and young adult (AYA) females with severe obesity. *Appetite, 99*, 211–218. https://doi.org/10.1016/j.appet.2016.01.020

Grisanti, R., & Weatherby, D. (2008). *Implementing functional diagnostic medicine into your clinic.* Functional Medicine University. Retrieved from http://www.functionalmedicine.net/pdf/lesson3_insider_guide.pdf

Grundy, S. M. (1998). Multifactorial causation of obesity: Implications for prevention. *American Journal of Clinical Nutrition, 67*(3 Suppl), 563S–572S.

Hamilton, M., Healy, G., Dunstan, D., Zderic, T., & Owen, N. (2008). Too little exercise and too much sitting: Inactivity physiology and the need for new recommendations on sedentary behavior. *Current Cardiovascular Risk Reports, 2*(4), 292–298. https://doi.org/10.1007/s12170-008-0054-8

Han, T. S., & Lean, M. E. J. (2016). A clinical perspective of obesity, metabolic syndrome, and cardiovascular disease. *JRSM Cardiovascular Disease, 5*, 1–13. https://doi.org/10.1177/2048004016633371

Hughes, K. (2014). *A case study discussion of the new era of applying the functional medicine model to patient care when managing detox-related health concerns.* The Institute for Functional Medicine. Retrieved from http://congress.metagenics.com.au/postcongress/media/presentation-slides/3-kristi-hughes-functional-medicine.pdf

Hyman, M. (2007). Systems biology, toxins, obesity, and functional medicine. *Alternative Therapies in Health and Medicine, 13*(2), 134–139.

Hyman, M. (2010). Environmental toxins, obesity, and diabetes: An emerging risk factor. *Alternative Therapies in Health and Medicine, 16*(2), 56–58.

Jones, D., & Quinn, S. (2016). *Introduction to functional medicine* (1st ed.). Gig Harbor, WA: The Institute for Functional Medicine. Retrieved from https://p.widencdn.net/wzl55z/Intro_Functional_Medicine

Lambert, E. A., Straznicky, N. E., Dixon, J. B., & Lambert, G. W. (2015). Should the sympathetic nervous system be a target to improve cardiometabolic risk in obesity? *American Journal of Physiology: Heart and Circulatory Physiology, 309*(2), H244–H258. https://doi.org/10.1152/ajpheart.00096.2015

Levi, J., Segal, L. M., Rayburn, J., & Martin, A. (2015). *The state of obesity: Better policies for a healthier America: 2015.* Obesity Policies Series: Trust for America's Health and the Robert Wood Johnson Foundation. Retrieved from http://stateofobesity.org/files/stateofobesity2015.pdf

Ley, R. (2009). Obesity and the human microbiome. *Current Opinion in Gastroenterology, 26*(1), 5–11. https://doi.org/10.1097/MOG.0b013e328333d751

Martínez-Martínez, L. A., Mora, T., Vargas, A., Fuentes-Iniestra, M., & Martínez-Lavín, M. (2014). Sympathetic nervous system dysfunction in fibromyalgia, chronic fatigue syndrome, irritable bowel syndrome, and interstitial cystitis: A review of case-control studies. *Journal of Clinical Rheumatology, 20*(3), 146–150. https://doi.org/10.1097/RHU.0000000000000089

McGrady, A. (2010). The effects of biofeedback in diabetes and hypertension. *Cleveland Clinic Journal of Medicine, 77*(Suppl 3), S68–S71. https://doi.org/10.3949/ccjm77.s3.12

McGrady, A., & Moss, D. (2013). *Pathways to illness, pathways to health.* New York, NY: Springer.

Monteiro, R., & Azevedo, I. (2010). Chronic inflammation in obesity and the metabolic syndrome. Mediators of Inflammation, Vol. 2010, Article ID 289645. doi:10.1155/2010/289645

Neilsen. (2016). *The total audience report: Q1 2016.* Nielsen.com. Retrieved from http://www.nielsen.com/us/en/insights/reports/2016/the-total-audience-report-q1-2016.html

Nesse, R., & Stearns, S. (2008). The great opportunity: Evolutionary applications to medicine and public health. *Evolutionary Applications,* 1(1), 28–48. https://doi.org/10.1111/j.1752-4571.2007.00006.x

Physical Activity Council. (2016). *2016 participation report* (1st ed.). Physical Activity Council. Retrieved from http://www.physicalactivitycouncil.com/pdfs/current.pdf

Pratt, M., Norris, J., Lobelo, F., Roux, L., & Wang, G. (2012). The cost of physical inactivity: Moving into the 21st century. *British Journal of Sports Medicine, 48*(3), 171–173. https://doi.org/10.1136/bjsports-2012-091810

Randall, S., & Ford, H. (Eds.). (2011). *Long term conditions: A guide for nurses and health professionals.* Chichester, West Sussex: Wiley-Blackwell

Speakman, J. (2013). Evolutionary perspectives on the obesity epidemic: Adaptive, maladaptive, and neutral viewpoints. *Annual Review of Nutrition, 33*(1), 289–317. https://doi.org/10.1146/annurev-nutr-071811-150711

United States Department of Health and Human Services. (2012). *What are the health risks of overweight and obesity?* Retrieved from https://www.nhlbi.nih.gov/health/health-topics/topics/obe/risks

United States Department of Health and Human Services & United States Department of Agriculture. (2015). *Dietary guidelines for Americans, 2015–2020* (8th ed.). Retrieved from https://health.gov/dietaryguidelines/2015/guidelines/chapter-2/current-eating-patterns-in-the-united-states/

United States Department of State. (n.d.). *Infectious and chronic disease.* Retrieved from http://www.state.gov/e/oes/intlhealthbiodefense/id/index.htm

Valavanis, J. K., Mougiakakou, S. G., Grimaldi, K. A., & Nikita, K. S. (2010). A multifactorial analysis of obesity as CVD risk factor: Use of neural network based methods in a nutrigenetics context. *BMC Bioinformatics, 11,* 453. https://doi.org/10.1186/1471-2105-11-453

Williamson, D. F., Thompson, T. J., & Anda, R. F. (2002). Body weight and obesity in adults and self-reported abuse in childhood. International Journal of Obesity, 26(8), 1075–1082. doi:10.1038/sj.ijo.0802038.

Wooley, J. D., Gorno-Tempini, M. L., Werner, K., Rankin, K. P., Ekman, P., Levenson, R. W., et al. (2004). The autonomic and behavioral profile of emotional dysregulation. *Neurology, 63*(9), 1740–1743.

World Health Organization. (1992). *Twenty steps for developing a healthy cities project.* Geneva, Switzerland: World Health Organization, Regional Office for Europe.

World Health Organization. (2003). *Diet, nutrition, and the prevention of chronic diseases: Report of a joint WHO/FAO expert consultation.* Geneva, Switzerland: World Health Organization. Retrieved from http://www.who.int/dietphysicalactivity/publications/trs916/en/gsfao_introduction.pdf

World Health Organization. (2011). *Global status report on non-communicable diseases 2010.* Geneva, Switzerland: World Health Organization.

World Health Organization. (2013). *Global action plan for the prevention and control of NCDs 2013–2020.* Geneva, Switzerland: World Health Organization. Retrieved from http://www.who.int/nmh/events/ncd_action_plan/en/

World Health Organization. (2015). *Non-communicable diseases: Fact sheet.* Geneva, Switzerland: World Health Organization. Retrieved from http://www.who.int/mediacentre/factsheets/fs355/en/

World Health Organization. (2016a). *Management of non-communicable diseases.* Geneva, Switzerland: World Health Organization. Retrieved from http://www.who.int/ncds/management/en/

World Health Organization. (2016b). *Non-communicable diseases and their risk factors.* Geneva, Switzerland: World Health Organization. Retrieved from http://www.who.int/ncds/en/

World Health Organization. (2016c). *Controlling the global obesity epidemic*. Geneva, Switzerland: World Health Organization. Retrieved from http://www.who.int/nutrition/topics/obesity/en/

World Health Organization. (2017). *Obesity and overweight: Fact sheet*. Geneva, Switzerland: World Health Organization. Retrieved from http://www.who.int/mediacentre/factsheets/fs311/en/

Young-Hyman, D. L., Peterson, C. M., Fischer, S., Markowitz, J. T., Muir, A. B., & Laffel, L. M. (2016). Depressive symptoms, emotion dysregulation, and bulimic symptoms in youth with type 1 diabetes: Varying interactions at diagnosis and during transition to insulin pump therapy. *Journal of Diabetes Science and Technology, 10*(4), 845–851. https://doi.org/10.1177/1932296816645118

Chapter 4
Religion, Spiritual Practices, and Well-Being

Abstract Religion, medicine, and healing have been connected in most cultures and eras. The development of scientific medicine in the nineteenth and twentieth centuries produced a practical divorce between medical care and religion. However, over four decades of research has shown that religious adherence, attendance at services, beliefs, spiritual practices, and sense of purpose in life can all impact health and longevity. This chapter explores the general impact of religion and spirituality on health, reviews research on specific elements of religious engagement and their effects on health, and examines the approaches of two Christian churches that have placed special emphasis on health and healing. The chapter also introduces religious and spiritual practices commonly used for comfort, consolation, and well-being.

Keywords Religion · Spirituality · Religious practices · Health · Well-being

Introduction

In January 1998, the American researcher Paul Lehrer carried his physiological monitoring equipment to Japan and visited groups of Zen Buddhist meditators in their monastic settings. His goal was to monitor the physiology, especially the cardiac activity and respiration, of monks during sitting meditation. Zen meditation typically includes various forms of slow paced breathing, and Lehrer's previous research had convinced him that the regular practice of paced diaphragmatic breathing, especially at specific breathing frequencies, could have beneficial effects for health and well-being.

Lehrer was aware that some research studies conducted on Zen monks had shown reduced levels of heart disease compared to the general population although slow breathing was only one factor that might account for that difference (Lehrer, Sasaki, & Saito, 1999). Zen monks eat no fish or meat, and this might aid cardiac health via lower serum lipids. Nevertheless, Lehrer hypothesized that the slow breathing during meditation might also be a factor in heart health, serving to produce higher heart rate variability. Higher variability in heart rate is correlated with better cardiac health and better health overall (Lehrer & Gevirtz, 2014; McCraty & Shaffer, 2015).

© Springer International Publishing AG, part of Springer Nature 2018   59
A. McGrady, D. Moss, *Integrative Pathways*,
https://doi.org/10.1007/978-3-319-89313-6_4

Lehrer found that during meditation many of the monks were breathing in the range of three to nine breaths per minute, approximately the optimal rate identified in Lehrer's previous research as producing higher heart rate variability. This slower breathing increased heart rate variability overall and shifted the largest portion of heart rate oscillations into the low frequency spectral band of heart rate variations. There are several schools in Zen Buddhism, each with variations in its approach to meditation, and the monks Lehrer studied in Japan followed the Rinzai and Soto traditions. Rinzai Zen monks breathed at slower rates than monks in the Soto Zen tradition and showed a higher amplitude of the low frequency heart rate variability during the slow breathing while meditating. Rinzai Zen places greater emphasis on breath control in meditation than does Soto Zen.

Some monks, however, including one Rinzai master, were breathing much slower, at rates as low as one breath per minute, and the largest portion of heart rate variation shifted even further into the very low frequency range. Cardiac rhythm irregularities also increased during these segments of very slow breathing.

Lehrer became concerned about the potential adverse heart health implications of these observations and wondered if the meditation practices might in some cases undermine the health of the heart. He sought out a senior monk among the Rinzai practitioners and described his observations of variable cardiac rhythm and possible adverse cardiac consequences of the very slow breathing during Zazen meditation. The monk stated: "This is not a health club" (Lehrer, personal communication). The monks' purpose in spending extended hours meditating was neither to enhance their health nor prolong their life span. For both Soto and Rinzai Zen, there is no goal beyond being fully present within the practice of sitting meditation itself.

This story presented here, of Dr. Lehrer and his research on meditating monks, is intended to remind the reader that the first objectives of religious and spiritual traditions are usually not to extend life or improve health. Religious practices variously emphasize reaching salvation, surrendering to the spirit, becoming close to God, achieving enlightenment, or awakening spiritually. Nevertheless, many religions and spiritual traditions currently address health and healing and even assign it a role of importance. In addition, many denominations and religious movements have proposed beneficial dietary and lifestyle guidelines, provided beneficial social supports through church communities, combated health destructive practices, and offered forms of direct spiritual healing. The purpose of this chapter is to examine the variety of ways in which religions, religious communities, spiritual practices, and religious/spiritual beliefs serve to support and optimize health. The chapter will also take a closer look at two Christian movements originating in nineteenth century America that placed central emphasis on health and healing.

The Historical Connection between Religion and Medicine

Harold Koenig has shown that throughout recorded history, religion and medicine have usually been intertwined, and physical disease has often been understood at least partly in spiritual terms. In his *Handbook of Religion and Health*, Koenig,

McCullough, and Larson (2012) provided a detailed outline of the historical overlap between religion and medicine. A few examples will suffice here: In Mesopotamia between 3200 and 1025 BC, medicine was based on a mixture of spiritual and natural explanations for disease (Koenig, 2012a). Between 2300 and 1700 BC, Hindu priests in India served as physicians and used rituals of dancing, incantations, and amulets to cure disease (Koenig, 2012a). In the fourth century BC, Greek priests presided at healing temples dedicated to the man-god Asclepius, where they induced their patients into a trance-like "temple-sleep" to produce healing (Agogino, 1965). In the medieval period, priests and monks provided the majority of care for the sick, through both ritualized prayers and herbal medicine. Duffy (2009, p. 164) published an example of a medieval prayer for relief from fevers, "through the thousand names of the lord." The clergy also drew on the traditions of Hippocrates and Galen and provided herbs and herbal draughts to be taken orally for various maladies (Goldiner, 2012). Christ remained the medieval exemplar for healing by words or touch. Throughout the medieval era, many individuals suffering with illness traveled to shrines commemorating various saints. At these sites, healing often took place through touching a *reliquary* containing hair, blood, or clothing of the saints (Goldiner, 2012). During the twelfth century, the Alexian brothers, a monastic order, began to care for the sick and the poor in Western Europe and provided care for many during the plagues of the twelfth to the fifteenth centuries (Koenig et al., 2012, p. 36).

The Modern Separation of Religion and Medicine

Since the advent of modern scientifically based medicine and the modern hospital, however, the domains of church and health care have been separated. Clergy have been welcome in church settings, as chaplains, to provide religious guidance and consolation to soothe those facing illness or death. Churches have also supported modern hospitals and provided patient care. But the clergy were no longer central to any diagnostic or treatment functions, which were assigned to the scientist-practitioners called physicians, who utilize laboratory testing and imaging studies to identify biological mechanisms and diagnose disease.

Yet, emerging research since the 1970s has shown that religious affiliation, religious practices, and spiritual experiences can have a profound impact on physical and mental health. As Koenig (2012b) has shown, there has been exponential growth in the publication of peer reviewed articles on spirituality and health from 1973 to the present. Involvement in religion and spirituality is correlated with a "wide variety of indicators of health and well-being" (Park et al., 2013, p. 828). This chapter, organized around a series of questions, will address the positive role that religious adherence, church participation, and specific religious/practices can play in health.

- How can we define religion and spirituality?
- Does regular participation in activities of a church, synagogue, or temple make a difference in health and well-being?
- Does the social support associated with church participation make a difference in health?

- Do religious belief and religious activities impart a sense of purpose in life and does this impact health?
- Is there a *dark side* to be considered in the effects of religious thinking and activities on health?
- By what means do religious engagement and religion-based variables affect health?
- How do churches directly support health and healing?
- Are there some religions or religious ways of life that impact more on health and well-being than do others?
- What religious and spiritual practices are commonly used for comfort, consolation, and palliation of suffering?

Definitions of Religion and Spirituality

First, some definition of key terms is imperative to keep this discussion more specific and clear. In recent years, many definitions have been published for *religion* and *spirituality,* and there is often overlap between the definitions of the two words. The National Cancer Institute, in an online monograph on spirituality in cancer care (2015), defined religion as "a specific set of beliefs and practices associated with a recognized religion or denomination." The same document described spirituality as "encompassing experiential aspects, whether related to engaging in religious practices, or to acknowledging a general sense of peace and connectedness." Some form of spirituality is found in all cultures, so it may be regarded as a universal dimension of humanity.

Harold Koenig provided more complex and lengthy definitions of both religion and spirituality as follows:

Religion "Involves beliefs, practices, and rituals related to the transcendent, where the *transcendent* is God, Allah, HaShem, or a Higher Power in Western traditions, or to Brahman, manifestations of Brahman, Buddha, Dao, or ultimate truth/reality in Eastern traditions… Religions usually have specific beliefs about life after death and rules about conduct within a social group" (2012b, p. 2).

Spirituality "Spirituality is distinguished from all other things—humanism, values, morals, and mental health—by its connection to that which is sacred, the transcendent. The transcendent is that which is outside of the self, yet also within the self… Spirituality includes both a search for the transcendent and the discovery of the transcendent…" (2012b, p. 3).

Koenig points out that the definitions of religion and spirituality indicate a considerable overlap. Many though not all persons seek and often find their spirituality through participation in organized religion. Others adhere to the rote beliefs and rules of organized religion, but evidence little experience of the spiritual or the transcendent. Finally, there are many, increasingly so today, who reject organized religion yet seek and find spiritual experiences outside of churches and organized religious activity.

Handwritten annotations: RELIGION BLUE ZONES; is it religion or connection to others

Regular Participation in Activities of a Church, Synagogue, or Temple and Effects on Health and Well-Being

> "A large body of research has emerged showing that attendance at religious services has an inverse relationship with coronary heart disease (CHD). Persons who attend services regularly are less likely to contract or die from CHD and suffer lower prevalence of other diseases."

A large body of research has emerged showing that attendance at religious services has an inverse relationship with coronary heart disease (CHD). Attendance is an external measure, which may not entirely reflect inward engagement and participation in religious and spiritual experiences. Nevertheless, attendance does correlate with measures of health. Persons who attend services regularly are less likely to develop CHD or die from CHD and suffer lower prevalence of other diseases. Hummer, Rogers, Nam, and Ellison (1999) analyzed data from the United States Health Interview Survey and found that persons who attended services more than once per week were 1.87 times less likely to die of cardiovascular causes in a given time period than persons who did not attend at all. This effect was still significant after controlling for age, gender, education, and ethnicity. Oman, Kurata, Strawbridge, and Cohen (2002) studied residents of Alameda County, California, and found that persons with infrequent attendance (less than weekly) at religious services suffered higher mortality from cardiovascular disease. Hummer et al. (1999) reported similar findings on religious attendance and diabetes. Persons who never attended services were 3.76 times more likely to die of diabetes and the complications of the disease.

Banerjee, Boyle, Anand, Strachan, and Oremus (2014) reported on a Canadian sample including over 5000 residents of Saskatchewan. In their sample, attendance at religious services was associated with lower prevalence of CHD, but this association was not statistically significant, once demographic, socioeconomic, and health behavior variables were controlled. In other words, some other factors associated with church attendance, such as decreased alcohol use and smoking, seemed to predict the health benefits. They did find a statistically significant lower prevalence of diabetes and hypertension in church attenders. Of interest, is that Banerjee found that even attending services 3–12 times per year was associated with lower prevalence of CHD than in non-attenders.

Both Hummer et al. (1999) and Oman et al. (2002) found that church attendance increased social connections and led to improved health behaviors: less smoking, more exercise, and less alcohol use. Yet in their research, church involvement was still a significant predictor of longevity when the effects of social connections and health behaviors were subtracted. Hummer, Ellison, Rogers, Moulton, and Romero (2004) also reported that the beneficial effects of attendance at religious services are strong across specific religious denominations. The later study attributes the effect to social integration, social regulation, and psychological resources. For Hummer et al. (2004), social integration refers to the social connections gained through church activities, social regulation refers to behavioral regulation through church and religious influences, including reduced smoking and alcohol use, and psychological resources indicates acquisition of coping skills and strategies.

Koenig (2008, p. 132) has pointed out, however, that religious involvement predicts future increases in social support, faster resolution of depression, and reductions in smoking and alcohol consumption. These corollary variables may account for many of the positive effects of religious involvement on health. Koenig, McCullough, and Larsen (2012, p. 100) pointed out that many religious institutions directly encourage and arrange socialization among members, thereby increasing the size of social networks, the numbers of social contacts, and satisfaction with social supports.

Social Support Associated with Church Participation and Health

"... individuals who are regularly involved in church activities report more social ties and connections, more friendship networks, and experience more social integration and social support in their communities."

Ellison and Hummer (2010) cited extensive research indicating that individuals who are regularly involved in church activities report more social ties and connections, more friendship networks, and experience more social integration and social support in their communities. These variables are likely to account for a significant portion of the links between religious involvement and health.

Galloway and Henry (2014) examined the impact of social connectedness and spiritual perspectives on depression and perceived health in a rural Colorado population. In their study, social connectedness had significant positive impact on reducing depression and improving perceived health. The instrument Galloway and Henry used to measure depression assesses the nine primary symptoms of major depression in the DSM-IV criteria (American Psychiatric Association, 2000). The more socially connected persons felt, the more they perceived themselves as physically and mentally healthy. Spiritual perspective, which in their study meant how much participants held spiritual beliefs and values and participated in spiritually related activities, did not independently predict either depression or perceived health.

A study by Morton, Lee, and Martin (2016) sought to control several variables that might mediate the effects of religiosity or religious engagement on health. Their study showed that religious engagement was predictive of reduced mortality risk, but much of the effect could be accounted for by religious supports, emotionality, and lifestyle factors (specifically diet and exercise). On the other hand, church activity independently predicted reduced mortality, and not all of this effect could be accounted for by religious supports, emotionality, or behavioral change.

Religious Belief and Religious Activities Produce a Sense of Purpose in Life and Health

Religious beliefs and religious orientation in life can produce a belief in a mission and meaning larger than the self. Emmons, Cheung, and Tehrani (1998) asked people what they were striving for in their lives. Those persons who reported more forms of spiritual striving also reported more sense of purpose in life, greater life satisfaction, and higher levels of personal well-being. As human beings advance in the life cycle into old age, there are more challenges to general well-being. Having a sense of purpose in life and relatively low levels of depression are important for a positive sense of well-being in the elderly (Dixon, 2007). Dixon also showed that a perception of *mattering to others*, especially friends and family, are critical to well-being in later life.

Mahoney et al. (2005) identified another phenomenon called "sanctification" that supports a sense of meaning and purpose in life. Sanctification refers to developing a sense of the sacred in everyday life. Broadly, when human beings have a "well-organized set of personal strivings," then their strivings contribute a sense of meaning to life and facilitate well-being. Further when human beings perceive their strivings as having a spiritual dimension, or a spiritual value, the struggles take on additional meaning. The research by Emmons et al. (1998) supports the concept of sanctification. These authors found that when strivings are perceived as religious or spiritual, they take on certain attributes—importance, investment, and social support—which lead to a meaningful life and positive psychological adjustments to change.

Hill and Turiano (2014) analyzed the Midlife in the United States (MIDUS) database and explored the effects that having a purpose in life had on longevity. The authors found that having a greater purpose in life serves as a "buffer against mortality risk" throughout adult life. This effect did not depend on age nor on retirement status. The effect of having a sense of meaning and purpose was robust and could not be explained by other variables such as positive relationships with others or positive/negative affect.

"Participants who scored higher on sense of purpose showed several differences: lower levels of functional disability, better performance on cognitive tasks, better self-rated health, and fewer depressive symptoms."

Windsor, Curtis, and Luszcz (2015) investigated a sample of older adults (Mean age 77.06 years) examining whether having a sense of purpose in life buffered against the effects of aging. Participants who scored higher on sense of purpose showed several differences: lower levels of functional disability, better performance on cognitive tasks, better self-rated health, and fewer depressive symptoms. Higher sense of purpose was associated with increased probability of survival, but this relationship attenuated with time. Their conclusion was that having a sense of purpose in life buffers against some of the effects of aging, but the buffering erodes in the oldest-old population. However, this study did not specifically study religion or spirituality-based purpose in life.

Considerations About the **Dark Side** *of Religious Thinking and Activity and Health*

According to Pargament, Koenig, and Perez (2000), many older persons mention religion as a resource for coping with the stress of life. Among certain groups—the elderly, minorities, and persons facing a life-threatening crisis—religion is cited more frequently than any other resource as a support. The same authors, however, have shown that religious coping has both positive and negative dimensions; to this end, they developed a psychological instrument called the RCOPE to assess the variety of forms of religious coping. Benevolent religious reappraisals re-define a current stressor in positive religious terms, for example, concluding that a particular situation is part of God's plan, that it may bring me closer to God, or that God may be trying to strengthen me in this situation. On the other hand, a stressor may be perceived as evidence that a punishing God is causing this situation because of my sins, or punishing me because of my lack of devotion, or that in some way I deserve this situation. Or, the stressful event may be perceived as the work of the devil. The authors concluded that religion has its dark side, and several negative forms of religious coping can amplify distress. The larger part of what the authors labeled as negative religious coping involved cognitive appraisals, such as interpreting a painful event as a result of God's punishing me for my sins. With positive religious coping, stress can lead to "stress-related growth," but that poor physical health was correlated with specific forms of negative religious coping.

Tarakeshwar et al. (2008) utilized the RCOPE developed in the Pargament et al. (2000) study and studied 170 patients with advanced cancer. They found that positive religious coping was associated with better overall quality of life, and greater use of negative religious coping was related to poorer overall quality of life. Kapogiannis, Berbey, Zamboni, Krueger, and Grafman (2009) utilized functional MRI to identify neural correlates of both positive and negative religious cognitions. They found that negative religious cognitions mobilized different brain structures and networks than did positive cognitions. The researchers presented pairs of statements to the research participants and found that statements about God's love mobilized activity in the right middle frontal gyrus, while statements about God's anger mobilized activity within the left middle temporal gyrus. Their findings were not easy to interpret; further research is clearly needed to understand the significance of the neural correlates of religious coping and religious experiences. Nevertheless, their research suggests that the two dimensions of God's presence or absence in the world, and God's love or anger were important, producing diverging correlates in brain activity.

In summary, the impact of religious and spiritual cognition on health and well-being is complex and depends on the individual person's beliefs and cognitions/coping. Negative beliefs and cognitions produce adverse effects on quality of life and divergent changes in neuronal processing. Religious coping is a neurophysiological process, with the potential to produce both adverse and positive effects on health and well-being.

Mechanisms by Which Religious Engagement and Religion-Based Variables Affect Health

Hill and Pargament (2003) have applied attachment theory to understanding peoples' experience of religion. They suggested that persons who experience a "secure connection with God," will also show less distress in stressful situations, and more confidence in coping with life. They cited a number of studies which support this thesis. People who report a closer connection to God, also show less depression, better self-esteem, less loneliness, more "relational maturity," and better psychosocial competence (Hill & Pargament, 2003, p. 66).

What does the Hill and Pargament study signify for religion and health? The application of attachment theory to religious engagement might imply a personified deity, which is not a part of some religious traditions including many strains of Buddhism and Hinduism. We might speculate, however, that the attachment may not be to a personal deity, but rather to an historical figure in the tradition, a present-day spiritual teacher, or a glorified saint or devotee. Many traditional Catholics develop an intense religious attachment to Mary the mother of Jesus, and this author has interacted with Sufis who focused their awareness on their spiritual guide while conducting self-piercings. The power of attachment can be mobilized by any relationship within the spiritual life of the individual.

Jackson and Bergeman (2011) developed a *resiliency* framework to understand the effects of religion/spirituality on well-being. They emphasized the building of adaptive resources and an enhanced sense of personal control that can be utilized in times of need. They utilized a sample of 539 adults ages 31–88 in northern Indiana and examined how much the effects of religion/spirituality on subjective well-being could be accounted for by an increased sense of perceived control. They examined three different dimensions related to religion—religious practices, daily spiritual experiences, and religious/spiritual coping—and examined each in relation to level of perceived control and subjective well-being. They explored these variables across three age groups: early mid-life (ages 31–49), later mid-life (ages 50–59), and later life (ages 60 and above). Interestingly, the relationship of perceived control to each dimension of religion varied by age group. Perceived control did not mediate the effects of religious practices on subjective well-being in the two mid-life groups, but did in later life. Perceived control did mediate the effects of daily spiritual experiences on well-being in the entire sample, and when analyzed separately had a significant mediating effect in the two older age groups. Similarly, perceived control mediated the effects of religious and spiritual coping on well-being in the full sample, and in the two older groups of participants. The authors concluded that an enhanced sense of personal control partially accounted for the impact of religion/ spirituality on well-being, and that this effect is strongest in later life.

In summary, the beneficial health effects of religious and spiritual engagement may be partially accounted for by the development of a strong attachment bond with God or with a religious figure, creating more positive mood and self-esteem and better "relational maturity." Religious engagement may also build resiliency, including a stronger sense of personal control in life, with particular benefit in later life.

Churches' Active Support of Health and Healing Today

Many mainstream churches combine pastoral care with denominational support for skilled mainstream medical and nursing care. Consequently, many major health institutions continue to bear names with resonance in church history, such as Jewish Children's, Mount Sinai, Beth Israel, Presbyterian, Adventist, Lutheran, Mercy, and Trinity. Religious health initiatives are often ecumenical, crossing religious lines in productive ways. The Alexian Brothers Health systems trace back to those medieval Alexian Monks who provided care for the sick in the twelfth century. Recently in Illinois, a division of the Adventist Health System operating four hospitals joined with Alexian Brothers Health Systems with its five hospitals to form Amita, an integrated care system for suburban Chicago (Schorsch, 2015). Other examples of religious organizations continuing to support health care, often in areas neglected by for-profit systems, include the Salvation Army which provides rehabilitation programs for substance abusers, and Goodwill Industries and other like-minded ministries that employ developmentally disabled persons who otherwise would languish without productive activity in their lives.

Many Christian churches in the United States and globally now endorse various forms of faith healing, healing prayer, and the active role of Christians in healing one another. The Christian Pentecostal movement emerged in the early 1900s and hearkened back to the emphasis on spiritual gifts and healing, of the early Christian era (Hummel, 1986). Initially that movement was dismissed by many mainstream churches. Since the 1950s and 1960s, however, the related charismatic movement has spread within mainstream Protestant, Catholic, and Orthodox churches, leading to the presence of healing prayer circles in many churches, the laying of hands on the sick and troubled, and a greater emphasis on the role of Christ and Christians in healing (Brown, 2011). The renewed emphasis on healing in many mainstream churches parallels the popular interest in the emergent research on the healing power of prayer. The actual scientific research attempting to measure the empirical effects of prayers for healing is inconsistent with many contradictions, but figures such as Larry Dossey (1993, 1996, 1997) received a wide and positive popular response, supporting renewed emphasis in churches on healing prayer.

> "Parish nursing follows a holistic model, integrating nursing care and health education with spiritual education and spiritual guidance."

Many churches today, across denominations, offer parish nursing services. The parish nursing movement was initiated by a Lutheran minister in Chicago, Granger Westberg, to revive the traditional role of Christian religious orders in healing (Westberg & Westberg McNamara, 1990). The role of the parish nurse or faith community nurse continued a nineteenth century tradition of the *deaconess*, a role for women in churches that developed in Kaiserswerth, Germany, and spread to the United States through Lutheran influences (Lutheran Deaconess Association, 2017). Deaconesses were often trained as nurses and staffed many "deaconess hospitals." Today, there are over 15,000 nurses in the parish nursing role, primarily in the United States but also in many other countries (Ziebarth, 2014, p. 1818). Although the parish nurses are primarily in Christian and Jewish congregations, there are Muslim parish nurses and some in other faith traditions. Parish nurses take on many roles, engaging in health and wellness education, promoting adequate nutrition, assisting church members to access adequate medical care, and conducting blood pressure clinics after church services to accomplish early identification of undetected cases of hypertension.

Parish nursing follows a holistic model, integrating nursing care and health education with spiritual education and spiritual guidance. The parish nurse also serves a role in assessing church members' medical problems and needs, providing referrals for medical care, and facilitating transportation and financial support for health care as needed. Optimally, the parish nurse is also integrated closely into a pastoral team (Roberts, 2014). The American Nursing Association has recognized *faith community nursing* as a specialty nursing practice and defined it as follows: "…the specialized practice of professional nursing that focuses on the intentional care of the spirit as part of the process of promoting holistic health and preventing or minimizing illness in a faith community" (American Nurses Association, 2012, p. 1).

Comparison of the Impact of Two Churches on Health and Well-being

> "The studies reported that Adventist men lived 7.3 years longer and Adventist women live 4.4 years longer than other Californians, and linked a number of dietary practices to reduced incidences of specific diseases."

This section will introduce two churches, both originating in nineteenth century America, which placed greater emphasis on health and healing than most mainstream church organizations. The two movements, the Seventh Day Adventist Church and the Church of Christ, Scientist, developed distinctly different theology, and sharply different strategies for promoting the health of their followers.

The Seventh Day Adventist Church Founded in the modern era, the Seventh Day Adventist Church has had a remarkable history of breakthrough initiatives for healthy lifestyle. The church was officially organized with a set of beliefs including a belief in a holistic human nature, with an indivisibility of body, mind, and spirit. In 1866, the first Adventist health care facility (called a "sanitarium") opened in Battle Creek, Michigan, and emphasized lifestyle change: proper nutrition, exercise, and "sanitation." John Harvey Kellogg was an early Adventist health advocate, who initiated the practice of consuming cereal products at breakfast.[1] The core health message today of Seventh Day Adventists advocates vegetarianism and the keeping of a work-free Sabbath and discourages alcohol, tobacco, and street drug use.

Researchers associated with Loma Linda University have conducted a series of large scale health studies comparing the health and disease patterns of over 30,000 Adventist Californians and non-Adventist Californians. The studies reported that Adventist men lived 7.3 years longer and Adventist women lived 4.4 years longer than other Californians and linked a number of dietary practices to reduced incidence of specific diseases. The first Adventist health study, which enrolled 34, 1092 participants, documented a substantial increase in life expectancy (up to an extra 10 years) for those following Adventist lifestyle guidelines (Fraser & Shavlik, 2001). The second Adventist health study, which recruited 96,469 participants, showed reductions in cardiovascular mortality, non-cardiovascular non-cancer mortality, renal mortality, and mortality from endocrine disease (Orlich et al., 2013). A number of valuable links were found between specific dietary practices and health. For example, older women in the groups eating nuts several times a week reduced risk of inflammatory disease mortality by between 32 and 51% with a dose-specific link between quantity consumed and reductions in mortality (Gopinath et al., 2011). Similar dose-related benefits were found for consumption of polyunsaturated fatty acids (Gopinath et al., 2011).

Today, the Adventists operate a large number of hospitals, health clinics, and lifestyle centers. The Loma Linda Medical School and Medical Center in California are the largest in North America, and the Adventist Health System is the largest not-for-profit Protestant health care system in the United States.

The Adventist CHIP program Currently, the Adventists also have adopted the *Complete Health Improvement Program (CHIP)* program worldwide, a large-scale program, staffed by trained facilitators and volunteers, to retrain individuals worldwide in well-lifestyle. (The program was initiated by Hans Diehl and influenced by Nathan Pritikin; it was earlier known as the Coronary Health Improvement Program). The CHIP program emphasizes a whole-food, plant-based eating pattern, daily physical activity, reduced use of addictive substances, and stress management. Aldana et al. (2006) reported on a randomized clinical trial studying a cohort of 348 middle-aged adults in the Rockford, Illinois area. Those assigned to the lifestyle

---

[1] *The Road to Wellville (Beacon Communications/Columbia Pictures)* was a 1994 comedy lampooning the medical practices and elaborate therapeutic devices of Dr. Kellogg although many of his interventions anticipated practices widely used by holistic health advocates today.

modification condition attended a 40-hours educational course over a 4-week period. Changes in nutrition, physical activity behavior, and several chronic disease risk factors were assessed at baseline and again at 6 months. Three-hundred and eighteen participants returned at 6 months for follow-up. Participants in the intervention group showed significant improvement in several physical activity and nutrition variables, and significant reductions in body mass index, weight, body fat, systolic and diastolic blood pressure, and resting heart rate.

A longer term study by Kent et al. (2013) followed a cohort of 284 individuals in New Zealand, who received a 30-day lifestyle modification program, delivered by volunteers. One-hundred and six persons (37% of the original cohort) returned for a three-year follow-up. Participants who entered the program with elevated biometrics at intake, maintained clinically significant reductions in body mass index, diastolic blood pressure, total cholesterol, and triglycerides after 3 years. Sixty-seven percent of those who returned for follow-up also reported continued compliance with lifestyle modifications.

In summary, the theology and values of the Seventh Day Adventist church emphasize the total human being, body, mind, and spirit, and the organization has sustained an emphasis on lifestyle changes for total wellness. The Adventist church has supported a number of hospitals and health centers and has now adopted the Complete Health Improvement Program to advanced community-based change in lifestyle worldwide.

"Christian Science proclaims that illness is essentially mental in nature, and can therefore be corrected by prayer rooted in an understanding of spiritual life. Christian Science also believes that since the true reality is spiritual, the mainstream medical emphasis on the body, and on physical and biochemical causes, may reinforce illness."

Christian Science The Church of Christ, Scientist, began in approximately the same time period as the Seventh Day Adventist movement, yet adopted a vastly different theological and practical path. While the Adventists emphasized the holistic nature of human being, mind, body, and spirit, the founder of Christian Science, Mary Baker Eddy, emphasized the spiritual nature of reality and the relationship of God as divine love to every human being. She rested the body of her practices on an inward spiritual devotion, a turning to prayer, and an openness to divine Mind. Eddy suffered a life-threatening injury in 1866, and on reading in the Bible an account of Jesus healing a man, experienced a physical healing that proved to be transformative. She turned her attention to a study of biblical texts, and then articulated a systematic approach to spiritual healing. Soon she developed a career as a spiritual healer or *practitioner* and published a formulation of her approach in 1875, *Science and Health, with Key to the Scriptures* (Eddy, 1994). She later stated that her intent was to "reinstate primitive Christianity and its lost element of healing" (Eddy, 1895, p. 17).

Christian Science proclaims that illness is essentially mental in nature and can therefore be corrected by prayer rooted in an understanding of spiritual life. Christian Science also believes that since the true reality is spiritual, the mainstream medical emphasis on the body, and on physical and biochemical causes, may reinforce illness (Committee on Publication, 1989). While Christian Scientists respect the humanitarian motives of physicians and mainstream medical personnel, their own approach to healing is based on a devotional life and a cultivation of religious studies. Christian Science practitioners devote themselves full time to a healing ministry as their vocation and spend their hours in prayer. This *is* their healing practice. A Christian Science practitioner clarified that the practice is not so much a matter of petitioning God to heal the sick, but of entering into a spiritual communion with and acknowledgement of God's healing love (Eric Nelson, Personal communication, August 2017).

Any student of this faith may offer healing to others, but those practitioners listed in the Church's official directory must complete a primary class instruction on Christian Science, attend an annual orientation, and engage in ongoing studies in Christian Science. The Church also provides for the training of Christian Science nurses, who provide spiritual reassurance and basic home care, including bathing the patient, dressing wounds, assistance with mobility, and preparation of food (Christian Science Journal, 2017). The Christian Science nurses do not undergo conventional medical training and do not make diagnoses, dispense medication, or conduct physical therapy.

Because Christian Science believes that spirit and love are the only reality, the Christian Science approach emphasizes a commitment to living out Christianity rather than the adoption of a particular lifestyle as a basis of health. Nevertheless, Christian Science followers are taught that alcohol, smoking, and social drugs enslave persons, impair their ability to understand their relationship to God. Christian Science followers are advised to find satisfaction through coming to know God's love and care. Foregoing alcohol, tobacco, and drugs is part of the general movement to end any trust in matter and material things (First Church, n.d.). In this way, the Church of Christ, Scientist does guide its followers to reduce known health risk behaviors.

There is no organized effort to utilize methodologically rigorous empirical research to document the effects of Christian Science healing, as there are in the Seventh Day Adventist community. The primary evidence for the efficacy of Christian Science healing comes from personal testimonies, most published in Christian Science periodicals. The Committee on Publication (1989) of the church estimated that 53,900 testimonies of Christian Science healings were published between 1900 and 1989 and investigated 7154 testimonies published between 1969 and 1988. Over 80% of these testimonies documented the healing of a medical disease. The church requires letters from three persons who have witnessed the healing or can vouch for the testifier's integrity. The evidence for specific diagnoses and corroborating medical testing is often lacking, in part because many Christian Science members seek a healing and do not participate in mainstream medical care.

Nevertheless, the Committee on Publication (1989) reported that 2337 of the healings involved medically diagnosed conditions, ranging from 27 healings of cancer, 42 of tumor, 68 of tuberculosis, 38 of pneumonia, 88 of heart disease, and so on. In several cases, bone fractures were depicted by successive X-rays to have healed within a day, or even between the first and second X-ray in a hospital emergency room (Committee on Publication, 1989).

What happens in a Christian Science healing? Healing in Christian Science may be gradual or immediate. Christian Scientists describe it as the outward effect of divine love felt and experienced. A Christian Science practitioner and writer discussed with the author the process of Christian Science healing, using an example from his own life. Although he did not consider himself obese, there was a time when he wasn't feeling good about himself and decided to lose some weight (Eric Nelson, personal communication, January 2017). Rather than evaluating the types or volume of food he was eating, he decided instead to pray about the situation, which, as he described it, involved a conscious willingness to see himself as God saw him.

What came to mind was that God, divine Mind, did not see him as a glutton and, by association, neither should he. It was then that a familiar citation from Mary Baker Eddy's book, Science and Health, came to mind: "We ought to weary of the fleeting and false, and to cherish nothing which hinders our highest selfhood" (Eddy, 1994, p. 68).

Without setting specific goals, his eating habits changed and his weight decreased. When a friend asked how he had been able to lose the weight, he explained, paraphrasing Mary Baker Eddy, "I decided to stop harboring any thought about myself that would hinder my highest selfhood, including the notion that I was a glutton." The healing that took place wasn't so much about weight loss as it was exchanging, through prayer, a less matter-based view of himself for a more divinely inspired one.

Conclusion

The examples of the Seventh Day Adventist church and the Church of Christ, Scientist provide illustrative examples showing the diversity of religious approaches to healing. The Seventh Day Adventist approach is compatible with the evolving mainstream medical emphasis on lifestyle medicine, but adds the elements of religious prescription and community support for lifestyle change. The Christian Science approach highlights the phenomenon that unexplained healings do occur, often with no physical explanation. Whether the active ingredient is placebo, belief, or spiritual grace is not a scientific question, but the Christian Science practitioners regularly provide either emotional comfort or physical healing for their patients. For over a century, a large number of Christian Science followers worldwide have found sufficient relief from this prayer-based healing practice to sustain the movement.

Religious and Spiritual Practices Commonly Used for Comfort, Consolation, and Palliation of Suffering

Medical professionals, counselors, and researchers realize or are aware that human beings worldwide engage in religious and spiritual practices for comfort, consolation, and palliation of suffering. The empirical research on specific health effects of prayer and spiritual practices is highly inconsistent, yet every day and throughout the world human beings turn to prayer and other spiritual practices for solace. This use of religious and spiritual practices seems to increase in frequency with aging, illness, and encounters with death. As human beings face discouragement and loss of strength and vitality, they struggle with how to understand and accept their lives in this time of darkness or decline. Palliative care specialists and chaplains observe that their patients study religious scriptures, discuss religious beliefs and spiritual insights, and pray as they struggle with pain, illness, and the meaning of their living and dying (Steinhorn, Din, & Johnson, 2017). What are some of these practices that the average person can learn and employ for self-care?

Reading/studying spiritual texts Human beings engage in reading and study of sacred scriptures, seeking guidance in their struggles. Many report a sense of greater acceptance for their current suffering, or the emergence of a different understanding of their current situation after reading the Christian Bible, Jewish scriptures, or texts from other spiritual traditions. Religious insights reframe personal problems and the stories in sacred texts provide encouragement by the examples of characters from other eras, who have also suffered and often found meaning in the struggles. For those persons who have grown uncomfortable with their religious upbringings and traditions, it is often easier to find more comfort in reading texts from other cultural and spiritual traditions. Those in the Judaeo-Christian tradition often read the biblical book of the psalms that provide much guidance for coping in the face of suffering, yet the Koran and the four noble truths of Buddhism also offer pathways to discover relief from suffering.

Spiritual discussions Many persons engage in spiritual discussions, sharing their own thoughts about their religious studies and listening to the thoughts and reactions of others. The discussions provoke the same kinds of reframing of personal suffering and emotional release, as reading spiritual texts. But the discussions can also bring direct encouragement from others, or a sense of empowerment by observing others gaining strength over misfortunes. These dialogues are sometimes informal among friends and family, sometimes dialogues with pastors, rabbis, spiritual teachers and chaplains, and sometimes classes and discussion groups organized within church, temple, or other formal religious settings. However, as discussed earlier in the section on the *dark side* of spirituality, spiritual discussions are most beneficial for health and well-being if they are positive, emphasizing God's abiding love and caring for human beings, or some other positive spiritual message. If spiritual discussion emphasizes divine punishment, God's anger, or personal blame for illness, this tends to undermine well-being (Pargament et al., 2000).

Prayer Prayer can consist of repetition of ritualized prayers memorized in child-hood religious training, but often consists of a quiet conversation with God, a saint, or a religious figure. Prayers can be petitions, pleas for intercession, help, or comfort, exclamations of thanksgiving, or expressions of awe and wonder for a spiritual experience, whether a sunset, the birth of a baby, or a sense of spiritual renewal. Prayers are most often verbal, but many persons find their prayer life becomes more intense and inspirational when they utilize visualization. Human beings can engage in quiet inward prayers or spoken prayers in myriad forms, alone and in groups, perhaps contributing not only to connectedness with a higher power but also adding to the social support described above.

Meditation Meditation describes a more systematic form of prayer, which may or may not have a specific religious focus. Today, mindfulness meditation is among the most commonly used meditation practices. Mindfulness meditation was developed from Buddhist Vipassana meditation, later promoted by Jon Kabat-Zinn (1990, 2006) as an intervention for medical and emotional disorders, as well as for positive well-being. Mindfulness meditation is a process of heightening awareness, learning to pay attention to everything that enters one's awareness, in a particular way, without judging, without self-criticism, and with acceptance. Mindfulness meditation often begins with cultivating an awareness of one's own breathing and progresses to a deep sense of acceptance for the here and now, for this moment; however, it emerges for the individual. Once cultivated in meditation, mindfulness also becomes an attitude of life, in which one cultivates in each moment throughout the day an open appreciation and acceptance, to "see a world in a grain of sand, and a heaven in a wild flower, hold infinity in the palm of your hand, and eternity in an hour" (William Blake, *Auguries of Innocence*). Meditation is also one of the most widely researched spiritual practices, with documented health benefits for many medical and emotional disorders (Horowitz, 2010).

Silence and solitude One of the lessons of most spiritual traditions is to utilize spiritual practices to escape everyday absorption in the busyness of life, and to discover an inward stillness. In the modern world, where human beings are surrounded by urban noise, social media stimulation, and the wired technology of cell phones, texting, and emails, life stress is compounded by constant over-stimulation. In his memoir, *Memories, Dreams, and Reflections,* Carl Jung wrote of the dawning new technologies:

> Mostly, they are deceptive sweetenings of existence, like speedier communications which unpleasantly accelerate the tempo of life and leave us with less time than ever before. *Omis festinato ex parte diabolic est*—all haste is of the devil, as the old masters used to say. (Jung, 1961, p. 236)

Spending time in solitude and in silence can facilitate reflection and deepen spiritual awareness. Psalm 46 advises the individual to cultivate stillness: "Be still and know that I am God" (Psalm 46:10, New International Version). Many spiritual centers provide organized retreats that include times of silence and times of solitude, so rare in life for many people. A spiritual teacher and guide is usually available to assist participants who experience unexpected emotional releases during unaccustomed silence.

Fasting Many spiritual traditions prescribe fasting for several hours or even days as a spiritual discipline. For Roman Catholics, Anglicans, and those in many other Christian churches, the season of Lent traditionally included restriction of full meals and omission of meat on certain days, and for Muslims the holy days of Ramadan are a time of extended fasting. As silence is a withdrawal from the distracting bustle of life, fasting is a withdrawal from the mindless grasp of appetites, and the assumption that one needs to satisfy each craving. There is a kind of dawning freedom in not eating for a time, and combining the fast with silence, solitude, and new awareness. In Christian monastic traditions, fasting took on many meanings, but often served as a voluntary tool to cultivate discipline and temperance (Berghuis, 2007). St. Benedict, the sixth century founder of the Benedictine order of monks, wrote that a monk's life should always be "like a Lenten observance" (Benedict, 1975, pp. 87–88). The health benefits from fasting are also apparent, when we see how emotional dysregulation and mindlessness, lacking awareness of the actual drivers of our hunger, often drives unhealthy eating.

Yoga Yoga in India is an inseparable component of spiritual practices within the traditions of Hinduism, the Jain religion, and Buddhism. Many Westerners practice yoga for physical fitness, but yoga can also be a spiritual practice for Westerners. Graceful disciplined movement, paced breathing, and meditative silence are all aspects of yoga that enhance spiritual awareness. There is a growing body of research on the health benefits of yoga, with increasing methodological rigor. Riggins (2013) reviewed a range of research reports and concluded that yoga's health effects have been supported for many chronic health conditions, including cancer, cardiovascular disease, obesity and diabetes, arthritis, and chronic pain.

Singing or listening to spiritual music Both singing and listening to sacred music are part of most spiritual traditions. The kinds of spiritual *feeling* differs from one musical tradition to another, but music typically brings the body and emotions into spiritual practices, whether the music is activating and mobilizing in the form of Christian rock music, a mournful expression of suffering in traditional African-American spirituals, or the deeply spiritual chanting in a Buddhist temple. Spirituality and religious awareness are not just cognitive experiences; they can absorb the entire human being, body, mind, emotions, and spirit, and music moves human beings out of the simply cognitive realm into a more fully absorbing experience.

Worship services Worship services, at their best, provide a medium to guide the human being into a heightened spiritual experience. Church traditions, East and West, utilize tools such as liturgical music, sacred dance, candles, incense, the imagery of sacred icons, religious art, and spiritual teaching in sermons or homilies. However, religious rituals at their worst can become overly routinized and unhelpful for those participating. This is why movements of renewal have been needed periodically, historically, to stir up tired routines, transform the patterns of worship, and restore genuine spiritual experiences.

Maybe some true defining jou "*Maybe some true defining jou*"

Conclusion: Religious Practices and Spiritual Disciplines

This last section has necessarily been a brief review of commonly used spiritual practices. Bellous and Scinos (2009) have emphasized that human beings differ substantially in the ways that they experience and express spirituality. They describe four styles of experiencing spirituality: word-centered, emotion-centered, symbol-centered, and action-centered. Spiritual practices that are based on words will open rich experiences for one person yet miss another. Providing resources and learning opportunities for persons with each style will increase the possibility that all persons will achieve a full spiritual development.

Readers may read further about religious practices, spiritual disciplines, and relief from everyday suffering and burdens by turning to the works of:

- Richard Foster (1998), who in his book *Celebration of Discipline*, described spiritual disciplines rooted in the Quaker tradition
- Tony Jones (2005), who in his book *The Sacred Way: Spiritual Practices for Everyday Life*, sifts through millennial wisdom to describe practices useful for the average person today
- Harold Kushner (1981), who in his book *When Bad Things Happen to Good People*, utilized biblical scriptures to address the issues so many human beings deal with in times of suffering and loss
- The Dalai Lama (2002), who in his book, *How to Practice: The Way to a Meaningful Life*, formulates many life principles and practices from Buddhism, in his own perspective

References

Agogino, G. A. (1965). The use of hypnotism as an ethnologic research technique. *Plains Anthropologist, 10*, 31–36.

Aldana, S. G., Greenlaw, R. L., Saiberg, A., Merrill, R. M., Ohmine, S., & Thomas, C. (2006). The behavioral and clinical effects of therapeutic lifestyle change on middle-aged adults. *Preventing Chronic Disease, 3*(1), A05.

American Nurses Association. (2012). *Faith community nursing: Scope and standards of practice* (2nd ed.). Silver Spring, MD: Author.

American Psychiatric Association. (2000). *The diagnostic and statistical manual of mental disorders* (4th ed.). Washington, DC: Author.

Banerjee, A. T., Boyle, M. H., Anand, S. S., Strachan, P. H., & Oremus, M. (2014). The relationship between religious service attendance and coronary heart disease and related risk factors in Saskatchewan, Canada. *Journal of Religion and Health, 53*(1), 141–156. https://doi.org/10.1007/s10943-012-9609-6

Bellous, J. E., & Scinos, D. M. (2009). Spiritual styles: Creating an environment to nurture spiritual wholeness. *International Journal of Children's Spirituality, 14*(3), 213–224. https://doi.org/10.1080/13644360903086471

Benedict. (1975). *The rule of St. Benedict* (transl. A. C. Meisel & M. L. del Mastro). New York, NY: Image/Doubleday.

Berghuis, K. (2007). *The development of fasting from monasticism through the reformation to the modern era. Christian fasting: A theological approach.* Bible.org. Retrieved from https://bible. org/seriespage/chapter-4-development-fasting-monasticism-through-reformation-modern-era#P1100_411069

Brown, C. G. (2011). *Global Pentecostal and charismatic healing.* Oxford: New York, NY.

Christian Science Journal. (2017). *Christian Science Journal Directory.* Retrieved from https:// journal.christianscience.com/directory

Committee on Publication. (1989). *An empirical analysis of medical evidence in Christian Science testimonies of healing.* Boston, MA: The First Church of Christ, Scientist.

Dalai Lama. (2002). *How to practice: The way to a meaningful life.* New York, NY: Pocket Books.

Dixon, A. L. (2007). Mattering in the later years: Older adults' experiences of mattering to others, purpose in life, depression, and wellness. *Adultspan Journal, 6*(2), 83–95.

Dossey, L. (1993). *Healing words: The power of prayer and the practice of medicine.* New York: HarperOne.

Dossey, L. (1996). *Prayer is good medicine: How to reap the healing benefits of prayer.* San Francisco: Harper.

Dossey, L. (1997). The return of prayer. *Alternative Therapies in Health and Medicine, 3*(6), 10–17, 113–120.

Duffy, E. (2009). Two healing prayers. In M. Rubin (Ed.), *Medieval Christianity in practice* (pp. 164–170). Princeton, NJ: Princeton University Press.

Eddy, M. B. (1895). *Manual of the mother church: The First Church of Christ, Scientist.* Boston, MA: Joseph Armstrong Publishers.

Eddy, M. B. (1994). *Science and health, with key to the scriptures.* Boston, MA: The First Church of Christ, Scientist.

Ellison, C. G., & Hummer, R. A. (2010). *Religion, families, and health: Population-based research in the United States.* New Brunswick, NJ: Rutgers University Press.

Emmons, R. A., Cheung, C., & Tehrani, K. (1998). Assessing spirituality through personal goals: Implications for research on religion and subjective well-being. *Social Indicators Research, 45*(1/3), 391–422.

First Church of Christ, Scientist, Riverside. (n.d.). *Questions and answers.* Retrieved from http:// christianscienceinriverside.org/index.php?pr=Questions#drugs

Foster, R. (1998). *Celebration of discipline: The path to spiritual growth* (3rd ed.). San Francisco, CA: Harper Collins.

Fraser, G. E., & Shavlik, D. J. (2001). Ten years of life: Is it a matter of choice? *Archives of Internal Medicine, 161*(13), 1645–1652.

Galloway, A. P., & Henry, M. (2014). Relationships between social connectedness and spirituality and depression and perceived health status of rural residents. *Online Journal of Rural Nursing and Health Care, 14*(2), 43. Retrieved from http://rnojournal.binghamton.edu/index.php/RNO/article/view/325

Goldiner, S. (2012). Medicine in the middle ages. In *Heibrunn timeline of art history.* New York: The Metropolitan Museum of Art, 2000-2017. Retrieved from http://www.metmuseum.org/toah/hd/medm/hd_medm.htm

Gopinath, B., Buyken, A. E., Flood, V. M., Empson, M., Rochtchina, E., & Mitchell, P. (2011). Consumption of polyunsaturated fatty acids, fish, and nuts and risk of inflammatory disease mortality. *American Journal of Clinical Nutrition, 93*(5), 1073–1079.

Hill, P. C., & Pargament, K. I. (2003). Advances in the conceptualization and measurement of religion and spirituality: Implications for physical and mental health research. *American Psychologist, 58*(1), 64–74.

Hill, P. L., & Turiano, N. A. (2014). Purpose in life as a predictor of mortality across adulthood. *Psychological Science, 57*(7), 1482–1486.

Horowitz, S. (2010). Health benefits of meditation: What the newest research shows. *Alternative and Complementary Therapies, 16*(4), 223–228. https://doi.org/10.1089/act2010.16402

Hummel, C. E. (1986). Worldwide renewal: The charismatic movement. *Christianity Today, 9.* Retrieved from http://www.christianitytoday.com/history/issues/issue-9/worldwide-renewal-charismatic-movement.html

Hummer, R. A., Ellison, C. G., Rogers, R. G., Moulton, B. E., & Romero, R. R. (2004). Religious involvement and adult mortality in the United States: Review and perspective. *Southern Medical Journal, 97*(12), 1223–1230.

Hummer, R. A., Rogers, R. G., Nam, C. B., & Ellison, C. G. (1999). Religious involvement and US adult mortality. *Demography, 36*(2), 273–285.

Jackson, B. R., & Bergeman, C. S. (2011). How does religiosity enhance well-being? The role of perceived self-control. *Psychology of Religion and Spirituality, 3*(2), 149–161. https://doi.org/10.1037/a0021597

Jones, T. (2005). *The sacred way: Spiritual practices for everyday life.* Grand Rapids, MI: Zondervan.

Jung, C. G. (1961). *Memories, dreams, and reflections* (transl. by R. Winston & C. Winston). New York, NY: Vintage.

Kabat-Zinn, J. (1990). *Full catastrophe living: Using the wisdom of your body and mind to face stress, pain, and illness.* New York, NY: Delacorte.

Kabat-Zinn, J. (2006). *Mindfulness for beginners: Reclaiming the present moment* (Educational CD). Louisville, CO: Sounds True.

Kapogiannis, D., Berbey, A. K., Zamboni, G., Krueger, F., & Grafman, J. (2009). Cognitive and neural foundations of religious belief. *Proceedings of the National Academy of Sciences of the United States of America, 106*(12), 4876–4881. https://doi.org/10.1073/pnas.0811717106

Kent, L., Morton, D., Hurlow, T., Rankin, P., Hanna, A., & Diehl, H. (2013). Long term effectiveness of the community-based Complete Health Improvement Program (CHIP) lifestyle intervention: A cohort study. *BMJ Open, 3*(11), e003751. https://doi.org/10.1136/bmjopen-2013-003751

Koenig, H. G. (2008). *Medicine, religion, and health: Where science and spirituality meet.* West Conshohocken, PA: Templeton Press.

Koenig, H. G. (2012a). *Medicine and religion: Twin healing traditions.* Catholic Exchange. Retrieved from http://catholicexchange.com/medicine-and-religion-twin-healing-traditions

Koenig, H. G. (2012b). Religion, spirituality, and health: The research and clinical implications. *International Scholarly Research Network, ISNR Psychiatry,* Article ID 278730, 1–33. https://doi.org/10.5402/2012/278370.

Koenig, H. G., McCullough, M. E., & Larson, D. B. (2012). *Handbook of religion and health* (2nd ed.). New York, NY: Oxford University Press.

Kushner, H. S. (1981). *When bad things happen to good people.* New York, NY: Shocken Books.

Lehrer, P. M., & Gevirtz, R. (2014). Heart rate variability biofeedback: How and why does it work. *Frontiers in Psychology, 5,* 756. https://doi.org/10.3389/fpsyg.2014.00756

Lehrer, P. M., Sasaki, Y., & Saito, Y. (1999). Zazen and cardiac variability. *Psychosomatic Medicine, 61,* 812–821.

Lutheran Deaconess Association. (2017). *History of deaconesses and parish nurses.* Retrieved from http://www.thelda.org/assets/docs/history_deacs_nurses.pdf

Mahoney, A., Pargament, K. I., Cole, B., Jewell, T., Magyar, G. M., Tarakeshwar, N., et al. (2005). A higher purpose: The sanctification of strivings in a community sample. *International Journal for the Psychology of Religion, 15*(3), 239–262. https://doi.org/10.1207/s15327582ijpr1503_4

McCraty, R., & Shaffer, F. (2015). Heart rate variability: New perspectives on physiological mechanisms, assessment of self-regulatory capacity, and health risk. *Global Advances in Health and Medicine, 4*(1), 46–61. https://doi.org/10.7453/gahmj.2014.073

Morton, K. R., Lee, J. W., & Martin, L. R. (2016). Pathways from religion to health: Mediation by psychosocial and lifestyle mechanisms. *Psychology of Religion and Spirituality, 9*(1), 106–117.

National Cancer Institute. (2015). *Spirituality in cancer care—For health professionals* (PDQ®). Retrieved from http://www.cancer.gov/about-cancer/coping/day-to-day/faith-and-spirituality/spirituality-hp-pdq#section/_4

Oman, D., Kurata, J. H., Strawbridge, W. J., & Cohen, R. D. (2002). Religious attendance and cause of death over 31 years. *International Journal of Psychiatry in Medicine, 32*(1), 69–89.

Orlich, M. J., Singh, P. N., Sabaté, J., Jaceldo-Siegl, K., Fan, J., Knutsen, S., et al. (2013). Vegetarian dietary patterns and mortality in Adventist Health Study 2. *JAMA Internal Medicine, 173*(13), 1230–1238. https://doi.org/10.1001/jamainternmed.2013.6473

Pargament, K. I., Koenig, H. G., & Perez, L. M. (2000). The many methods of religious coping: Development and initial validation of the RCOPE. *Journal of Clinical Psychology, 56*, 519–543.

Park, N. S., Lee, B. S., Sun, F., Klemmack, D. L., Roff, L. L., & Koenig, H. G. (2013). Typologies of religiousness/spirituality: Implications for health and well-being. *Journal of Religion and Health, 52*, 828–839. https://doi.org/10.1007/s10943-011-9520-6

Riggins, L. (2013). Understanding the health benefits of yoga and implications for public health. *Health Education Monograph Series, 30*(1), 46–53.

Roberts, S. T. (2014). Parish nursing: Providing spiritual, physical, and emotional care in a small community parish. *Clinical Nursing Studies, 2*(2), 118–122. https://doi.org/10.5430/cns.v2n2p118

Schorsch, K. (2015). *Alexian, Adventist have a new name for their joint venture.* Crain's Chicago Business. Retrieved from http://www.chicagobusiness.com/article/20150413/NEWS03/150419957/alexian-adventist-have-a-new-name-for-their-joint-venture

Steinhorn, D. M., Din, J., & Johnson, A. (2017). Healing, spirituality, and integrative medicine. *Annals of Palliative Medicine, 6*(3), 237–247. https://doi.org/10.21037/apm.2017.05.01

Tarakeshwar, N., Vanderwerker, L. C., Paulk, E., Pearce, M. J., Kasl, S. V., & Priferson, H. G. (2008). Religious coping is associated with the quality of life of patients with advanced cancer. *Journal of Palliative Medicine, 9*(3), 646–657.

Westberg, G., & Westberg McNamara, J. (1990). *Parish nurse: Providing a minister of health for your congregation.* Minneapolis, MN: Augsburg Books.

Windsor, T. D., Curtis, R. G., & Luszcz, M. A. (2015). Sense of purpose as a psychological resource for aging well. *Developmental Psychology, 51*(7), 976–986.

Ziebarth, D. (2014). Evolutionary conceptual analysis: Faith community nursing. *Journal of Religion and Health, 53*(6), 1817–1823. https://doi.org/10.1007/s10943-014-9918-z

Chapter 5
Complementary and Integrative Medicine for the Pathways Model

Abstract This chapter will describe the emergence of the complementary and alternative medicine (CAM) movement historically, and the current drive toward integrating complementary therapies and mainstream medicine into a comprehensive integrative medicine. The five domains of complementary medicine are defined; emphasis is placed on therapies with a strong evidence base. The second part of the chapter will summarize applications of complementary medicine to some of the disorders on which this book is focused. The chapter closes with discussion of continuing obstacles in creating access to complementary and integrative clinical practice, and challenges in design and implementation of research studies.

Keywords Complementary and alternative medicine · Integrative medicine · Biologically based therapies · Mind-body therapies · Energy therapies · Manipulation and body-based therapies and whole medical systems

Part I: Historical Origins of Complementary and Integrative Medicine

Alternatives to mainstream and conventional medicine are not new. The father of Western medicine, the Greek physician Hippocrates, who lived in the fifth century BC, is quoted as saying, "It is far more important to know what person the disease has, than what disease the person has."

Ayurveda, the traditional medicine of India, dates back 3000–5000 years, prior to written records, with information passed from person to person by word of mouth. Ayurvedic medicine developed an elaborate system for understanding the person, the person's *doshas* (the patterns of energy and movement in this person's organism), the balance of energies in the chakras, and the contribution of these factors to health and disease (Halpern, 2011). Ayurveda focuses treatment on appropriate interventions to strengthen the person, rather than targeting the illness (Frawley & Ranade, 2001; Ninivaggi, 2010). Similarly, the major intent of Ayurveda is not

© Springer International Publishing AG, part of Springer Nature 2018
A. McGrady, D. Moss, *Integrative Pathways*,
https://doi.org/10.1007/978-3-319-89313-6_5

exclusively on treatment, but on prevention and on improving mental and physical health (Mishra, Singh, & Dagenais, 2001).

The practices of Ayurveda mainly consist of diet, lifestyle, along with herbal remedies, massage, and yoga, and prioritize maintaining the *dosha* equilibrium (Chopra & Doiphode, 2002). The Ayurvedic products are composed of herbs only or a combination of herbs, metals, minerals, and other substances in a practice termed rasa shastra (National Center for Complementary and Integrative Health, 2014). The most prominent mind-body component of Ayurveda is meditation (Sharma & Clark, 2012).

Traditional Chinese Medicine (TCM) is another system of medicine that dates back more than 3000 years. It attempts to explain illness based on disruptions of energy (or *qi*) in the body, and loss of harmony between the person's outer and inner worlds. It is a patient-centered approach, relying on a complicated diagnostic framework. Interventions consist of acupuncture, believed to rebalance the energy within the body, herbal compounds, Chinese massage, and Qigong (Thie, 2007). Medical Qigong is conducted by a skilled master practitioner to heal others. In contrast, western practices of Qigong consist of exercises done by individuals to enhance their own health and well-being. Research continues to delve into the effectiveness of TCM. Up to 2015, there were 1270 clinical trials of all components of TCM. Over 505 were acupuncture trials and 35% were herbal medicines. Most were classified as "small" enrolling fewer than 100 subjects (Chen et al., 2017).

The Emergence of Holistic, Patient-Centered, Person-Centered, Complementary, Alternative, and Integrative Health Care

If we fast-forward to the late twentieth century, the holistic health movement emerged in the 1970s, from many sources, including sources within medicine itself. The concept of holistic health emphasizes paying attention to the whole person— body, mind, and spirit. Harold Koenig, a Duke University-based researcher, expressed the importance of a holistic point of view:

> "Patients want to be seen and treated as a whole person, not as diseases. A whole person is someone whose being has physical, emotional, and spiritual dimensions. Ignoring any of these aspects of humanity leaves the person incomplete and may even interfere with healing" (Koenig, 2000)

In June 1975, the first National Conference on Holistic Health was held at the University of California, San Diego School of Medicine (Ralph & Taylor, 2013), leading to the founding of the American holistic medical Association in 1978. (http://www.healthy.net/scr/PractitionerSearch.aspx?AssocId=36).

In 1977, George Engel published an article in *Science,* calling for a new *biopsychosocial* medicine (Engel, 1977). Engel asserted that many of the complaints presented by human beings to clinicians today are caused either by various psychosocial stressors or have been aggravated by them. A disorder may have a strong genetic basis; it may be visible in laboratory tests and imaging scans. Yet the basis for the current exacerbation, bringing the patient into contact with the provider with heightened complaints, is often a maladaptive stress response due to job, marital conflict, or existential crisis. A medical system that views all problems only through a biomedical lens misses the most critical factors shaping the course of the disease and the ebb and flow of symptoms. Worse, an excessive focus on biomedical variables in treatment may miss the healing resources within each organism, within each person.

Along with a holistic viewpoint, a variety of alternative treatments emerged. Acupuncture gained considerable attention after Richard Nixon's 1971 visit to China because James Reston, a New York Times journalist covering the Nixon visit, received acupuncture for postoperative pain following an appendectomy in Beijing (Reston, 1971). Other alternative therapies, naturopathy, chiropractic, and osteopathy, had been present throughout the twentieth century, but gained adherents in the 1970s (Baer, 1992). This upsurge in the use of alternative medicine was observable across the Western world (Albrecht, Fitzpatrick, & Scrimshaw, 2000).

Since the 1970s, consumers have steadily increased their usage of alternative health practices. An initial study conducted by Eisenberg and colleagues in 1990 reported that one in three Americans surveyed had utilized at least one "unconventional therapy" in the preceding year (Eisenberg et al., 1993). A later study by Eisenberg and colleagues in 1998 showed even more widespread acceptance and use of alternative therapies by the general public, and about half paid for services themselves (Eisenberg et al., 1998). Eisenberg's data showed that by 1997, 42.1% of the population had used at least one of the 16 alternative therapies studied, and that consumers made 629 million visits to alternative practitioners in 1997, more than to primary care physicians!

Furthermore, an international study in 2012, based on a meta-analysis of 49 studies conducted in 15 countries, showed that this trend toward increased use of alternative therapies is evident worldwide (Harris, Cooper, Relton, & Thomas, 2012).

Usage of alternative medicine continued to grow, often without regard to any research basis for the alternative therapies. For the average citizen, it is challenging to discriminate among the various alternative therapies marketed in health fairs, health food stores, and through pyramid marketing schemes. As dietary supplements became more commercialized, and the internet evolved into a forum for marketing, it became even more difficult to discriminate between the attractive online presentations for useless techniques and the more credible evidence-based complementary interventions.

Further, many users of alternative therapy don't inform their physicians of their use of these therapies, which results in a lack of coordination of simultaneous care. It is important to keep in mind as there are risks of interactions among prescribed medicines, dietary supplements, and herbal medicines, when providers are not in communication. Eisenberg's 1998 study found that only 39.8% of usages of alternative therapies were reported to physicians. Further, a 2008 study in cancer patients reported that between 40 and 77% of those patients who used CAM therapies did not inform their physicians of the CAM use. Patient's explanations for their unwillingness to disclose use include: (1) expectancy that physicians will react negatively (2) the belief that CAM therapies are natural and benign and therefore do not need to be disclosed, and (3) the failure of the physician to ask about CAM (Vishal, Mishra, & Raychaudhuri, 2011). Trends in use of complementary therapies were summarized in 2015. The most commonly used approaches were non-vitamin, non-mineral dietary supplements. The use of yoga, Tai Chi, and Qigong have increased steadily from 2002, 2007 until 2012, but yoga accounts for the majority of the increase in prevalence (Clarke, Black, Strussman, Barnes, & Nahin, 2015).

Federal Support for Alternative Health Care

The federal government was late to support alternatives to mainstream medicine. Finally, in 1991, a department was founded within the National Institutes of Medicine, with the unfortunate name, The Office for the Study of Unconventional Medical Practices, with an initial budget of two million dollars (Talesnik, 2016). In 1992, the office was renamed the Office of Alternative Medicine, and in 1998 it became the National Center for Complementary and Alternative Medicine (NCCAM). For 16 years, NCCAM oversaw a growing research budget and sponsored a series of critical meeting reflecting the slow acceptance of complementary and alternative therapies into the mainstream. In 2014, NIH took another significant step, in renaming NCCAM as the National Center for Complementary and Integrative Health (NCCIH), placing an emphasis on the integration of complementary and alternative care with mainstream medicine. This organization, part of the National Institutes of Health funds research, maintains databases and reviews evidence. It interacts with the FDA to provide recommendations for safety of interventions for providers and consumers. In addition, information is summarized, packaged, and presented in a format understandable by the lay public.

The vision of an integrated and integrative medicine was expressed beautifully by Cummings and Cummings:

> "The patient of the future will encounter an integrated system of behavioral and medical care, involving a partnership of behavioral practitioners, physicians and nurses, in 'one house' and 'one system.'" (Cummings & Cummings, 2000)

This seamless integration of the many streams of health care under one umbrella remains a dream, but in many settings that dream is slowly becoming a reality.

Terminology

"The patient of the future will encounter an integrated system of behavioral and medical care, involving a partnership of behavioral practitioners, physicians and nurses, in 'one house' and 'one system'" (Cummings & Cummings, 2000).

In this section, we will provide definitions of those various movements that have emerged since the 1970s in the United States and the developed world, each of which captures one facet of the vision of an integrative comprehensive health care for the whole person.

Holistic health is an approach to health care that emphasizes attending to the whole human being, body, mind, and spirit. Holistic care also emphasizes drawing on the body's own inner resources for healing.

Patient-centered care is an approach to health care that promotes active participation in all health care decisions by the patient and his/her family. The Institute of Medicine emphasizes that patient-centered care "gives patients abundant opportunities to be informed and involved in medical decision-making, and guides and supports those providing care in attending to their patients' physical and emotional needs, and maintaining or improving their quality of life to the extent possible" (Institute of Medicine, 2001, p. 49). One of the hallmarks of patient-centered care is enhanced communication between physician and patient.

Person-centered care is an approach that claims to go beyond patient-centered care, by adapting a more holistically focused view of the human person's health over the life span. Starfield (2011) asserted that patient-centered care focused too much on managing a disease present at a specific medical visit and proposed that "person-focused care is provided to patients over time independent of care for particular diseases."

Complementary therapies are non-mainstream health care interventions that are compatible with and easily combined with mainstream medical care. In most cases, complementary therapies also work through mechanisms that make sense in the paradigms of Western science. Examples of complementary therapies that are easily integrated in medical settings, and which rely at least in part on neurophysiological mechanisms that can be measured scientifically are biofeedback, meditation, massage, some herbal medicines and supplements, and hypnosis.

> *"Integrative medicine* is the effort to combine evidence-based complementary therapies (those complementary therapies whose efficacy is supported by outcomes research) with mainstream health care, in a reasonably seamless process with coordination of mainstream and complementary care."

Alternative therapies are interventions that are usually used instead of rather than in conjunction with mainstream medicine. In many cases, alternative therapies also seem to rely on mechanisms and explanatory theories that are not easily understood in the paradigms of Western science. Today, many once alternative therapies are being combined with mainstream medicine. In past years, for example, acupuncture was regarded as *alternative* because it was frequently practiced independently of mainstream health care, and the traditional explanations of the mechanism for acupuncture's effects relied on concepts such as qi (the life force) and meridians, alien to Western science. Today, acupuncture is practiced in many medical settings, integrated with mainstream interventions, and extensive scientific research has pursued scientific explanations for acupuncture's effects, through fMRI, PET, and other methodologies (Chernyak & Sessler, 2005; Towler, Molassiotis, & Brearley, 2013).

Integrative medicine is the effort to combine evidence-based complementary therapies (those complementary therapies whose efficacy is supported by outcomes research) with mainstream healthcare, in a reasonably seamless process with coordination of mainstream and complementary care.

The Five Domains of Complementary and Alternative Medicine

During the years of growing support for complementary and alternative medicine, NCCAM adopted a classification of complementary and alternative therapies into five domains: biologically based therapies, mind-body therapies, energy therapies, manipulation and body-based therapies, and whole medical systems (National Library of Medicine, 2003). This chapter will focus primarily on the mind-body therapies, and especially on those with the most credible evidence base. The authors advocate that the best of the complementary therapies, as proven in the crucible of outcomes research, be made more accessible to patients within a comprehensive integrative health care system. There are many well-documented complementary therapies that should be integrated within every primary care setting, as well as in specialty care.

Mind-Body Therapies

Mind-body therapies consist of interventions that utilize some kind of mental practice or mental activity to modify the body. Elmer Green and his associates at the Menninger Clinic articulated the psychophysiological principle, which states that: "Every change in the physiological state is accompanied by an appropriate change in the mental-emotional state, and conversely, every change in the mental-emotional state, conscious or unconscious, is accompanied by an appropriate change in the physiological state" (Green, Green, & Walters, 1970).

Mind and body are one, and a variety of mental and behavioral practices can be utilized to produce health-enhancing changes in the body. Widely used mind-body medicine therapies include: meditation, hypnosis, biofeedback, imagery training, art, music, and dance therapy, and prayer and mental healing.

Meditation Meditation is the oldest mind-body technique. The history of meditation in India, for example, goes back at least three to five millennia before the common era. Archeologists in the Indus valley have studied wall paintings of sitting meditators dating to between 3500 and 5000 BCE. Hindu scriptures dating back at least to 1500 BCE describe yogic meditation techniques (Khalsa, 2004).

"Mind and body are one, and a variety of mental and behavioral practices can be utilized to produce health-enhancing changes in the body."

Meditation involves the use of any of a wide variety of mental and behavioral practices to transform and shape awareness in a positive manner, producing personal self-control, spiritual awakening, and enhanced health. Sat Bir Khalsa defined meditation broadly as:

...the sustained control of mental attention in a relaxed and passive manner ... any behavior in which the mind is so absorbed ... That only the pure experience of the present moment exists. (Khalsa, 2004)

There are several kinds of meditation practices, including concentrative meditation, awareness meditation, and expressive meditation.

Transcendental meditation (TM) is a form of concentrative meditation and has been widely utilized since the 1970s in the West for spiritual growth and awareness, as well as health and wellness. Practitioners of TM used a mantra, a Sanskrit syllable received from their original trainer, and chanted this mantra as the vehicle to concentrate their mind. Herbert Benson coined the term relaxation response to describe the stress-erasing effects of transcendental meditation and promoted the use of a secular form of mantra meditation for health and wellness (Benson, 1975). Benson taught naïve meditators to select a word such as "one," "peace," or another word or phrase of personal significance, and say this mantra repeatedly in synchrony with one's breathing.

One advantage of mantra meditation is that it is easier for persons with anxiety or distracted thoughts to stay with an audible repetition of a sound. Benson conducted extensive research on transcendental meditation and documented beneficial physiological effects, reversing the effects of stress in body and mind.

Zen meditation is an awareness-based meditation and has gained wide acceptance in the West since the 1950s and 1960s (Suzuki, 1956). The American counterculture figure Alan Watts popularized "The Way of Zen" in his 1957 book of the same name. Thich Nhat Hanh is a Vietnamese Zen teacher, now living in the United States, who serves as a link between Zen practices and contemporary mindfulness practices.

> "Mindfulness involves cultivating the skill of bringing one's entire attention to the present experience, by observing events unfold from moment to moment. In mindfulness, the individual suspends judgment and evaluation, accepting whatever arises in awareness."

Jon Kabat-Zinn (1990) introduced the next wave in the use of meditation for physical and emotional health, the mindfulness movement. He drew on Buddhist "vipassana" meditation, an awareness-oriented meditative approach, and developed a simple practice called mindfulness. Mindfulness involves cultivating the skill of bringing one's entire attention to the present experience, by observing events unfold from moment to moment. In mindfulness, the individual suspends judgment and evaluation, accepting whatever arises in awareness. Mindfulness can be practiced as a meditative technique or utilized as a coping strategy, providing a way to mindfully encounter the stresses and strains of life.

Today, mindfulness is the most widely practiced meditation technique; it has been adapted to be used as a clinical intervention applied to health and mental health problems (Baer, 2003). Several structured mindfulness-based approaches have been developed, including mindfulness-based stress reduction (MBSR), mindfulness-based cognitive therapy (MBCT), dialectical behavior therapy (DBT), and acceptance and commitment therapy (ACT). The empirical research on mindfulness is extensive, showing benefit for anxiety, depression, inattention, insomnia, and a host of other disorders. A recent meta-analysis reviewed the research on mindfulness-based interventions and concluded that mindfulness is "promising for the mental health and quality of life of primary care patients" (Demarzo et al., 2015, p. 573). The incorporation of mindfulness into psychiatric practice initially met with resistance. But more recently the understanding that meditation can be adjunctive to medication management and to the psychotherapies with positive results has led to increased integrative care of persons with mental and emotional illness (McGee, 2008).

Hypnosis Hypnosis is widely used in medical and mental health circles. The hypnosis division of the American Psychological Association defines hypnosis as "A state of consciousness involving focused attention and reduced peripheral awareness characterized by an enhanced capacity for response to suggestion" (Division 30, http://www.apadivisions.org/division-30/about/index.aspx). Human beings vary greatly in their hypnotizability, their ability to enter into a hypnotic state, receive hypnotic suggestions, and show positive effects.

"Research has documented the efficacy of hypnosis in the treatment of pain, anxiety, and depression. It is also used to facilitate behavioral change, especially with health risk behaviors, such as cigarette smoking, nutritional choices, and substance use."

Historically, hypnosis dates back to the charismatic Franz Anton Mesmer (1734–1815), a German physician, who developed hypnotic techniques but attributed them to "animal magnetism." Mesmer's followers discarded the theory of magnetism, but rapidly extended the techniques and applications of hypnosis. James Braid, a Scottish physician, proposed the name of hypnosis or *neurohypnology* and promoted its use especially for nervous disorders (Braid, 1843).

Today, there is a multiplicity of hypnotic approaches and applications. Hypnosis is used to deepen and enhance psychotherapy, including the use of both age regressions to explore or resolve past trauma, and age progressions to anticipate and facilitate positive attitudes. Research has documented the efficacy of hypnosis in the treatment of pain, anxiety, and depression. It is also used to facilitate behavioral change, especially with health risk behaviors, such as cigarette smoking, nutritional choices, and substance use. Elkins (2016) has summarized the current state of clinical applications of hypnosis, and the evidence base for their efficacy.

Biofeedback Biofeedback is a technique that guides an individual to learn how to change his or her own physiology to produce improved health and performance (Moss & Shaffer, 2016). Biofeedback utilizes electronic instruments to measure an individual's physiology and feedback instantaneous information about that physiology, allowing the individual to gain greater awareness and control over the body's responses.

Biofeedback is a relatively recent development, emerging from several lines of research in the 1960s, including operant conditioning studies on animals and humans, cybernetics (information science) and systems theory, polysomnography, physiological psychology, and medicine. A key conference in 1969 brought together laboratory researchers with gurus from the emerging human potential movement at the Surfrider Inn in Santa Monica. This meeting of the white coated lab scientists and the white robed gurus highlighted the emerging promise on this self-regulation process and selected the name *biofeedback* to describe it. The conference also founded a professional society to promote this new biofeedback paradigm, the Biofeedback Research Society (today known as the Association for Applied Psychophysiology and Biofeedback). A second professional association, the International Society for Neurofeedback and Research, emerged to focus on brain-focused feedback training or neurofeedback.

Today's biofeedback instruments measure muscle activity, skin temperature, electrodermal activity (ambient electrical activity in the skin), respiration, heart rate, heart rate variability, blood pressure, brain electrical activity, and blood flow (Shaffer & Moss, 2006). In each case, if the practitioner can measure a bodily process accurately, and feedback information to the trainee, the trainee can modify that bodily process in beneficial ways. Through biofeedback training, anxious patients learn to slow and smooth their breathing and reduce anxiety; headache patients learn to reduce muscle tension and slow excessive nervous activation in their brains, reducing the frequency and severity of headaches. In neurofeedback clinics across the country, children and adults learn to correct abnormal activation patterns in frontal areas of their brains and reduce the symptoms of attention deficit hyperactivity disorder.

"Through biofeedback training, anxious patients learn to slow and smooth their breathing and reduce anxiety; headache patients learn to reduce muscle tension and slow excessive nervous activation in their brains, reducing the frequency and severity of headaches."

When biofeedback is utilized to control and modify brain activity it is called neurofeedback. Neurofeedback primarily utilizes the EEG- and EEG-based feedback to train modifications on electrical; activation patterns in the cortex. The fMRI has also been used to provide feedback based on neuro-imaging of brain structures and networks.

Biofeedback has been researched in thousands of empirical studies, showing its therapeutic benefit for a wide range of medical and mental health disorders, from attention deficit hyperactivity disorder to anxiety to depression to fibromyalgia to traumatic brain injury. A recent publication, from Tan, Shaffer, Lyle, and Teo (2016) reviewed the extensive body of outcomes research on biofeedback and neurofeedback and rated the level of evidence to show efficacy for the use of biofeedback and neurofeedback with a wide range of disorders. Current research shows the greatest evidence for the efficacy of biofeedback for the following disorders: alcohol/substance use disorders, anxiety disorders and post-traumatic stress disorder (PTSD), arthritis, asthma, attention deficit hyperactivity disorder (ADHD), autism, "chemo-brain," constipation, depression, diabetes mellitus (glycemic control), erectile dysfunction, fecal incontinence, fibromyalgia, headache, essential hypertension and prehypertension, insomnia, irritable bowel syndrome, motion sickness, chronic muscle pain, preeclampsia, Raynaud's disease, tinnitus, traumatic brain injury, and urinary incontinence (Tan et al., 2016).

Imagery Pioneers in the application of imagery to twentieth and twenty-first century medical problems acknowledge their indebtedness to centuries of Greek sleep/dream healers, medieval wise women, indigenous healers, and faith healers, who cultivated the use of imagery and visions for healing (Achterberg, 1985). In the 1970s, imagery emerged in a variety of circles in clinical medicine and research, as a powerful tool for healing. The oncologist Carl Simonton and his wife Stephanie Mathews-Simonton published accounts of their cancer patients' drawings. They suggested that guiding their patients from dark pessimistic images of their disease to more hopeful images of their immune system triumphing over cancer cells appeared to facilitate longer survival (Simonton, Matthews-Simonton, & Creighton, 1978). Jeanne Achterberg and Frank Lawlis studied the imagery of these cancer patients scientifically and showed that measurable qualities in the patients' imagery were of prognostic value for the patient's survival (Achterberg & Lawlis, 1980).

Meanwhile, medical practitioners experimented with imagery techniques as interventions to assist their patients with pain, illness, and emotional distress. Irving Oyle, a general practice physician, combined his interests in psychology, parapsychology, and medicine to develop a panoply of relaxation and visualization techniques, eliciting greater self-awareness and clinical improvements in a wide range of disorders (Rossman, 2000). Martin Rossman, influenced by Oyle and the Simontons, proceeded to develop a number of imagery and visualization techniques to assist human beings with both medical and emotional suffering (Rossman, 2000).

In the same time period, laboratory research provided documentation for the power of imagery to modify physiology and reduce pain and suffering. The emerging field of psychoneuroimmunology (PNI) systematically studied the adverse effects of stress on human physiology, and conversely the positive impact of imagery, relaxation, and other psychological interventions to elicit changes in the nervous system and the immune system.

Janice Kiecolt-Glaser and colleagues directed an elegant series of experiments showing the effects of stress on the immune system, both acutely and long term. Medical students, married couples during conflict and caregivers of persons with dementia have been the focus of her research. In each case, psychological stress was associated with significant, measurable changes in immune reactions (Fagundes, Glaser, & Kiecolt-Glaser, 2013; Kiecolt-Glaser, Derry, & Fagundes, 2015). On the other hand, research in PNI has measured the powerful positive effects that guided imagery, hypnosis, and other PNI interventions can have on the immune system and illness. Trakhtenberg (2008) reviewed decades of research and concluded that guided imagery can reduce stress and distress and elicit more effective immune system function.

Part II: Application of CIM Therapies to Mental and Emotional Disorders

The next part of this chapter considers the specific applications of complementary and integrative medicine (CIM) to some of the disorders that are the focus of this book, but there is no attempt to provide comprehensive discussion of all of the therapies, nor of all the disorders. Emphasis is placed on reviews of the literature and meta-analysis of data where those are available. Some citations were located from the NCCIH databases since those documents are updated frequently based on recent research. The abbreviation for the complementary/integrative therapies from this point on is CIM.

People with chronic illness utilize complementary therapies for several reasons. First, patients seek help because standard medical interventions are not sufficiently effective or have serious side effects. Some patients wish a holistic approach to their illness, instead of relying only on pharmacological solutions for their pain and suffering. Other patients desire to be active participants in their health care, so they choose interventions where they have more responsibility for their illness, such as relaxation, meditation, and yoga.

Providers must become knowledgeable in CIM therapies that are relevant to their practice. For example, physicians specializing in pain management need to update themselves frequently on mind-body therapies and acupuncture. The medical providers who manage patients with cancer or gastrointestinal problems will have to answer questions about herbal products and supplements (National Center for Complementary and Integrative Health, 2014).

"Some patients wish a holistic approach to their illness, instead of relying only on pharmacological solutions for their pain and suffering. Other patients desire to be active participants in their health care ..."

Analyzing the literature on the effects of CIM therapies on disorders relevant to this book immediately highlights the difficulties in reaching valid conclusions. Often, the CIM studies have included more than one intervention so it is difficult to ascertain the efficacy of each therapy, such as when biofeedback is combined with relaxation (biofeedback-assisted relaxation) or acupuncture offered with meditation (Fraser, Matsuzawa, Lee, & Minen, 2017). Multiple outcomes are studied and sometimes, the intervention has no benefit on the primary outcome, but is associated with major effects on secondary outcomes, such as personal suffering or better coping with the illness. The putative benefit that is most important to the patient with uncontrolled back pain may not even be measured in a study which focuses only on pain relief (Hsu, Bluespruce, Sherman, & Cherkin, 2010).

The study of herbal products and supplements is particularly difficult. Over-the-counter herbal products may contain varying amounts of the active ingredient and different combinations of the active and inactive components. For example, the portion of the plant that is used in the preparation may vary and plants grown in American soil may not have the same chemical makeup or effects as the same plant grown, for example, in Japanese soil.

Designing active controls for CIM research is much more challenging than instituting a randomized controlled trial of a new medicine. In this age of social media, and the internet, patients know what to expect with biofeedback, yoga, and even pictures of needle placement for acupuncture are easily available. Therefore, reasonable active controls require exceptional acuity on the part of the researcher, who is all too aware that the project is likely to be criticized and the efficacy of the intervention downplayed because of the lack of double blind conditions. Efforts to study integrative care at the medical centers where it exists is also difficult for several reasons. Clinical productivity may not be compatible with research design or the organization's compensation schedule is focused on patient care and teaching, with research holding a distant third in priority (Verhoef, Mulkins, Kania, Findlay-Reece, & Mior, 2010).

Despite all of the above, patients will continue to seek CIM, providers will offer various types with and without confirmatory evidence and researchers will diligently work on better experimental designs. Chronic illnesses, both mental and physical have been and continue to be the primary types of disorders for which patient seek CIM. Sometimes, the benefits are general, such as a greater sense of well-being, a spiritual awakening, or less irritability.

General Benefits

"The basic food groups: carbohydrates, fats, protein and minerals are all necessary for survival and inadequate amounts of any of these major groups will affect physical and emotional health. Our nutritional balance of these substances allows the cells in the body to regenerate, thus sustaining life ..."

Higher nutrient intake is correlated with better mental health and may be considered in treatment of people with mood disorders. As has been described elsewhere in this volume, individuals who have limited resources or who are not eating enough will suffer not only physically but also mentally. In one study, Davison and Kaplan (2012) studied the impact of poor nutrition on overall psychiatric health. They assessed psychiatric health through the global assessment of function (GAF), in addition to scoring depression inventories in adults with mood disorders. They found that severity of nutritional deficiencies correlated with emotional health. The basic food groups: carbohydrates, fats, proteins, and minerals are all necessary for survival and inadequate amounts of any of these major groups will affect physical and emotional health. The nutritional balance of these substances allows the cells in the body to regenerate, thus sustaining life; secondly, what we eat is a major determinant in resistance to disease (Karren, Smith, Hafen, & Jenkins, 2010).

Patients suffering with health conditions seek help to decrease the emotional pain or the physical pain even as they realize that their illness is not curable. The meta-analysis by Grossman, Niemann, Schmidt, and Walach (2004) summarized the application of complementary therapies in patients who were suffering with chronic illness and found that patients benefited by experiencing a growing sense of self-efficacy, less personal suffering, and finding meaning in their suffering. The increased sense of internal control emerges from a greater ability to relax, feeling more energetic and experiencing more positive emotions (Hsu et al., 2010).

Specific Disorders Treated with CIM Therapies

Attention Deficit Hyperactivity Disorder (ADHD) Supplements, mind-body therapies, and physical activity have been tested in children with ADHD. Addition of omega-3-fatty acids to the diet produced only a modest improvement in symptoms but a statistically significant outcome (Bloch & Qawasmi, 2011). Polyunsaturated fatty acid administration also achieved statistical significance in improving pediatric ADHD. Another relevant symptom in children with ADHD is difficulty falling asleep, so in the same study melatonin was tested for its effect on sleep latency and found to be effective in reducing the time expended before falling asleep (Bloch & Mulqueen, 2014).

From the mind-body class, mindfulness has shown promise in modulating the symptoms of ADHD. Meditation training provided to adolescents and adults with ADHD was associated with improvement in the domains of processes related to attention and other symptoms of the disorder. Participants were better able to regulate emotional state, demonstrated less reactivity, were more attentive, and showed less excessive activity. The parts of the brain associated with these functions demonstrated changes that coincided with the behaviors observed (Baijal & Gupta, 2008).

A review of studies of neurofeedback treatment for pediatric ADHD yielded enough evidence of significant improvements in attention and decreases in hyperactivity that this intervention was considered "probably efficacious" in one study (Lofthouse, Arnold, Hersch, Hurt, & DeBeus, 2011) and "efficacious and specific" in a later review (Tan et al., 2016). Two studies that contributed to these ratings were conducted in 2nd and 4th grade school children within the school setting. Significant improvements using standardized assessment tools completed by parents and teachers were observed (Steiner, Frenette, Rene, Brennan, & Perrin, 2014a, 2014b). Steiner et al. (2014a, 2014b) confirmed that the benefits achieved by the children were sustained at 6 months follow-up. It is important to note that measurement of long-term effects of the CIM therapies is critical since patients often seek these therapies for chronic, not acute illnesses. Regarding ADHD, the effects of medication are well documented, but many parents become concerned about maintaining stimulant medication for months and years. In contrast, long-term training and use of neurofeedback carries very low risk and no side effects to our knowledge.

Aerobic exercise is usually considered a standard lifestyle recommendation. It is included here because of the documented effects of physical activity on symptoms of ADHD. A systematic review and meta-analysis was conducted using data from publications reporting the effects of 6–10 weeks of structured aerobic exercise program. Findings were summarized as a moderate to large effect on attention, hyperactivity, impulsivity, anxiety, and executive function. The same review also identified yoga as improving core symptoms of ADHD although the number of studies of yoga were much fewer than for exercise (Cerrillo-Urbina et al., 2015).

Anxiety The anxiety disorders, primarily generalized anxiety disorder (GAD), panic disorder, and phobias, are the most common psychiatric disorders. Burden of disease and functional impairment vary from mild to severe and incapacitating with reduced quality of life. Patients miss work, fail their classes, and interact poorly with others. Anxiety also has physical manifestations such as gastrointestinal discomfort, tightness in muscles, shortness of breath, and these experiences are uncomfortable and further increase anxiety. It is not unexpected that these patients would seek CIM therapies, in particular the mind-body therapies, herbs, and supplements. It must be recalled that anxiety is a chronic illness and short-term benefits, although providing some relief for patients, must be put into the context of a disorder usually beginning in childhood or adolescence and continuing into adulthood.

"Mindfulness has been recommended as a first line intervention for anxiety with very low risk and rare side effects, assuming that the patient is not severely compromised at the time of entry into treatment ..."

A review of herbal therapy and supplements used for anxiety showed that extracts of passion flower or kava and combinations of l-lysine and l-arginine were effective. The potential serious side effects associated with kava were recorded but the authors stated that at low doses, kava is safe (Lakhan & Vieira, 2010). However, NCCIH repeated the FDA warning for liver damage caused by kava and no longer supports the use this substance even at low doses. Sarris, McIntyre, and Camfield (2013) found that 13 herbs had some effect in reducing anxiety in adults. Chamomile extract resulted in modest anxiety reduction in those with mild to moderate anxiety (Amsterdam et al., 2009). A literature review was conducted on the effects of herbs in GAD and summarized the effects of herbals such as kava and passion flower as helpful short term, but not enough data is available on long-term benefits (Asher, Gerkin, & Gaynes, 2017).

Mindfulness has been recommended as a first line intervention for anxiety because of very low risk and rare side effects, assuming that the patient is not severely compromised at the time of entry into treatment (Asher et al., 2017). Goyal et al. (2014) performed a meta-analysis on the effects of mindfulness meditation. The level of evidence for decreased anxiety and depression with mindfulness was deemed to be moderate. No evidence was reported that meditation was better than other active treatments, such as drugs. However, if the effects are equivalent, patients may choose the non-chemical intervention and the one where they can take some responsibility for their own care. Meditation will usually have additional benefits such as increasing the sense of well-being; it can be continued for years with no side effects.

A 2016 review of three decades of outcome studies on the use of biofeedback for anxiety concluded that general biofeedback is efficacious for student anxiety, anxiety accompanying medical disorders, and anxiety disorders (Moss, 2016).

CIM therapies of the mind-body class can easily be combined with standard psychological therapy to increase its effectiveness. For example, hypnosis was shown to increase the positive effects of cognitive behavioral therapy for patients with anxiety. The patient is engaged in two active therapies and may have homework in CBT to document negative thoughts during a stressful event and counter them. In addition, the patient is reinforcing the suggestions obtained during hypnosis to relax and not over react to stressful situations (Vickers & Zollman, 1999). Yoga in combination with CBT was more effective at reducing panic than CBT alone. Yoga alone was associated with decreases in anxiety from severe to mild-moderate levels (Field, 2016).

A meta-analysis by Cuijpers et al. (2014) found that relaxation was equal to cognitive behavioral therapy in patients with generalized anxiety disorder in the short term, while CBT was superior in the longer term. This meta-analysis gathered data from 41 studies involving over one thousand patients. Even with these large numbers available for analysis, the authors admitted that the results are difficult to interpret. Relaxation is often a part of CBT and the "relaxation" studies sometimes included other components such as exposure and instructions to improve sleep. Another challenge in interpretation of the studies was that most of the trials used waiting list controls while others designed different types of active controls.

Depression In a review of the types of disorders for which patients most commonly seek the CIM therapies, major depression was the most common diagnosis (Freeman, Fava, et al., 2010). Some patients cannot tolerate standard treatment with the serotonin reuptake inhibitors (SSRI) because of weight gain and effects on sexuality, and accordingly seek a complementary therapy. Several interventions in various categories of CIM hold promise, including omega-3 fatty acid, St. John's Wort, folate, S-adenosyl L methionine from the herbs and supplements class, acupuncture from the traditional Chinese medicine class, light therapy from the phototherapy class, mindfulness from the mind-body category, and physical exercise.

Participation in trials of saffron (the stigma and petal parts of the plant) was offered to patients with mild to moderate depression. Saffron stigma produced decreased depressive mood in patients similar to that of Fluoxetine. Saffron petal showed a significant decrease in Hamilton Rating Scale for Depression scores (a standard assessment tool for depression) compared to placebo (Dwyer, Whitten, & Hawrelak, 2011). A review of clinical evidence supported the use of herbal substances formulated as medicines (phytomedicines) for depression. A high level of evidence was found for *Hypericum perforatum* (St. John's Wort) for depression and

Piper methysticum (passion flower) for anxiety disorders (Sarris, Panossian, Schweeitzer, Stough, & Scholey, 2011). However, it must be considered that side effects of *Piper methysticum* are common when it is used with other medications (birth control pills, warfarin, some HIV drugs, etc.) so the prescribing physician must be knowledgeable about potential dangers of medicine/herb interactions and be able to elicit information about herbal use from patients.

S-adenosyl methionine has shown efficacy in improving mood in individuals with a diagnosis of depression when compared to placebo, and it may be more beneficial in males than females. However, there is some conflicting research stating that S-adenosyl methionine is no more effective than placebo (Karas Kuželički, 2016). Sarris et al. (2016) reviewed the literature on the use of supplements as adjunctive treatments to standard antidepressant therapy in major depression, particularly omega-3, vitamin D methylfolate, and SAMe (S-adenosylmethionine). They concluded that these supplements could be used in combination with antidepressants for additional benefit. Augmentation may be necessary if medication produces only minimal effects, the depression is treatment resistant, and the patient declines ECT or side effects of medication are not tolerable. Nutraceuticals (standardized pharmaceutical grade nutrients) may enhance effects of antidepressants by affecting the same pathway or mechanism, or medicine-nutrient combinations may work through different pathways (Freeman, Mischoulon, et al., 2010; Wani, Bhat, & Ara, 2015). Two herbals have also been combined in efforts to reduce depressive symptoms in patients with major depression. St. John's Wort and passion flower in combination were reported to be synergistic in achieving improved mood in depressed patients (Fiebich, Knorle, Appel, & Weiss, 2010).

Sarris et al. (2011) reviewed the literature and concluded that St. John's Wort and kava have strong research support. However, there are concerns in combining medication and some herbal products because of safety issues. These authors reiterate the need for an integrative approach for treatment of mental health disorders.

Acupuncture for depression

"Acupuncture was provided to depressed pregnant women and the positive results highlighted the benefits of acupuncture in improving mood without the potential for negative effects on the developing fetus ..."

MacPherson et al. (2013) used the Patient Health Questionnaire (PHQ-9_ as an assessment tool and offered ten sessions of acupuncture or mental health counseling to patients who scored in the depressive range. They found that the PHQ-9 scores decreased at 3 months for both counseling and acupuncture and the benefits continued at 6 months for the acupuncture group. This study is titled as a "primary care study," but patients were referred to acupuncture by their primary care physicians; the service was not done in primary care. This observation raises the question of which patients are most likely to accept a referral. Patients who follow through on a referral may have different personality characteristics from patients who do not and therefore may be more likely to respond.

Acupuncture was provided to depressed pregnant women and the positive results highlighted the benefits of acupuncture in improving mood without the potential for negative effects on the developing fetus (Manber et al., 2010). Based on the Hamilton Rating Scale for Depression, the results for acupuncture were greater than nonspecific acupuncture (random placement of needles) and massage. Pregnant women suffering from depression cannot safely take many of the antidepressants without risk of harming the baby. Yet the untreated depression itself may impede the woman from taking care of herself, keeping appointments, maintaining nutrition or being physically active, all of which have potentially harmful effects on mother and fetus.

A common challenge in depression is insomnia or early awakening which results in depressed persons feeling fatigued during the day. Acupuncture improved sleep quality and shorted the time necessary to fall asleep when combined with standard treatment in depressed adults (Dong et al., 2017).

Other interventions for depression: Music therapy and yoga Music is often a mood enhancer in individuals of all ages, in healthy people, those who suffer with depression, and others with chronic medical illnesses (Codding & Hanser, 2007). There are only a small number of studies of music effects on clinical depression. Music is enjoyable, transports the patient into another world, free of pain and worry, and mood improves possibly due to a direct effect or resulting from the relaxing effect of soothing, calming music, or perhaps because the patient is resting comfortably at the time of listening to music (Maratos, Gold, Wang, & Crawford, 2008). The practice of yoga, particularly the breathing components, was found to reduce depression scores and the improvement was consistent at the 1-year follow-up (Field, 2016).

Most psychiatrists would agree that the benefits and risks of medical management in patients with depression, particularly those patients with other medical conditions or during pregnancy must be carefully weighed. Decisions about medication and supplementation with CIM therapies must be made with full understanding on the part of the patient. Education of pregnant women is critical with specification of risks in a manner that is not frightening, but allows for a intentional decision.

Physical Disorders

Just as patients with mental disorders frequently seek CIM, patients suffering from chronic physical problems (particularly pain) are among the most likely to seek CIM treatment in addition to medication. Widespread benefits from Reiki were reported by McManus (2017) in patients with a broad range of chronic physical illnesses. Reiki was more effective than progressive relaxation, placebo, sham Reiki, and rest. Pain decreased in addition to reduced depressive and anxious symptoms. There was a shift to internal locus of control (patients feeling more powerful in making decisions and action) and an increase in self-esteem.

Chronic Pain: Headache

Mind-body therapies Several reviews and meta-analyses are available on the topic of CIM interventions for chronic headache. A recent summary review of the literature describing the effects of several CIM therapies for primary migraine and tension headache found the overall quality of the evidence to be low to moderate. Nonetheless, five CIM therapies were found to have a positive effect on reducing pain: acupuncture, massage, yoga, biofeedback, and meditation (Millstine, 2017). Combining CBT, relaxation, and biofeedback with pharmacotherapy was reported to reduce the frequency of days of headache as measured by self-report and better quality of life, compared to either behavioral or pharmacotherapy alone (Sullivan, Cousins, & Ridsdale, 2016). Although the primary outcome measure was headache, subjects also reported decreased anxiety and improved mood.

> "Relaxation training decreased pain in college students with chronic pain and the students also reported being better able to manage the pain when it occurred …"

In another study, active self-care and complementary medicine interventions including self-hypnosis and autogenic training were designed to enhance coping skills and lessen pain in patients with chronic migraine and tension headaches. Relaxation training decreased pain in college students with chronic pain and the students also reported being better able to manage the pain when it occurred. The intervention was intensive and required subjects to practice the relaxation skills every day and maintain records of medication use, pain, and relaxation practice (Lee, Crawford, Teo, & Spevak, 2014).

Acupuncture for headache Crawford and Kim (2016) compared acupuncture with routine care for patients with frequent tension-type headaches. The same endpoint of pain reduction was achieved in both acupuncture and routine care, but more patients reduced frequency by 50% as a result of acupuncture than with routine care. Linde et al. (2005) reported on the effects of 12 sessions of acupuncture over 8 weeks. Based on headache diaries, the number of days that patients suffered with headache decreased more after acupuncture than in wait list controls. However, there were no differences in outcome between patients in the actual and sham acupuncture groups. This and similar studies have raised the question of the placebo effect in acupuncture. Information about the correct positioning of the acupuncture needles is not as easily found on the internet, compared to the type of biofeedback recommended for specific illness, for example; however, beliefs about efficacy and trust in the practitioner may influence perceived benefit of the CIM therapies similarly to the placebo effect of medication.

Massage for headache Massage therapy was found more effective than no treatment in relieving the intensity, duration, and frequency of tension-type headache pain (Wahbeh, Elsas, & Oken, 2008). In another study, massage did not result in a change in average intensity of migraine headache, but participants reported significant decreases in migraine frequency (Chaibi, Tuchin, & Russell, 2011).

Other interventions for headache include butterbur and Tai Chi (National Center for Complementary and Alternative Medicine, 2012). Butterbur extract (Petadolex) was associated with improvement in frequency and intensity of pain in sufferers of migraine. A 15-week program in Tai Chi was compared to an equal time control group in patients with tension-type headache and resulted in improvement in frequency of these headaches.

Chronic Pain: Low Back Pain

Yoga An extensive review of the body of research on yoga and low back pain summarized the quality of evidence supporting yoga for therapy of low back pain and found it to be moderate (Chou et al., 2017). Lyengar yoga, which is more physical than yoga primarily focused on breathing, was compared to physical exercise. Both groups improved but the Lyengar yoga was associated with greater reduction in pain and an increase in flexibility (Field, 2016). In a randomized controlled trial of yoga, physical therapy, and education, the detailed protocol was published first (Saper et al., 2014). The outcome study then reported similar benefits at 52 weeks in comparison to patients in the education control group. The active group patients reduced pain and improved function and in addition lowered their use of pain medication (Saper et al., 2017). This study, funded by NCCIH, specifically recruited participants of lower socioeconomic status and enrolled a racially diverse group of patients. The degree of improvement was correlated with the number of sessions of either yoga or physical therapy that the group members attended. Based on that finding, it is important to consider which therapy will be easier or harder to maintain once patients complete the study. Yoga, once learned, can be practiced by patients in their own homes, alone or with others, does not require equipment, and has no corresponding transportation costs.

Other Interventions for low back pain Mindfulness from the mind-body class of therapies and acupuncture from traditional Chinese medicine were evaluated as having moderate strength of evidence and low to moderate benefit, respectively (Chou et al., 2017). Guidelines from the Center for Complementary Medicine and from the American Pain Society rated massage, relaxation, and acupuncture as valid therapies for low back pain (Chou et al., 2009; National Center for Complementary and Alternative Medicine, 2010a). The level of evidence for CBT or progressive relaxation was stated as "fair" for relaxation while the benefit was "substantial." Further, the evidence for acupuncture was stated as "fair" and the observed benefit was "moderate." Low back pain is common, creates disability and a high burden of disease. Medical management often produces less than optimal benefits and puts the person at risk for addiction to narcotics. Complementary interventions have an important role to play in overall management of back pain. The actual pain may not be the major factor responsible for the disability so pain relief should not be the only variable measured in outcome studies. Secondary outcomes, such as positive mood, greater sense of wellness, or improvement in other physical conditions unrelated to back pain but contributing to non-functionality, should also be considered (Hsu et al., 2010).

Other Pain Conditions: Fibromyalgia and Osteoarthritis of the Knee

Fibromyalgia is a musculoskeletal disorder characterized not only by pain but also by negative mood state, often with comorbid depression and mental confusion. Acupuncture was associated with a clinically significant improvement in symptoms of fibromyalgia in comparison to controls. The main outcome measure was the Fibromyalgia Impact Questionnaire (Martin-Sanchez, Torralba, Díaz-Domínguez, Barriga, & Martin, 2009). An 8-week regimen of 16 sessions of 17-point acupuncture was associated with improved mood in patients with fibromyalgia and the benefit was sustained at follow-up at 1 and 2 months after the end of active therapy (Singh et al., 2006).

An Ayurvedic compound, alfapin, was tested in a double blind randomized placebo controlled trial in patients with osteoarthritis of the knee. Aflapin is a compound derived from *Boswellia serrata* gum resin and is reported to be fast acting. Significant reductions in pain scores and improved physical functioning were reported in patients given aflapin compared to controls (Vishal et al., 2011).

Cardiovascular Problems

Essential hypertension Resperate is an FDA-approved device that assists individuals to pace their breathing. It is easy to learn and can be used at home. Regular practice of paced, slow breathing has been shown to decrease both systolic and diastolic blood pressure. The most appropriate candidates for this intervention are patients with mild hypertension or high blood pressure uncomplicated by diabetes or heart disease (Cernes & Zimlichman, 2017). Other forms of biofeedback, including heart rate variability, thermal, and sEMG (muscle biofeedback) combined with relaxation have been used in patients with essential hypertension. Decreases in both systolic and diastolic blood pressure have been documented (Tan et al., 2016).

"The combination of qigong and blood pressure medication produced the maximum benefit compared to medication alone or Qigong alone ..."

There have been multiple trials of transcendental meditation (TN) in patients with essential hypertension. A study of TM in African-American men and women produced positive results in clinically and statistically significant decreases in blood pressure (Schneider,

Alexander, Staggers, Orme-Johnson, et al., 2005; Schneider, Alexander, Staggers, Rainforth, et al., 2005). Another trial in individuals over the age of 55 years produced similar benefits to participants (Schneider et al., 2012).

Qigong was compared to exercise, no intervention, and antihypertensive drugs in an extensive review using 20 trials containing over 2000 patients. Qigong was superior to no treatment, better than exercise in decreasing systolic blood pressure only and more effective in lowering diastolic blood pressure than some antihypertensives. The combination of qigong and blood pressure medication produced the maximum benefit compared to medication alone or Qigong alone (Xiong, Wang, Li, & Zhang, 2015).

"Nutrition and diet are well known to contribute to the health of the cardiovascular system. Lower mortality was found in those individuals who kept to a diet of low saturated fats, high intake of fruits, vegetables, whole grains legumes, and nuts ..."

Coronary heart disease Alexander et al. (2012) designed a two-part study in African-American men and women patients who had at least one coronary artery with more than 50% stenosis. First, subjects were randomized to either TM or to health education and completed either program. Then patients were followed for an average of 5 years. The TM group sustained a significant risk reduction of 48% in mortality, non-fatal heart attack and non-fatal stroke. The authors postulated that decreased blood pressure and, from the psychological domain, less anger expression may be elements in the pathways responsible for the effects of TM in this study. Similarly to other studies, adherence to regular practice of TM was necessary to obtain maximum benefits.

Nutrition and diet are well known to contribute to the health of the cardiovascular system. Lower mortality was found in those individuals who kept to a diet of low saturated fats, high intake of fruits, vegetables, whole grains legumes, and nuts (Freeman et al., 2016).

Sleep Disorders

Insomnia Black, O'Reilly, Olmstead, Breen, and Irwin (2015) reported on the effects of a 6-weeks trial of mindfulness meditation compared to sleep hygiene recommendations. The Pittsburgh Sleep Quality Index was used to track progress. Participants practiced mindfulness for 2 hours per week while the sleep hygiene group had the same number of contact hours but consisting of education instead of mindfulness. Significantly greater improvements were noted the mindfulness awareness group, compared to the sleep hygiene group, in sleep quality, and daytime functioning. The mindfulness awareness group also showed significantly greater secondary benefits including decreases in fatigue severity and decreases in interference in functioning caused by fatigue and depressive symptoms.

The relaxation therapies, particularly progressive relaxation, were recommended as "standard treatment" by the American Academy of Sleep Medicine which means that there was a high-level evidence to support the use of relaxation in treatment of insomnia (Morgenthaler et al., 2006). The results of a national survey of relaxation and other complementary therapies in insomnia led Bertisch, Wells, Smith, and McCarthy (2012) to recommend wider use. Compared to the potential for abuse of medications used to treat insomnia and the risk of side effects, relaxation, once learned, has no side effects and can be continued throughout the person's life span.

The use of melatonin in treatment of insomnia has been controversial with variable results reported in controlled studies. The results of the meta-analysis carried out by Van Geijlswijk, Korzilius, and Smits (2010) were summarized as follows: Melatonin is effective as a phase re-setter in delayed sleep phase disorder (individuals have difficulty falling asleep and waking up in the morning) and in insomnia due to circadian rhythm disorders. Melatonin shortened the time required to fall asleep and decreased daytime sleepiness.

Summary

"Healthy adults will seek massage, mindfulness, and herbal products to enhance well-being and sometimes as preventatives. In addition, those who are ill will search diligently for alternative forms of help in managing symptoms when cures are not available."

The evaluation of the effectiveness of the CIM therapies presents challenges to the researcher, the educator, and the clinician. Healthy adults will seek massage, mindfulness, and herbal products to enhance well-being and sometimes as preventatives. In addition, those who are ill will search diligently for alternative forms of help in managing symptoms when cures are not available. A sense of control, mutual decision-making with the provider, and a desire for holistic health will continue to motivate patients. Keeping current with research in order to answer patients' questions is time consuming and frustrating for health care providers who are bombarded with information from pharmaceutical representatives, yet receive little education about the myriad of complementary interventions.

Understanding the literature on herbal medicine is perhaps the most difficult because different parts of the plant are used in clinical trials, and plants grown in the United States may be different than those plants grown in other parts of the world. The FDA regulates supplements and herbs, but the guidelines are much less strict than those for medications (NIH 2014). The contribution of placebo effects is considered to be a negative in research as it confounds analysis. However, as pointed out by Thibault and Raz (2017) the placebo effect can contribute in a positive way to effectiveness; clinical practice should not seek to eliminate it.

CIM therapies are often tested in combination, since multi-modal treatment is cost- and time-effective, so research conducted in the clinical (real) setting cannot be used to determine specific effects of each component of the package. In some studies of anxiety disorders, for example, some patients may also have a physical condition which affects the anxiety and therefore the response to treatment. Characteristics of generalized anxiety disorder are quite different from panic disorder although both are listed in the anxiety disorder category. Recommending mindfulness or biofeedback to patients with either GAD or panic requires understanding of the difference between the two categories and offering instructions specific to each disorder. The field of neuroscience is beginning to contribute to our understanding of some of the CIM therapies, but progress is slow, research is costly, and results often equivocal. Hopefully, integrative medicine centers and academic health centers will collaborate to empower research to answer basic questions and create the future of complementary medicine.

References

Achterberg, J. (1985). *Imagery in healing: Shamanism and modern medicine*. Boston, MA: Shambhala.

Achterberg, J., & Lawlis, G. F. (1980). *Bridges of the bodymind: Behavioral approaches to health care*. Champaign, IL: Institute for Personality and Ability Testing.

Albrecht, G. L., Fitzpatrick, R., & Scrimshaw, S. C. (2000). *The handbook of social studies in health and medicine*. Thousand Oaks, CA: Sage.

Alexander, C. N., Grim, C. E., Gaylord-King, C., Kotchen, T., Kotchen, J. M., Nidich, S., et al. (2012). Stress reduction in the secondary prevention of cardiovascular disease: Randomized, controlled trial of transcendental meditation and health education in Blacks. *Circulation. Cardiovascular Quality and Outcomes, 5*(6), 750–758.

American Psychological Association (APA). *Division 30, Society of Psychological Hypnosis*. Retrieved from http://www.apadivisions.org/division-30/about/index.aspx

Amsterdam, J. D., Li, Y., Soeller, I., Rockwell, K., Mao, J. J., & Shults, J. (2009). A randomized, double-blind, placebo-controlled trial of oral Matricaria recutita(chamomile) extract therapy for generalized anxiety disorder. *Journal of Clinical Psychopharmacology, 29*(4), 378–382. https://doi.org/10.1097/JCP.0b013e3181ac935c. PubMed PMID: 19593179; PubMed Central PMCID: PMC3600416.

Asher, G. N., Gerkin, J., & Gaynes, B. N. (2017). Complementary therapies for mental health disorders. *Medical Clinics of North America, 101*(5), 847–864. https://doi.org/10.1016/j.mcna.2017.04.004. Epub 2017 Jun 20. Review. PubMed PMID: 28802467.

Baer, H. (1992). The potential rejuvenation of American naturopathy as a consequence of the holistic health movement. *Medical Anthropology, 8*, 151–168.

Baer, H. (2003). Mindfulness training as a clinical intervention: A conceptual and empirical review. *Clinical Psychology: Science and Practice, 10*(2), 125–143.

Baijal, S., & Gupta, R. (2008). Medication-based training: A possible intervention for attention deficit hyperactivity disorder. *Psychiatry, 5*(4), 48–55.

Benson, H. (1975). *The relaxation response*. New York: William Morrow.

Bertisch, S. M., Wells, R. E., Smith, M. T., & McCarthy, E. P. (2012). Use of relaxation techniques and complementary and alternative medicine by American adults with insomnia symptoms: Results from a national survey. *Journal of Clinical Sleep Medicine, 8*(6), 681–691. https://doi.org/10.5664/jcsm.2264. PubMed PMID: 23243402; PubMed Central PMCID: PMC3501665.

Black, D. S., O'Reilly, G. A., Olmstead, R., Breen, E. C., & Irwin, M. R. (2015). Mindfulness meditation and improvement in sleep quality and daytime impairment among older adults with sleep disturbances: A randomized clinical trial. *JAMA Internal Medicine, 175*(4), 494–501. https://doi.org/10.1001/jamainternmed.2014.8081

Bloch, M. H., & Mulqueen, J. (2014). Nutritional supplements for the treatment of attention-deficit hyperactivity disorder. *Child and Adolescent Psychiatric Clinics of North America, 23*(4), 883–897. https://doi.org/10.1016/j.chc.2014.05.002

Bloch, M. H., & Qawasmi, A. (2011). Omega-3 fatty acid supplementation for the treatment of children with attention-deficit/hyperactivity disorder symptomatology: Systematic review and meta-analysis. *Journal of the American Academy of Child and Adolescent Psychiatry, 50*(10), 991–1000. https://doi.org/10.1016/j.jaac.2011.06.008

Braid, J. (1843). *Neurypnology or the rationale of nervous sleep considered in relation with animal magnetism illustrated by numerous cases of its successful application in the relief and cure of disease.* London: John Churchill.

Cernes, R., & Zimlichman, R. (2017). Role of paced breathing for treatment of hypertension. *Current Hypertension Reports, 19*, 45. https://doi.org/10.1007/s11906-017-0742-1

Cerrillo-Urbina, A. J., García-Hermoso, A., Sánchez-López, M., Pardo-Guijarro, M. J., Santos Gómez, J. L., & Martínez-Vizcaíno, V. (2015). The effects of physical exercise in children with attention deficit hyperactivity disorder: A systematic review and meta-analysis of randomized control trials. *Child: Care, Health and Development, 41*(6), 779–788. https://doi.org/10.1111/cch.12255. Epub 2015 May 18. Review. PubMed PMID: 25988743.

Chaibi, A., Tuchin, P. J., & Russell, M. B. (2011). Manual therapies for migraine: A systematic review. *Journal of Headache and Pain, 12*(2), 127–133.

Chen, J., Huang, J., Li, J. V., Lv, Y., He, Y., & Zheng, Q. (2017). The characteristics of TCM clinical trials: A systematic review of ClinicalTrials.gov. *Evidence-based Complementary and Alternative Medicine: eCAM, 2017*, 9461415. https://doi.org/10.1155/2017/9461415

Chernyak, G. V., & Sessler, D. L. (2005). Perioperative acupuncture and related techniques. *Anesthesiology, 102*, 1031–1049.

Chopra, A., & Doiphode, V. V. (2002). Ayurvedic medicine. Core concept, therapeutic principles, and current relevance. *Medical Clinics of North America, 86*(1), 75–89, vii. Review. PubMed PMID: 11795092.

Chou, R., Deyo, R., Friedly, J., Skelly, A., Hashimoto, R., Weimer, M., et al. (2017). Nonpharmacologic therapies for low back pain: A systematic review for an American College of Physicians Clinical Practice Guideline. *Annals of Internal Medicine, 166*, 493–505. https://doi.org/10.7326/M16-2459

Chou, R., Qaseem, A., Snow, V., Casey, D., Cross, J. T., Jr., Shekelle, P., et al. (2009). Diagnosis and treatment of low back pain: A joint clinical practice guideline from the American College of Physicians and the American Pain Society. *Annals of Internal Medicine, 147*(7), 479–491.

Clarke, T. C., Black, L. I., Strussman, B., Barnes, P. M., Nahin, R. L. (2015). Trends in the use of complementary health approaches among adults: United States, 2002-2012. *National Health Statistics Reports, (79)*, 1–16.

Codding, P., & Hanser, S. (2007). Music therapy. In: Complementary and alternative treatments in mental health care. In M. I. Weintraub, R. Mamtani, & M. S. Micozzi (Eds.), *Complementary and integrative medicine in pain management* (pp. 41–68). New York: Springer.

Crawford, P., & Kim, M. (2016). Acupuncture for frequent tension-type headaches. *American Family Physicians, 94*(3), 208–209B.

Cuijpers, P., Sijbrandij, M., Koole, S., Huibers, M., Berking, M., & Andersson, G. (2014). Psychological treatment of generalized anxiety disorder: A meta-analysis. *Clinical Psychology Review, 34*(2), 130–140. https://doi.org/10.1016/j.cpr.2014.01.002

Cummings, N., & Cummings, J. (2000). *The essence of psychotherapy: Reinventing the art in the age of data.* San Diego, CA: Academic Press.

Davison, K. M., & Kaplan, B. J. (2012). Nutrient intakes are correlated with overall psychiatric functioning in adults with mood disorders. *Canadian Journal of Psychiatry, 57*(2), 85–92.

Demarzo, M. M., Montero-Marin, J., Cuijpers, P., Zabaleta-del-Olmo, E., Mahtani, K. R., Vellinga, A., et al. (2015). The efficacy of mindfulness-based interventions in primary care: A meta-analytic review. *Annals of Family Medicine, 13*, 573–582. https://doi.org/10.1370/afm.1863

Dong, B., Chen, Z., Yin, X., Li, D., Ma, J., Yin, P., et al. (2017). The efficacy of acupuncture for treating depression-related insomnia compared with a control group: A systematic review and Meta-analysis. *BioMed Research International, 2017*, Article ID 9614810, 11 pages, 2017. https://doi.org/10.1155/2017/9614810.

Dwyer, A. V., Whitten, D. L., & Hawrelak, J. A. (2011). Herbal medicines, other than St. John's Wort, in the treatment of depression: A systematic review. *Alternative Medicine Review, 16*(1), 40–49.

Eisenberg, D. M., Davis, R. B., Ettner, S. L., Appel, S., Wilkey, S., Van Rompay, M., et al. (1998). Trends in alternative medicine use in the United States, 1990-1997: Results of a follow-up national survey. *Journal of the American Medical Association, 280*(18), 1569–1575.

Eisenberg, D. M., Kessler, R. C., Foster, C., Norlock, F. E., Calkins, D. R., & Delbanco, T. L. (1993). Unconventional medicine in the United States. Prevalence, costs, and patterns of use. *New England Journal of Medicine, 328*(4), 246–252.

Elkins, G. (Ed.). (2016). Handbook of medical and psychological hypnosis: Foundations, applications, and professional issues. New York, NY: Springer.

Engel, G. L. (1977). The need for a new medical model. *Science, 196*, 129–136.

Fagundes, C. P., Glaser, R., & Kiecolt-Glaser, J. K. (2013). Stressful early life experiences and immune dysregulation across the lifespan. *Brain, Behavior, and Immunity, 27*(1), 8–12.

Fiebich, B. L., Knorle, R., Appel, K., & Weiss, G. (2010). Pharmacological studies in an herbal drug combination of St. John's Wort (Hypericum perforatum) and passion flower (Passiflora incarnate): In vitro and in vivo evidence of synergy between Hypericum and Passiflora in anti-depressant pharmacological models. *Fitoterapia, 82*(3), 474–480. https://doi.org/10.1016/j.fitote.2010.12.006

Field, T. (2016). Yoga research review. *Complementary Therapy Clinical Practice, 24*, 145–161.

Fraser, F., Matsuzawa, Y., Lee, Y. S. C., & Minen, M. (2017). Behavioral treatments for post-traumatic headache. *Curr Pain Headache Rep, 21*(5), 22. https://doi.org/10.1007/s11916-017-0624-x. Review. PubMed PMID: 28283812.

Frawley, D., & Ranade, S. (2001). *Ayurveda, nature's medicine*. Twin Lakes, WI: Lotus Press.

Freeman, M., Fava, M., Lake, J., Trivedi, M., Wisner, K., & Mischoulon, D. (2010). Complementary and alternative medicine in major depressive disorder: The American Psychiatric Association task force report. *The Journal of Clinical Psychiatry, 71*(6), 669–681.

Freeman, M. P., Mischoulon, D., Tedeschini, E., Goodness, T., Cohen, L. S., Fava, M., et al. (2010). Complementary and alternative medicine for major depressive disorder: A meta-analysis of patient characteristics, placebo-response rates, and treatment outcomes relative to standard antidepressants. *The Journal of Clinical Psychiatry, 71*(6), 682–688.

Freeman, A. M., Morris, P., Barnard, N., Esselstyn, C. B., Ros, E., Agatston, A., et al. (2016). Trending cardiovascular nutrition controversies. *Journal of the American College of Cardiology, 69*(9), 1172–1187. https://doi.org/10.1016/j.jacc.2016.10.086

Goyal, M., Singh, S., Sibinga, E. M. S., Gould, N. F., Rowland-Seymour, A., Sharma, R., et al. (2014). Meditation programs for psychological stress and well-being: A systematic review and meta-analysis. *JAMA Internal Medicine, 174*(3), 357–368. https://doi.org/10.1001/jamainternmed.2013.13018

Green, E., Green, A., & Walters, D. (1970). Voluntary control of internal states: Psychological and physiological. *Journal of Transpersonal Psychology, 2*, 1–26.

Grossman, P., Niemann, L., Schmidt, S., & Walach, H. (2004). Mindfulness-based stress reduction and health benefits. A meta-analysis. *Journal of Psychosomatic Research, 57*(1), 35–43.

Halpern, M. (2011). *Healing your life: Lessons on the path of Ayurveda*. Twin Lakes, WI: Lotus Press.

Harris, P. E., Cooper, K. L., Relton, C., & Thomas, K. J. (2012). Prevalence of complementary and alternative medicine (CAM) use by the general population: A systematic review and update. *International Journal of Clinical Practice, 66*(10), 924–939. https://doi.org/10.1111/j.1742-1241.2012.02945.x

Hsu, C., Bluespruce, J., Sherman, K., & Cherkin, D. (2010). Unanticipated benefits of CAM therapies for back pain: An exploration of patient experiences. *Journal of Alternative and Complementary Medicine, 16*(2), 157–163. https://doi.org/10.1089/acm.2009.0188

Institute of Medicine. (2001). *Crossing the quality chasm: A new health care system for the 21st century*. Washington, DC: National Academy of Sciences.

Kabat-Zinn, J. (1990). *Full catastrophe living: Using the wisdom of your body and mind to face stress, pain, and illness*. New York: Delta.

Karas Kuželički, N. (2016). S-Adenosyl methionine in the therapy of depression and other psychiatric disorders. *Drug Development Research, 77*, 346–356. https://doi.org/10.1002/ddr.21345

Karren, K. J., Smith, N. L., Hafen, B. Q., & Jenkins, K. J. (2010). *Mind/body health. The effect of attitudes, emotions and relationships*. New York: Benjamin Cummings.

Khalsa, S. B. (2004). Meditation: Elevating consciousness, improving health. *Biofeedback, 32*(3), 9–10.

Kiecolt-Glaser, J. K., Derry, H. M., & Fagundes, C. P. (2015). Inflammation: Depression fans the flames and feats on the heat. *American Journal of Psychiatry, 172*(11), 1075–1091.

Koenig, H. (2000). Religion, spirituality, and medicine: Application to clinical practice. *Journal of the American Medical Association, 284*(13), 1708. https://doi.org/10.1001/jama.284.13.1708-JMS1004-5-1

Lakhan, S. E., & Vieira, K. F. (2010). Nutritional and herbal supplements for anxiety and anxiety-related disorders: Systematic review. *Nutrition Journal, 9*, 42. https://doi.org/10.1186/1475-2891-9-42

Lee, C., Crawford, C., Teo, L., & Spevak, C. (2014). An analysis of the various chronic pain conditions captured in a systematic review of active self-care complementary and integrative medicine therapies for the management of chronic pain symptoms. *Pain Medicine, 15*(S1), S96–S103. https://doi.org/10.1111/pme.12357

Linde, K., Streng, A., Jurgens, S., Hoppw, A., Brinkhaus, B., Witt, C., et al. (2005). Acupuncture for patients with migraine: A randomized controlled trial. *Journal of the American Medical Association, 293*(17), 2118–2125.

Lofthouse, N., Arnold, E., Hersch, S., Hurt, E., & DeBeus, R. (2011). A review of neurofeedback treatment for pediatric ADHD. *Journal of Attention Disorders, 16*(5), 351–372. https://doi.org/10.1177/1087054711427530

MacPherson, H., Richmond, S., Bland, M., Brealey, S., Gabe, R., Hopton, A., et al. (2013). Acupuncture and counselling for depression in primary care: A randomised controlled trial. *PLoS Medicine, 10*(9), e1001518. https://doi.org/10.1371/journal.pmed.1001518

Manber, R., Schnyer, R., Lyell, D., Chambers, A., Caughey, A., Druzin, M., et al. (2010). Acupuncture for depression during pregnancy: A randomized controlled trial. *Obstetrics and Gynecology, 115*(3), 511–520.

Maratos, A., Gold, C., Wang, X., & Crawford, M. (2008). Music therapy for depression. *Cochrane Database of Systematic Reviews*, (1). Art. No.: CD004517. https://doi.org/10.1002/14651858.CD004517.pub2.

Martin-Sanchez, E., Torralba, E., Díaz-Domínguez, E., Barriga, A., & Martin, J. L. R. (2009). Efficacy of acupuncture for the treatment of fibromyalgia: Systematic review and Meta-analysis of randomized trials. *The Open Rheumatology Journal, 3*, 25–29. https://doi.org/10.2174/1874312900903010025

McGee, M. (2008). Meditation and psychiatry. *Psychiatry (Edgmont), 5*(1), 28–41.

McManus, D. E. (2017). Reiki is better than placebo and has broad potential as a complementary health therapy. *Journal of Evidence-Based Complementary & Alternative Medicine, 22*, 1051–1057. https://doi.org/10.1177/2156587217728644

Millstine, D. (2017). Complementary and integrative medicine in the management of headache. *British Medical Journal, 357*, 1805.

Mishra, L., Singh, B. B., & Dagenais, S. (2001). Healthcare and disease management in Ayurveda. *Alternative Therapies, 7*(2), 44–49.

Morgenthaler, T., Kramer, M., Alessi, C., Friedman, L., Boehlecke, B., Brown, T., et al. (2006). Practice parameters for the psychological and behavioral treatment of insomnia: An update. An American academy of sleep medicine report. *Sleep, 29*(11), 1415–1419. PubMed PMID: 17162987.

Moss, D. (2016). Anxiety and anxiety disorders. In G. Tan, F. Shaffer, R. Lyle, & I. Teo (Eds.), *Evidence-based treatment in biofeedback and neurofeedback* (3rd ed., pp. 27–31). Wheat Ridge, CO: Association for Applied Psychophysiology and Biofeedback.

Moss, D., & Shaffer, F. (2016). Foreword: Evidence-based practice in biofeedback and neurofeedback. In G. Tan, F. Shaffer, R. Lyle, & I. Teo (Eds.), *Evidence-based practice in biofeedback and neurofeedback* (3rd ed.). Wheat Ridge, CO: Association for Applied Psychophysiology and Biofeedback.

National Center for Complementary and Alternative Medicine. (2010a). Acupuncture and pain: Applying modern science to an ancient practice. *Complementary and Alternative Medicine, 2010*, 1–6.

National Center for Complementary and Alternative Medicine. (2012). *Headaches and complementary health approaches* (NCCIH Pub No.: D462).

National Center for Complementary and Integrative Health. (2014). *Using dietary supplements wisely, National Center for Complementary and Integrative Health* (NCCIH Pub No.: D426).

National Library of Medicine. (2003). *Complementary and alternative medicine*. Website of the National Library of Medicine, National Institutes of Health. Retrieved from https://www.nlm.nih.gov/tsd/acquisitions/cdm/subjects24.html

Ninivaggi, F. (2010). *Ayurveda: A comprehensive guide to traditional Indian medicine for the West*. Westport, CT: Praeger.

Ralph, S. S., & Taylor, C. M. (2013). *Sparks and Taylor's nursing reference diagnostic manual* (9th ed.). Philadelphia, PA: Lippincott, Williams, and Williams.

Reston, J. (1971, July 26). Now, about my operation in Beijing. *New York Times*.

Rossman, M. (2000). *Guided imagery for self-healing*. Novato, CA: New World Library.

Saper, R. B., Lemaster, C., Delitto, A., Sherman, K. J., Herman, P. M., Sadikova, E., et al. (2017). Yoga, physical therapy, or education for chronic low back pain: A randomized controlled non-inferiority trial. *Annals of Internal Medicine, 167*(2), 85–94.

Saper, R. B., Sherman, K. J., Delitto, A., Herman, P. M., Stevans, J., Paris, R., et al. (2014). Yoga vs. physical therapy vs. education for chronic low back pain in predominantly minority populations: Study protocol for a randomized controlled trial. *Trials, 15*, 67. https://doi.org/10.1186/1745-6215-15-67

Sarris, J., McIntyre, E., & Camfield, D. A. (2013). Plant-based medicines for anxiety disorders part 2: A review of clinical studies with supporting preclinical evidence. *CNS Drugs, 27*(4), 301–319. https://doi.org/10.1007/s40263-013-0059-9

Sarris, J., Murphy, J., Mischoulon, D., Papakostas, G., Fava, M., Berk, M., et al. (2016). Adjunctive nutraceuticals for depression: A systematic review and meta-analyses. *American Journal of Psychiatry, 173*(6), 575–587. https://doi.org/10.1176/appi.sjp.2016.15091228

Sarris, J., Panossian, A., Schweeitzer, I., Stough, C., & Scholey, A. (2011). Herbal medicine for depression, anxiety and insomnia: A review of psychopharmacology and clinical evidence. *European Neuropsycopharmacology, 21*(12), 841–860. https://doi.org/10.1016/j.euroneuro.2011.04.002

Schneider, R. H., Alexander, C. N., Staggers, F., Orme-Johnson, D. W., Rainforth, M., Salerno, J. W., et al. (2005). A randomized controlled trial of stress reduction in African Americans treated for hypertension for over one year. *American Journal of Hypertension, 18*(1), 88–98. https://doi.org/10.1016/j.amjhyper.2004.08.027

Schneider, R. H., Alexander, C. N., Staggers, F., Rainforth, M., Salerno, J. W., Hartz, A., et al. (2005). Long-term effects of stress reduction on mortality in persons ≥55 years of age with systemic hypertension. *The American Journal of Cardiology, 95*(9), 1060–1064. https://doi. org/10.1016/j.amjcard.2004.12.058

Schneider, R. H., Grim, C. E., Rainforth, M. V., Kotchen, T., Nidich, S. I., Gaylord-King, C., et al. (2012). Stress reduction in the secondary prevention of cardiovascular disease: Randomized, controlled trial of transcendental meditation and health education in blacks. *Circulation Cardiovascular Quality and Outcomes, 5*, 750–758. https://doi.org/10.1161/ CIRCOUTCOMES.112.967406

Shaffer, F., & Moss, D. (2006). Biofeedback. In C.-S. Yuan, E. J. Bieber, & B. A. Bauer (Eds.), *Textbook of complementary and alternative medicine* (2nd ed., pp. 291–312). Abingdon, UK: Informa Healthcare.

Sharma, H., & Clark, C. (2012). *Ayurvedic healing: Contemporary maharishi Ayurveda medicine and science*. London: Singing Dragon.

Simonton, O. C., Matthews-Simonton, S., & Creighton, J. (1978). *Getting well again*. Los Angeles, CA: J. P. Tarcher.

Singh, B. B., Wu, W., Hwang, S. H., Khorsan, R., Der-Martirosian, C., Vinjamury, S. P., et al. (2006). Effectiveness of acupuncture in the treatment of fibromyalgia. *Alternative Therapies in Health and Medicine, 12*(2), 34–41.

Starfield, B. (2011). Is patient-centered care the same as person-centered care? *The Permanente Journal, 15*(2), 63–69.

Steiner, N., Frenette, E., Rene, K., Brennan, R., & Perrin, E. (2014a). In-school neurofeedback training for ADHD: Sustained improvements from a randomized control trial. *Pediatrics Official Journal of the American Academy of Pediatrics, 33*(3), 483–492. https://doi. org/10.1542/peds.2013-2059

Steiner, N. J., Frenette, E. C., Rene, K. M., Brennan, R. T., & Perrin, E. C. (2014b). Neurofeedback and cognitive attention training for children with attention-deficit hyperactivity disorder in schools. *Journal of Developmental and Behavioral Pediatrics, 35*(1), 18–27. https://doi. org/10.1097/DBP.0000000000000009. PubMed PMID: 24399101.

Sullivan, A., Cousins, S., & Ridsdale, L. (2016). Psychological interventions for migraine: A systematic review. *Journal of Neurology, 263*(12), 2369–2377. https://doi.org/10.1007/ s00415-016-8126-z

Suzuki, D. T. (1956). *Zen Buddhism: Selected writings of D.T. Suzuki* (W. Barrett, Ed.). New York: Doubleday.

Talesnik, D. (2016, April 8). NIH's unconventional journey toward integrative health. *NIH Record, LXVIII* (8). Retrieved from https://nihrecord.nih.gov/newsletters/2016/04_08_2016/story3.htm

Tan, G., Shaffer, F., Lyle, R., & Teo, I. (Eds.). (2016). *Evidence-based treatment in biofeedback and neurofeedback* (3rd ed.). Wheat Ridge, CO: Association for Applied Psychophysiology and Biofeedback.

Thibault, R. T., & Raz, A. (2017). The psychology of neurofeedback: Clinical intervention even if applied placebo. *The American Psychologist, 72*(7), 679–688. https://doi.org/10.1037/ amp0000118. PubMed PMID: 29016171.

Thie, J. (2007). Chinese medical treatments. In J. H. Lake & D. Spiegel (Eds.), *Complementary and alternative treatments in mental health care* (pp. 169–194). Washington, DC: American Psychiatric Publishing, Inc..

Towler, P., Molassiotis, A., & Brearley, S. G. (2013). What is the evidence for the use of acupuncture as an intervention for symptom management in cancer supportive and palliative care: An integrative overview of reviews. *Supportive Care in Cancer, 21*, 2913–2923. https://doi. org/10.1007/s00520-013-1882-8

Trakhtenberg E.C. The effects of guided imagery on the immune system: a critical review. Int J Neurosci. 2008 Jun;118(6):839–55. doi:10.1080/00207450701792705. Review. PubMed PMID: 18465428.

Van Geijlswijk, I. M., Korzilius, H. P., & Smits, M. G. (2010). The use of exogenous melatonin in delayed sleep phase disorder: A meta-analysis. *Sleep, 33*, 1605–1614.

Verhoef, M. J., Mulkins, A., Kania, A., Findlay-Reece, B., & Mior, S. (2010). Identifying the barriers to conducting outcomes research in integrative health care clinic settings—A qualitative study. *BMC Health Services Research, 10*, 14. https://doi.org/10.1186/1472-6963-10-14

Vickers, A., & Zollman, C. (1999). ABC of complementary medicine: Herbal medicine. *British Medical Journal, 319*(7216), 1050–1053. Review. Erratum in: BMJ 1999 Nov 27;319(7222):1422.PubMed PMID: 10521203; PubMed Central PMCID: PMC1116847.

Vishal, A. A., Mishra, A., & Raychaudhuri, S. P. (2011). A double blind, randomized, placebo controlled clinical study evaluates the early efficacy of Aflapin® in subjects with osteoarthritis of knee. *International Journal of Medical Sciences, 8*(7), 615–622.

Wahbeh, H., Elsas, S.-M., & Oken, B. S. (2008). Mind–body interventions: Applications in neurology. *Neurology, 70*(24), 2321–2328. https://doi.org/10.1212/01.wnl.0000314667.16386.5e

Wani, A. L., Bhat, S. A., & Ara, A. (2015). Omega-3 fatty acids and the treatment of depression: A review of scientific evidence. *Integrative Medicine Research, 4*(3), 132–141. https://doi.org/10.1016/j.imr.2015.07.003

Xiong, X., Wang, P., Li, X., & Zhang, Y. (2015). Qigong for hypertension: A systematic review. *Medicine, 94*(1), e352. https://doi.org/10.1097/MD.0000000000000352

Chapter 6
A Pathways Approach to Chronic Pain

Abstract Chronic pain is a major cause of human suffering and impairment in function, affecting not only individuals, but also families, productivity in the workplace and society. Selected mechanisms involved in the transformation of acute pain into chronic debilitating pain are discussed. Two cases, one of a patient with chronic migraine and another case of a sufferer of back pain are presented in detail. The multi-level Pathways Model is applied to each case. The patient with migraine had a history of sexual abuse and met criteria for major depressive disorder. The example chosen for low back pain is that of a married man whose wife is emotionally and physically ill. He is stuck in past memories of a highly successful period of his life when he was a high school star athlete. Both patients were able to reduce pain, but perhaps even more importantly, they acquired healthier lifestyle behaviors, learned coping skills, and lessened symptoms of anxiety and depression. Although the interventions did not cure their pain, their suffering from chronic pain decreased and their ability to function in their personal world improved.

Keywords Chronic pain · Migraines · Back pain · Adverse life events · Central and peripheral sensitization · Pathways Model

The Case of Doreen

Doreen was a 40-year-old woman who taught at a local community college. She suffered with headaches from the time she was 6 years old. The headaches were well controlled with Tylenol (Acetaminophen) from the time of onset until puberty. At 12 years of age, Doreen experienced a distinct visual phenomenon of jagged lines followed by a severe headache and vomiting which lasted long enough to frighten her and her parents. She was hospitalized for 3 days and diagnosed with migraine headache with aura. Subsequently, headaches recurred monthly with her menstrual periods and sometimes at the time of mid-cycle ovulation. During the past 5 years, the headaches increased in frequency; she had a daily headache of mild to moderate pain, severe pain three to four times per week and incapacitating pain

© Springer International Publishing AG, part of Springer Nature 2018   111
A. McGrady, D. Moss, *Integrative Pathways*,
https://doi.org/10.1007/978-3-319-89313-6_6

at least 4 days a month. When those days coincided with scheduled classes, Doreen had to take sick time and missed class. According to her contract at the community college, if a professor cancels class, the students had to be provided with alternative assignments, but missing classes for any reason was strongly discouraged. Doreen came to us because her department chair at the community college advised her to apply for disability because of absenteeism.

Chronic Pain Chronic pain is a common disabling condition affecting millions of people around the world (Yaqub, 2015). Pain may have an identifiable original cause and initially respond to medical interventions, but often returns in another treatment-resistant form. Pain can emerge early in life, such as in childhood headache or functional abdominal pain, and it often resolves completely. In other cases, no cause is identified. Pain is considered chronic when it persists longer than 12 weeks (National Institutes of Health, 2011). Pain often prevents restorative sleep so patients feel fatigued and sluggish during the day, which interferes with effective functioning (Moldofsky, 2014). Experiencing pain for extended periods of time causes emotional suffering, and over time, psychological disorders emerge. Thus comorbid depression, anxiety, and sleep disorders are frequently part of the presentation of patients with chronic pain, making diagnosis and treatment more complex (Tietjen, Herial, Hardgrove, Utley, & White, 2007).

The Etiology of Chronic Pain

The etiology of certain types of chronic pain, specifically, migraine, chronic daily headache, and back pain (which are covered in this chapter), does include genetic underpinnings. So the family histories of headache patients provide important insights. Besides genetics, many psychological, environmental, and behavioral factors converge to increase frequency and intensity of headache. Migraine patients in particular may be sensitive to certain foods, weather changes, alcohol, and poor air quality in addition to stress (Murray, O'Neal, & Weisz, 2015; Prince, Rapoport, Sheftell, Tepper, & Bigal, 2004; Tietjen, Khubchandani, Ghosh, Bhattacharjee, & Kleinfelder, 2012).

Physical, emotional, or sexual abuse/maltreatment or combinations of adverse events are associated with chronic pain later in life, in particular headaches (Juang & Yang, 2014; Tietjen, 2016). Dysregulation of the hypothalamic-pituitary axis (HPA) is postulated to be one of the links between adverse childhood events and later mood disruption (Van Voorhees & Scarpa, 2004). The stress hormones (such as cortisol) that are usually protective in short-term stress become maladaptive if the hormones are overproduced or if the feedback loop (cortisol—negative feedback—hypothalamus, pituitary, adrenal cortex) fails to shut down the stress response (Shea, Walsh, MacMillan, & Steiner, 2004).

Further, two or more factors can overlap and increase the risk of acute pain becoming chronic. For example, feeling isolated or disconnected from others is associated with distress and poor sleep quality (Cacioppo, Hawkley, & Thisted, 2010; Kurina et al., 2011). For patients who are lonely and experiencing acute pain, the effects on sleep multiply the risk for pain becoming chronic (Christiansen, Larsen, & Lasgaard, 2016). Depression is frequently comorbid with chronic pain, loneliness, non-restorative sleep, and HPA dysregulation (Stetler & Miller, 2011; Vreeburg et al., 2009). Too often, the physician's standard recommendations for acute pain, namely to rest and restrict exercise are contraindicated when pain lingers and becomes chronic pain. Pharmaceutical pain management is essential in the treatment of severe acute pain; however, reliance on analgesics and particularly narcotics to control chronic pain does not provide long-term relief for the patient and increases risk for biological and psychological addiction, with accompanying serious consequences. Challenges in the treatment of chronic pain and the application of the Pathways Model will be discussed in the cases presented in this chapter.

The Impact of Stress on the Course of Headaches Current stress is a major factor in the onset and worsening of headache and contributes to a poorer response to medical treatment (Martin, 2016). In general, headache sufferers rate situations as more stressful, both the events recalled from the past and current stressors (Wittrock & Foraker, 2001). The way that patients reconstruct past stressful experiences matches their personal life schema; a once pleasant stimulus is reconfigured as negative if a headache develops later. Frequent pain understandably leads to fear and anxiety about the next headache; patients avoid situations and experiences that were once associated with pain (Norton & Asmundson, 2004). Fear, rumination about the effects of the injury that may have started the pain process, and anxiety involve multiple regions of the brain. With time, patients learn to anticipate pain and to have difficulty in uncoupling original pain stimuli from pain reactions; additionally, the scope of the learning broadens to include more stimuli, negative affect, and pain-related behaviors (Apkarian, 2008).

Peripheral and Central Sensitization A detailed explanation of the mechanisms underlying the phenomenon of the development of chronic intractable pain is beyond the scope of this book, so the reader is referred to a textbook of neuroscience such as Purves et al. (2012). But a basic understanding of peripheral and central sensitization is helpful for clinicians involved in the care of chronic pain patients since education of patients is an important component of each level of the Pathways Model. What follows is a brief summary of the highly complex process of transformation of acute or infrequent pain into a chronic condition.

Limited, short-term pain becomes chronic or intractable in discrete pathophysiological steps involving multiple nerve cells in the periphery and in the central nervous system (Voscopoulos & Lema, 2010). Primary pain neurons in the periphery can be altered in several ways, including release of substances from damaged tissues, such as prostaglandins, bradykinins, and peptides, abnormal excitability of the ion channels through which neurotransmitters pass, or by degeneration of the peripheral axon, so that receptors that normally are at the distal most point are now along the axon. Regarding this latter mechanism, pain can be generated at any point along the nerve where there is a receptor in addition to the nerve ending since the cell body is still intact and can continue to produce receptors. Finally, pain neurons are altered by excess release and contact with the stress neurotransmitter NE (nor-epinephrine), which activates the primary neuron; the pain neurons also gain greater sensitivity to NE because there are additional receptors on the cell membrane.

Central sensitization occurs concomitant with the peripheral effects described above. The central pain matrix neurons refer to all of the parts of the brain that partici-pate in processing incoming data from the periphery, activating memories of past pain, eliciting physiological and emotional responses, and forming cognitive schemas. Over time, non-pain stimuli can create a pain experience in the central pain matrix from sources not usually associated with transmission of the pain signal (allodynia); normal pain-sensitive neurons are maximally activated by low levels of stimuli or become spontaneously active. Neurotransmitters are also involved in the sensitization process; for example, excess substance P and glutamate (excitatory substances) are released, whereas normally inhibitory transmitters (glycine and GABA) are down regulated. The synapses that carry the neurotransmitter from one nerve cell to the next are struc-turally altered due to abnormal sprouting of the ends of the axons. Glial cells (astro-cytes and microglia) whose normal role is to maintain the integrity of the neuronal environment and support the matrix instead release proinflammatory substances and disrupt the delicate balance in the synapse (Elman & Borsook, 2016; Lu et al., 2016).

Description of the neuroscience of pain perception and amplification does not capture the emotional, cognitive, and behavioral dimensions of the pain experience for patients. Transformation of acute, episodic headache into chronic daily head-ache also involves parts of the brain which process emotion and behavior. The area of the brain that processes emotional stimuli takes on the role of amplifier of pain signals (Vachon-Presseau et al., 2016). These authors present a model in which the amygdala, hippocampus, and limbic system are essential contributors to develop-ment and maintenance of chronic pain. In vulnerable individuals, the normal inhibi-tion of strong emotional reactions to injury is not functional, culminating over time in enhanced emotional reactions to repeated pain and reorganization of the cortex. If we consider the definitive role of adverse childhood events on later pain condi-tions, a connection between brain areas that process highly emotional events and the pain circuitry is logical. Emotions potentially serve both adaptive and maladaptive roles. Primary emotions, such as anger, sadness, and fear, need to be identified and experienced because they are valuable for the purposes of motivation and adapta-tion. In contrast, secondary emotions such as depression and anxiety may result from suppressed primary emotions and actually interfere with adjustment to life changes and motivation for change (Lumley et al., 2011).

Based on current knowledge of the multidimensional aspects and complexity of chronic pain summarized above, effective treatment must also include behavioral, psychophysiological, and psychological components along with self-management training. Several reviews have summarized non-pharmacological evidence-based treatments for chronic pain. Among those interventions are relaxation therapy, bio-feedback, mindfulness, cognitive behavioral therapy, and exercise, all of which are included in the Pathways Model (Chiesa & Serretti, 2011; Eccleston et al., 2014;

Hayden, van Tulder, Malmivaara, & Koes, 2005; Monticone et al., 2015; Penzien, Irby, Smitherman, Rains, & Houle, 2015).

Using a resilience model as a way to help patients decrease pain emphasizes developing patients' ability to bounce back and move through the adversity of dealing with pain (Hassett & Finan, 2016). Interventions based on positive psychology include several areas of emphasis; they serve to decrease negative interpretations by patients of their capabilities and events and increase the use of positive, self-affirming behaviors. The influence of personality was highlighted in a unique study of motivation and relief seeking in normal individuals subjected to experimental pain. Those in a motivated state who scored higher on the personality trait of novelty seeking obtained more pain relief. Increased dopamine during times of high motivation leads to increased release of endogenous opioids (Becker, Gandhi, Kwan, Ahmed, & Schweinhardt, 2015). In contrast, low dopamine levels are associated with pain patients' greater sensitivity to emotional stimuli and less downstream inhibition of pain pathways (Borsook et al., 2016). Chronic pain and stress lessen dopaminergic transmission (situations usually classified as pleasant are interpreted as less pleasant or negative); in addition, avoiding pain becomes a priority over a potentially emotionally rewarding action (not bending over to pick flowers for fear of pain), so patients are exposed to fewer rewarding situations (Navratilova, Atcherley, & Porreca, 2015).

The Evaluation of Doreen

As the team took a detailed history, Doreen became impatient since she had told the story so many times before. She questioned why her history was not readily available since she had consulted several physicians at the same facility. Our response to Doreen was that we had accessed the history and the medication list from the electronic medical record, but we needed to review the information with her in person and we had additional questions. Doreen certainly met the diagnostic criteria for chronic headache; she described daily pain of mild to moderate intensity, punctuated with days of moderate to severe pain, and incapacitating pain 3–4 days per month. Food triggers were minimal: only nuts, some cheeses, and wine. One to two cups of coffee a day never presented a problem and sometimes a half cup of coffee decreased headache pain intensity.

Early Abuse History   As we progressed to the section of our interview focused on abuse history, Doreen stated that she did not see the relevance of these questions. We responded that it was part of her history and might be relevant to the present problems. Reluctantly, Doreen reported that she had been sexually abused by her older brother's friend. One of her previous therapists had helped her with that memory so she did not want to say any more about it. More candidly, she described the emotional abuse perpetrated by her dance teacher. As a child, Doreen had loved to dance. In high school, she was accepted to an excellent ballet school. Unfortunately, the teacher went from being demanding and strict to being an emotional abuser. All the girls were criticized and belittled, but Doreen in particular was a frequent target, possibly because she was the most naturally talented of her peers. Within 2 years, Doreen was beaten down emotionally and had lost confidence as a dancer and as a young woman. She gave up what she loved most, her dancing. The loss of sense of self and the unhappiness affected her school performance; she dropped from an A-B student to a C student. Doreen's mother openly expressed her disappointment that Doreen had stopped dancing, labeling her a quitter who couldn't take "a little criticism" and was "blowing this opportunity to train with a famous teacher." As Doreen described these interactions with her mother and recalled the dance teacher, she stopped abruptly, saying that her head was pounding and she could not continue any longer. That ended the session for that day.

> "When Darien began to talk about separating, Doreen almost felt relieved, telling herself that she couldn't keep up the life that many young couples take for granted. She believed Darien was "owed" a normal wife; he was a good man who only wanted normal things."

Impact of Pain on Marriage Doreen met Darien in college and they were married after both of them graduated. Although Darien had expressed understanding of the headaches when they were dating, he had not witnessed the days of pain that became obvious when living with Doreen. Darien wanted a partner who worked hard, saved money, and raised a family side by side with him; he was not expecting financial strains due to expenditures for co-pays and deductibles for doctor's visits, expensive medications, lost days of work, and frequent absences from social events. They were married for 5 years but had no children. When Darien began to talk about separating, Doreen almost felt relieved, telling herself that she was not able to keep up the life that many young couples take for granted. She believed Darien was "owed" a normal wife; he was a good man who only wanted normal things. Nonetheless, the divorce was another blow to her self-esteem. Her parents were cruel: "what was wrong with Doreen that she couldn't keep a great guy like Darien happy?" The day of the divorce proceedings, Doreen could hardly sit in the courtroom because her head was hurting so badly. She went directly from the courthouse to the emergency room, where fortunately she received an infusion of dihydroergotamine mesylate (DHE) which stopped the pain. She returned home late in the evening, a defeated woman.

Medication for Migraine Doreen was under the care of an excellent neurologist at the medical center. Medications at the start of intervention were: Imitrex (sumatriptan) injectable, 6 mg/0.5 mL subcutaneous solution, maximum allowed dose 2/24 hours twice per week; Sumatriptan oral tablet, 100 mg; Topiramate 100 mg b.i.d.; Venlafaxine ER 37.5 mg capsule 1 per day; Excedrin tablets 2–4 per day, almost every day; and Hydrocodone 5 mg/acetaminophen 325 mg every 6 hours; 10 tablets must last 30 days. Doreen had had occipital nerve blocks of the greater and lesser occipital nerve with minimal effects. Because of the lack of responsiveness, i.e., decreased pain, she was not a candidate for the next step in invasive treatment, nerve ablation. Despite medical management, Doreen experienced severe breakthrough headaches; after hours of intractable pain, she would drive to the emergency room for help. It is important to note that seeking relief becomes more and more complicated for the patient with chronic pain who has acute exacerbations. For example, frequent emergency room visits raise suspicion and patients may be labeled as merely drug seeking. Patients who have had years of headache often request drugs by name, stating that they know what works and what they need. However, physicians in the emergency room setting often resist these suggestions from patients, assuming that patients who name a desired medication are abusers. Increased knowledge of medication overuse in headache patients (Dodick & Freitag, 2006) further biases some physicians against a chronic headache patient presenting for care in the emergency setting. They assume that the patient takes multiple daily doses of over-the-counter analgesics, which are known to cause rebound headaches. Too often, the unspoken but understood message from the physician is "these headaches are your fault."

Pathways Level One: Breath, Movement and Education

Breath, Movement, and Education Pathways Level One activities emphasize self-directed behavioral and lifestyle changes. In her initial assessment, Doreen described rapid breathing and an uncomfortable feeling in her chest when she was in pain or when she felt anxious in a challenging situation. The basics of mindful breathing were explained and she practiced slow, mindful abdominal breathing with the provider. The second intervention—movement—was directed toward Doreen's sedentary lifestyle. She was fearful that exertion would worsen pain, which it had done in the past. So she was advised to walk a short distance every day, gradually to increase the distance up to one mile and not to speed up. After several weeks without problems, she was to increase her speed at the same distance, completing a mile in 15 minutes. She slowly increased her activity, eventually losing her fear of creating a headache beginning during exercise. Doreen began to feel some healthy excitement when she anticipated a walk, sometimes experiencing relief from a minor headache during or after her walk. From that time on, she walked at a nearby park year round, carrying hand weights for at least a mile, except on days where the headaches were severe or the weather was prohibitive.

Doreen responded well to the mindful breathing exercise and reported feeling calmer and more focused after minutes of slow breathing. However, she still expressed frustration about the chronicity of her pain; what used to be controllable with over-the-counter medicines was now barely controlled with powerful triptans and narcotics. The team utilized current neuroscience information to explain in lay person's terms the transformation of acute short-term pain into chronic daily pain.

The concept of pain sensitization was logical to Doreen and she now better understood the connection between the theory and our intervention plan.

Pathways Level Two: Relaxation, Exercise, Imagery, Communication, and Cognitive Restructuring

Relaxation Exercises Progressive muscle relaxation (PMR) (Davis, Eshelman, & McKay, 2008) instruction followed. The usual sequence for progressive muscle relaxation involves a sequence of tensing each muscle group, then releasing the tension, and focusing one's awareness on the contrast between tensing and releasing the muscles. Doreen feared that increasing muscle tension voluntarily would bring on a headache and she was reluctant to use it. The team explained that people voluntarily increase muscle tension many times during the day without causing pain. Nonetheless, the PMR exercise was modified to include very small increases in tension in the neck and face areas, with moderate increases in tension in the parts of the body where she rarely had pain (legs, torso, and arms). Calming imagery was introduced as an additional component in her relaxation. Doreen found this combination of slow breathing, muscle relaxation and imagery exercise very enjoyable and found several YouTube videos of beautiful scenery, which were calming. She bookmarked them for regular use and also found a downloadable relaxation phone app to use when she was away from home.

Despite some moderation in the headaches up to this point, Doreen believed that she was doomed to disability. There had been so many failed or partially successful treatments, including migraine medicines, antidepressants, herbals, nerve blocks, chiropractic, and massage. She had been in psychological therapy before, but the psychologist did not have much experience with patients suffering from chronic pain. Writing down her headaches in a log book as her psychologist requested reminded Doreen that she suffered so many days per month and was never totally free of pain. Some of her symptoms of depression decreased during prior therapy, but overall, Doreen had the feeling that the therapist did not "get it." She refused to keep a headache diary for us, even though a daily log is usually used as an important indicator of improvement (Andrasik, Lipchik, McCrory, & Wittrock, 2005).

Assertive Communication Improved, assertive communication was a major need for Doreen. She was reticent with others and spoke in a low voice most of the time. During her marriage, Doreen had deferred to her husband. She thought that since she was sometimes incapacitated with pain and spending so much money on her illness, she had no rights. Darien decided who they went out with and what they did and then often was angry that plans had to be cancelled because Doreen could not get out of bed. Her history with the dance teacher who criticized her without mercy had seriously damaged her self-esteem and she had yet to recover from that experience in her teen age years. In order to build assertiveness, Doreen was instructed to make one "I" statement a day about something she liked, appreciated, or believed in. For example, she could say to a colleague at the community college: "I find it easy to use the new textbook." To a neighbor she could state: "I am glad the sun came out." These simple "I" phrases, spoken by Doreen in a slightly louder voice than usual, could not be contradicted by others and gave her a sense that she had a right to an opinion and could say it out loud. This simple exercise gradually decreased the fear of criticism for her statements. Over time, the client is encouraged to make statements about slightly more controversial topics, such as a particular restaurant, a movie, or a book.

Pathways Level Three: Biofeedback and Psychotherapy

Biofeedback Biofeedback was introduced in order to give Doreen a sense of control over some aspects of her physiology. Heart rate variability (HRV) biofeedback supplemented mindful breathing and Doreen was shown the proof that her regular practice resulted in excellent coherence curves[1] on the computer screen. Thermal biofeedback allowed Doreen to learn to raise her finger temperature consistently from baseline temperatures in the low 80s (indicative of over activity of sympathetic nervous system and vasoconstriction of the blood vessels in the fingers) to 94°. Warmer hands are associated with decreased sympathetic activity and better blood flow to the fingers. A small hand thermometer was given to Doreen for home practice. Surface electromyography (SEMG), muscle biofeedback, was initiated to help Doreen decrease the tension in the forehead and neck areas (Penzien et al., 2015).

Psychotherapy During psychodynamic therapy, the memories of the sexual and emotional abuse that she had suffered as a young girl re-surfaced. In an attempt to clarify the relationship between early abuse and pain, Doreen was told that many women with migraine have been the victims of abuse. Instead of the desired effect, that is to increase understanding of the etiology of the headaches, Doreen was devastated by this information, sobbing for a long time. She stated:

> … you are telling me that the guy who touched me when I was a young girl and the horrible dance teacher are still present in my life and have cost me my marriage, and may ruin my career. The abusers controlled my whole life. I have taken medicines, had injections, had therapy, but NO—that is not enough. The pain has almost brought me to suicide and they continue to live; they probably have great families and terrific careers. The sexual abuser has never given me another thought and the dance teacher moved on to other students.
>
> Meanwhile I have lost so much. I feel furious and helpless at the same time. You have suggested that I express my anger. But then getting mad makes my head hurt more. You

---

[1] Coherence is a term introduced by the HeartMath Institute to describe a "physiological mode that encompasses a range of distinct but related phenomena, including synchronization, entrainment, and resonance, all of which emerge from the harmonious interactions of the body's subsystems" (McCraty, 2002, p. 24). Operationally, trainees earn high coherence scores by increasing overall heart rate variability (HRV), specifically by increasing the percentage of the total power of HRV falling within the low frequency range, that is, between 0.04 and 0.26 Hz in the HRV power spectrum.

want me to feel my feelings, but you are sending me into a trap because my pain becomes intolerable and I feel worse.

This was a critical session: a deep-seated anger surfaced, but suicidal thoughts wer also revealed and a desperation that could increase the risk for a suicide attempt The therapist spoke in a calm soft voice so that Doreen had to listen closely. The etiology of migraine is very complex. Contributing factors are genetics, hyper excitability of the brain, faulty neurotransmission, food sensitivities, environment and yes, a history of abuse contributes to the development of migraine.

Doreen's psychologist emphasized that she, Doreen, was now taking contro back from the headaches and from the people who had hurt her. She had already made progress; the severe vascular headaches that required Imitrex (sumatriptan had already decreased from 15 a month to 8 although the daily headaches contin ued. She had learned to pace her breathing, to relax her muscles, and to warm he hands. But Doreen said she could never regain the years lost to suffering. The improvement that she had achieved up to this point might not be enough to keep he job and make life worth living. Doreen's team worked with her to create a writte suicide prevention plan, with recommendations for managing fleeting passive thoughts, consistent passive thoughts, suicidal intent, suicidal plans, and moment of "beginning to take action" on suicidal thoughts. This session continued into the next hour, but at the end, Doreen agreed to the written prevention plan and took i with her. In truth, the team was concerned about Doreen's safety. At the case review meeting, the following day, the team also decided that they would ask Doreen for the names of two family members or close friends in case she did not show up for an appointment. Our 24-hours contact information would also be shared with these two people.

Over the next month, Doreen was seen twice a week, with phone calls between sessions. She began to speak about reclaiming her life, proving to her department chair that she could continue to teach. In the process of giving her two friends our phone numbers, she really talked to them. Of course, they knew that she had inca-pacitating headaches, but they did not know of her suffering as a child, as a teen, and now. Both friends overwhelmed Doreen with compassion and empathy. They told her that she had always been there for them and they were rock solid with her now. They volunteered to come to our office and be part of the therapy if necessary.

Progress in Treatment Treatment with the Pathways Model interventions lasted for 3 years during which time headache frequency and intensity gradually improved. The neurologist decreased *topiramate* slowly over 8 weeks to 25 mg b.i.d. and then eliminated it. The antidepressant *Venlafaxine* was maintained. The prescriptions for Imitrex injections and 100 mg tablets were continued. Excedrin use was gradually decreased as daily pain lessened; the goal was to use Excedrin no more than three times a week, not daily. Botox 1 unit by injection (chemode-nervation) was added quarterly. Dronabinal (a derivative of marijuana) 2.5 mg b.i.d. was added. Doreen practiced her relaxation skills (mindful breathing, imag-ery, and occasionally progressive relaxation) for 1 hour a day and continued to walk almost every day.

In the spring semester of the second year of treatment, Doreen did not have an incapacitating headache so she did not miss a single day of class. Her boss no longer talked about forcing her to apply for disability. The formerly daily headaches decreased to three per week; headaches requiring Imitrex, but not limiting function, decreased to three per month, a significant improvement.

Doreen reported meeting a wonderful guy (Jerodd), who had been hired at the school and with whom Doreen shared many interests. He loved the theater and the arts. Doreen told him about her dance background, and they decided that they would take lessons together and see if they liked it, while making sure that the activity did not increase headaches. The low impact dance routines were wonderful exercise for both of them, and they became excellent dancers. Jerodd accompanied Doreen to her last session where she proudly showed off her diamond engagement ring. Jerodd told us that he knew all about the headaches and what Doreen had been through in the past. He said that Doreen was the most courageous person that he had ever met and that he would love her for the rest of their lives.

Introducing Michael

Michael was a 43-year-old mortgage banker who worked in a large financial institution. He was college educated and also certified by the National Mortgage Lending Association. He came to us with complaints of "simple" chronic low back pain. He had heard about the efficacy of biofeedback and wanted to try it. Michael had been a very active athlete in high school, competing in three sports: baseball, basketball, and lacrosse. He had been named as a first team all-city athlete in basketball for three of his four high school years. His high school had won the state championship in baseball in his junior year and he received the most valuable player trophy. In college at a Division 3 school, he focused on basketball, but since there were no athletic scholarships, he worked several part-time jobs to pay most of his tuition. At graduation, there was only a relatively small outstanding loan to be repaid for tuition.

During the evaluation, the description of Michael's high school years took up much more time than customary in a psychological assessment of a 43-year-old man. The memories seemed fresh and full of detail, not merely a recounting of events that took place more than 20 years in the past. Back pain began in college after a hard fall in basketball practice; the college's health center physician prescribed ibuprofen 800 mg three times a day for 2 weeks, which eliminated the pain for the short term. Months later, pain of mild intensity returned, but Michael did not seek medical attention because he was working and focused on finishing his college degree. During his 30s, the pain worsened and he consulted his primary care doctor, then an orthopedic physician. The diagnosis was degenerative disc disease, more commonly referred to as lumbar facet joint osteoarthritis (Kalichman et al., 2008). In this condition, intervertebral discs and facet joints between the lumbar vertebra slowly deteriorate, resulting in nerve compression (Lewinnek & Warfield, 1986).

Pain and numbness in the lower back region ensues and becomes more and more frequent. Medications were meloxicam (Mobic) and cyclobenzaprine (Flexeril). Michael supplemented prescription medication with acetaminophen and ibuprofen. At intake, the most intense pain was rated as an 8 on a 10-point scale and average pain ranged from 3 to 4. There were some pain-free intervals most days.

Michael was married to Julianne and they had three children, ages 16, 12, and 8. The marriage was described as stable; the children had only the normal childhood illnesses, no emotional problems and were progressing appropriately in school. The 16-year-old and 8-year-old seemed to have some potential as athletes, which made Michael very happy. His job presented challenges, particularly during the time when accelerated mortgage lending in 2005–2007 was followed by a period of home owners failing to make payments and eventually losing their homes. But his bank and he had survived those years, and the mortgage banking industry had stabilized. His yearly evaluations from his supervisor were very good, but he had not been promoted on schedule last year. His boss expected employees at the manager level to stay later after the bank closed and Michael left exactly at 4 or earlier to drive his children to their practices and games.

The lifestyle assessment consisted of questions about nutrition, activity, sleep, and stress. Michael reported his activity levels as modest: his job involved sitting at a computer or desk most of the day, while outside of work he took care of the yard and garden. Several times a week, the evening meal was eaten at 8 p.m. because of his children's sports activities. He went to bed at midnight and set the alarm for 6 a.m. Sleep was not always continuous during the night with one to two awakenings.

The Pathways Model was described to Michael as a multidimensional treatment plan which assists patients not only with their physical complaints but also incorporates emotional, cognitive, and spiritual components. The Level I interventions recommended for Michael were mindful breathing, correction of posture, and improving sleep. The lifestyle coach explained the importance of good posture and effects of poor posture on maintenance of pain. Sleep hygiene recommendations were instituted, particularly changing Michael's eating schedule so that caloric intake was spread out during the day and the evening meal occurred earlier than 8 p.m. Interestingly, Michael resisted the suggestions except for the posture recommendations, often repeating, "This is about my back pain. I want to learn the biofeedback which I have heard is very helpful. I admit I am frustrated with *your* treatment plan."

Pathways Model in the Treatment of Michael

Pathways Level One It was explained to Michael that Pathways Level I is the foundation for the rest of the interventions. It was important that he master mindful breathing and consider making changes in his eating schedule. In addition, the idea that the model was the team's treatment plan had to be addressed. The team allocated time to affirming Michael's primary goal to decrease his pain, but promoting understanding that many other factors affect pain. It was also emphasized that all the interventions are evidence based. For example, the effects of mindful breathing were studied in patients with back pain, and the results were positive for both pain and functioning (Mehling, Hamel, Acree, Byl, & Hecht, 2005). Readings on healthy and unhealthy posture were recommended (McKenzie, 2011). Finally, Michael agreed that the breathing was of some help and he would try to adjust his eating schedule and to pay more attention to his posture.

Several weeks passed before the next appointment due to scheduling issues. When Michael arrived, he immediately complained that he received no benefit for his back pain so far. Michael's appointments were always on Monday mornings since he went to work at 10 a.m. and worked later on that day. During further discussion on activity the previous weekend, Michael surprised the team when he became tearful and stated,

> I have severe pain right now, but it is my own fault. I have been lying to you since the beginning. I am still very active physically, probably doing things that I shouldn't do. I am in an adult softball league, and we practice or play twice a week. During the winter months I play basketball with the guys every Sunday night. You will want me to give this up, but I can't do it. I have loved sports and physical activity since my high school days. Some of the guys whom I play with are guys that I grew up with, and with whom I won the state championship in baseball. I can't and won't give up this part of my life. But after a vigorous game, my back is on fire and I go home to lie down on ice. I slid hard into second base yesterday and that is why I am suffering this morning. I didn't sleep much last night. But I was called safe at second…

he concluded ruefully.

"I have severe pain right now, but it is my own fault. I have been lying to you since the beginning."

Chronic back pain is one of the more common and debilitating conditions, affecting the person suffering, their family, and workplace performance, and it contributes to the global burden of disease (Becker et al., 2015). Similarly to the detailed description of transformation of acute pain into chronic pain in headache, back pain often begins with a signal event, but over time, central sensitization takes place with disastrous sequelae (Woolf, 2011). In Michael's history, he reported falling hard on his back in college. Two weeks of a nonsteroidal anti-inflammatory agent eliminated the pain, but it returned months later as mild pain, then with increased frequency and intensity. Medical management had been the only approach utilized when Michael came to our clinic.

Michael's revelation of his activity seemed to lift a burden from him and, concomitantly, allowed the team to devise a better plan with posture a major target for intervention. Adjustments were necessary in Michael's standing, walking, and sitting postures. He was 6'2" and often walked or sat with shoulders turned in and his head lowered. The lifestyle coach recommended that Michael request an ergonomic evaluation of his office space. His bank manager was agreeable to this and proceeded to order a review of each person's working environment. Many changes could be made relatively quickly while others required expenditures for new chairs. With his new chair and desk set at the proper height and angle for him, Michael reported less pain at the end of the work day.

Pathways Level Two Progressive relaxation, a regular sequence of slowly tensing and relaxing muscle groups was instituted as the first Level Two intervention. A brief background on the six families of relaxation interventions was provided to Michael and progressive relaxation was chosen because of his problems with muscle tension (Bernstein, Carlson, & Schmidt, 2007; Smith, 2007). He accepted the rationale and practiced the skill with the therapist, reporting a sensation of relaxation in most of the muscle groups except for his back muscles.

Pathways Level Three Another surprise was in store for the team during the initial entry into formal psychotherapy, specifically supportive and cognitive behavioral therapy. Michael revealed that his wife Julianne suffered from serious depression. She was currently under the care of a psychiatrist, but was not receiving psychotherapy. She had been in therapy several times in her life, beginning at age 15, but it had not produced long-term benefits.

> I am bent over with responsibility when Julianne is non-functional. We keep a master schedule for the family and I organize it; there are car pools for sports, bus schedules, school events and family gatherings in different color pencils. Sometimes I am overwhelmed and feel that my family is riding on my back, but what can I do? I love Julianne and hope that she will have better times. Julianne's depression is not always severe; there are months where she does well and we enjoy activities as a family. The longest time without depression was three years, but right now, she is feeling bad and not doing much. She barely gets to work at her part-time job as a librarian. I have to carry the kids to all their games.

The team identified several cue words during this interchange: *on my back, bent over, carry,* and therefore decided that a change to a psychodynamic model was better suited to Michael's situation. However, when we entered into exploring potential conflict between his love for Julianne and the burdens imposed on him by her illness, Michael interpreted this as an attack on his wife. He reiterated that this was only about his back pain. Now, he wanted to take a break from the Pathways intervention plan and requested a referral to a sports medicine program.

   To our surprise, 6 months later, Michael returned to our clinic and reported a significant decrease in back pain. He had followed up with our referral to sports medicine. The sports medicine physician and the athletic trainer in her practice were described as "amazing." Michael told the team that *they* understood why he could never give up his sports activities. They did however agree with our analysis of Michael's unhealthy posture and recommended physical therapy performed by a trainer (Hayden et al., 2005). The reason that he returned was that the sports medicine physician told him that his stressors at home were affecting his pain, and although medical management had been effective, the pain would return if he did not delve into the psychological and emotional aspects of pain. He would follow through with our recommendations if we did not try to get him to stop playing sports (*we had never said this*). He also stated that he would never leave Julianne (*we had never suggested this either*).

The medical management plan designed by the sports medicine team comprised injections at the site of the pain including lumbar epidural corticosteroid injections (Injections and Implants for Back Pain Relief, 2017) to reduce joint swelling and inflammation as well as Hyalgan, a hyaluronic acid injection, to lubricate the facet joints by serving as a "synthetic" synovial fluid. Ibuprofen, a nonsteroidal anti-inflammatory drug (NSAID), was added three times daily 600–800 mg (Griffin, Tudiver, & Grant, 2002). The trainer worked with Michael to increase his flexibility and core strength, as well as his range of motion (Geneen et al., 2017). Michael was told that pre-exercise stretching was critical to prevent injury and to lessen the effects of heavy activity on his back muscles and joints (Yu & Hunter, 2015). The sports medicine physician did not advise him to curtail the physical activity that he loved, but suggested that Michael might also enjoy water sports, such as water volleyball, since these activities have less of a physical impact on his back (Yu & Hunter, 2015).

Cognitive behavioral therapy was instituted with a focus on identifying automatic thoughts and countering negative interpretations. The thoughts that came into Michael's mind were "I must do all this; there is no one else; I can't ask Julianne or my kids for help." It doesn't matter that I have not been promoted at work as long as my kids can get to practice and games. Progress in CBT was slow because Michael resisted any suggestions that were interpreted as critical of Julianne. The psychologist framed the automatic thoughts in a different way—what would it be like if you did not have to leave work right at 4 p.m. to get the kids to practice? Let's consider other sources of help and support in fulfilling day-to-day responsibilities.

A family therapy session was suggested, and Michael reluctantly agreed to only 1 hour. The intervention was conducted by our expert therapist with the psychologist who had been working with Michael present and involved in a minor way. It was obvious that the kids loved both of their parents equally but differently. Mom was a protected human being, frail, somewhat helpless and unable to cope. Their father was believed to be dynamic, successful and "amazing" in his athleticism. Both Michael and Julianne accepted these roles. The challenge presented to the family was to find ways to decrease the stress and responsibility on Michael, but he was not allowed to downplay any suggestion. This was brainstorming with no negative comments permitted. The oldest daughter said that she was 16 and could start drivers' education. The 8-year-old offered to go to the after school program with her friends and complete homework there. The 12-year-old who was playing three sports was glad to give up softball, which she had continued only to please her father, but softball was not her favorite sport. All three children would observe quiet time after 10 p.m., so that the home would be more conducive to sleep.

Julianne became tearful during this session and expressed her frustration with her own disability (that was her word). She was so proud of her kids that they were taking on tasks and removing some burdens from Michael, but for herself, this was the hand which she was dealt—chronic depression, similarly to her mother and her grandmother. Michael immediately reacted to the word "burden" and presumed that

Julianne felt attacked. He commented that the psychiatrist had told him that Julianne's depression was genetic and biological; she was trying as hard as she could. The family therapist mentioned that there was no criticism intended; all ideas were to be considered and discussed before any decisions were made. She returned the focus to Michael and his view of the suggested changes in the routine of the household. As long as no one asked any more of Julianne, Michael was OK with the ideas and was willing to try them.

Michael continued in our care for an additional 3 months. The most severe back pain now occurred less than once a week and he had more pain-free hours every day. The sports medicine program had corrected his posture for both basketball and soft-ball. He made those adjustments without noticing a decrease in his game performance. He stretched both before and after practice and games. After a long game, he came home and put a brace on and rested his back, so he no longer experienced hours of fiery pain. He used mindful breathing and progressive relaxation several times a week, most often during his lunch break at work.

True to their promises, the kids did assume more responsibility. The oldest daughter passed her driver's test and could take her brother and sister to some events. At our termination session with Michael, he walked in the door demonstrating excellent posture. He reported that Julianne had started attending some of his and the kids' games and was speaking to one or two of the wives or mothers also in attendance.

> Julianne and my kids are the best things that ever happened to me. I still enjoy my sports and time with the guys, but I don't suffer nearly as much as before. I have been staying later at work several days a week and my boss has noticed. He is talking about sending me for training for more complicated mortgage work. In the past I would have worried about how the kids would get to practice if I were away for a few days, but now I know that my oldest can handle it. Julianne is feeling better and volunteered to drive one of the car pools last week. She is amazing!

Summary

Multiple interventions from each of the Pathways levels were necessary to help Doreen and Michael decrease pain and regain control of their lives. Years of pain changes the brain itself, including neural pathways, sensitivity, and reactions to stress, particularly when there is a history of abuse. For Doreen, the critical point of intervention was the revelation of the abuse history and the role that it played in the etiology of migraine. A highly experienced mental health provider must be on board to deal with these issues, since not only the memories but also the association with years of pain may overwhelm the client and increase the risk for suicide. The provider must be equipped to gather an intervention team, deal with suicide risk, and monitor the patient closely for the time it takes to decrease risk. Michael presented with "simple back pain"; however, overuse, poor posture, and unacknowledged family issues impacted the pain pathways and heightened sensitivity. Trajectory through the levels of the Pathways Model was not linear, but accomplished over time. The involvement of sports medicine and a family therapist was necessary to achieve improvement. Suggestions particularly those related to reducing intense activity in sport or problems in the marriage were immediately rejected. Flexibility in the treatment plan, referral to other providers, and acceptance of the client goals which had not been in the therapist's original plan were critical to successful management of Michael's back pain.

References

Andrasik, F., Lipchik, G. L., McCrory, D. C., & Wittrock, D. A. (2005). Outcome measurement in behavioral headache research: Headache parameters and psychosocial outcomes. *Headache, 45*, 429–437.

Apkarian, A. V. (2008). Pain perception in relation to emotional learning. *Current Opinion in Neurobiology, 18*, 464–468.

Becker, S., Gandhi, W., Kwan, S., Ahmed, A. K., & Schweinhardt, P. (2015). Doubling your payoff: Winning pain relief engages endogenous pain inhibition. *eNeuro, 2*(4), pii: ENEURO.0029-15.2015. https://doi.org/10.1523/ENEURO.0029-15.2015

Bernstein, D. A., Carlson, S. R., & Schmidt, J. E. (2007). Progressive relaxation: Abbreviated methods. In P. M. Lehrer, R. L. Woolfolk, & W. E. Sime (Eds.), *Principles and practice of stress management* (3rd ed., pp. 88–124). New York: Guilford Press.

Borsook, D., Linnman, C., Faria, V., Strassman, A. M., Becerra, L., & Elman, I. (2016). Reward deficiency and anti-reward in pain chronification. *Neuroscience and Biobehavioral Reviews, 68*, 282–297.

Cacioppo, J. T., Hawkley, L. C., & Thisted, R. A. (2010). Perceived social isolation makes me sad: Five year cross-lagged analyses of loneliness and depressive symptomatology in the Chicago Health, Aging, and Social Relations Study. *Psychology and Aging, 25*, 453–463.

Chiesa, A., & Serretti, A. (2011). Mindfulness-based interventions for chronic pain: A systematic review of the evidence (structured abstract). *Journal of Alternative and Complementary Medicine, 17*(1), 83–93.

Christiansen, J., Larsen, F. B., & Lasgaard, M. (2016). Do stress, health behavior, and sleep mediate the association between loneliness and adverse health conditions among older people? *Social Science and Medicine, 152*, 80–86. https://doi.org/10.1016/j.socscimed.2016.01.020

Davis, M., Eshelman, E. R., & McKay, M. (2008). *The relaxation and stress reduction workbook.* Oakland, CA: New Harbinger Publications, Inc..

Dodick, D., & Freitag, G. (2006). Evidence-based understanding of medication-overuse headache: Clinical implications. *Headache, 46*(Supp 4), S202–S211.

Eccleston, C., Palermo, T. M., Williams, A. C., Lewandowski, H. A., Morley, S., Fisher, E., et al. (2014). Psychological therapies for the management of chronic and recurrent pain in children and adolescents (review). *Cochrane Database of Systematic Reviews, 5.* https://doi.org/10.1002/14651858.CD003968.pub4

Elman, I., & Borsook, D. (2016). Common brain mechanisms of chronic pain and addiction. *Neuron, 89*, 11–36.

Geneen, L. J., Moore, R., Clarke, C., Martin, D., Colvin, L. A., & Smith, B. H. (2017). Physical activity and exercise for chronic pain in adults: An overview of Cochrane Reviews. *Cochrane Database of Systematic Reviews, (4).*

Griffin, G., Tudiver, F., & Grant, W. (2002). Do NSAIDs help in acute or chronic low back pain. *American Family Physician, 65*(7), 1319–1322.

Hassett, A. L., & Finan, P. H. (2016). The role of resilience in the clinical management of chronic pain. *Current Pain and Headache Reports, 20*(6), 39.

Hayden, J., van Tulder, M. W., Malmivaara, A., & Koes, B. W. (2005). Exercise therapy for treatment of non-specific low back pain. *Cochrane Database of Systematic Reviews, 3*. https://doi. org/10.1002/14651858.CD000335.pub2

Injections and Implants for Back Pain Relief. (2017). *Resource document.* Arthritis Foundation. Retrieved June 20, 2017, from http://www.arthritis.org/about-arthritis/where-it-hurts/back-pain/treatment/back-pain-relief-injections.php

Juang, K. D., & Yang, C. Y. (2014). Psychiatric comorbidity of chronic daily headache: Focus on traumatic experiences in childhood, post-traumatic stress disorder and suicidality. *Current Pain and Headache Reports, 18*(4), 405.

Kalichman, L. L., Li, L., Kim, D. H., Guermazi, A., Berkin, V., O'Donnell, C. J., et al. (2008). Facet joint osteoarthritis and low back pain in the community-based population. *Spine, 33*(23), 2560–2565.

Kurina, L. M., Knutson, K. L., Hawkley, L. C., Cacioppo, J. T., Lauderdale, D. S., & Ober, C. (2011). Loneliness is associated with sleep fragmentation in a communal society. *Sleep, 34*(11), 1519–1526. https://doi.org/10.5665/sleep.1390

Lewinnek, G. E., & Warfield, C. A. (1986). Facet joint degeneration as a cause of low back pain. *Clinical Orthopaedics and Related Research, 213*, 216–222.

Lu, C., Yang, T., Zhao, H., Zhang, M., Meng, F., Fu, H., et al. (2016). Insular cortex is critical for the perception, modulation, and chronification of pain. *Neuroscience Bulletin, 32*(2), 191–201.

Lumley, M. A., Cohen, J. L., Borszoz, G. S., Cano, A., Radcliffe, A. M., Porter, L. S., et al. (2011). Pain and emotion: A biopsychosocial review of recent research. *Journal of Clinical Psychology, 67*(9), 942–968.

Martin, P. R. (2016). Stress and primary headache: Review of the research and clinical management. *Current Pain and Headache Reports, 20*(7), 45.

McCraty, R. (2002). Heart rhythm coherence—An emerging area of biofeedback. *Biofeedback, 30*, 23–25.

McKenzie, R. (2011). *Treat your own back* (9th ed.). Raumati Beach, New Zealand: Spinal Publications New Zealand Ltd.

Mehling, W. E., Hamel, K. A., Acree, M., Byl, N., & Hecht, F. M. (2005). Randomized, controlled trial of breath therapy for patients with chronic low-back pain. *Alternative Therapies, 11*(4), 44–52.

Moldofsky, H. (2014). *Pain and insomnia: What every clinician should know.* Retrieved August 31, 2014, from http://www.medscape.org/viewarticle/494872

Monticone, M., Cedraschi, C., Ambrosini, E., Rocca, B., Fiorentini, R., Restelli, M., et al. (2015). Cognitive-behavioural treatment for subacute and chronic neck pain. (review). *Cochrane Database of Systematic Reviews, 5*. https://doi.org/10.1002/14651858.CD010664.pub2

Murray, K. A., O'Neal, K., & Weisz, M. (2015). Dietary suggestions for migraine prevention. *American Journal of Health-System Pharmacy, 72*, 519–521.

National Institutes of Health. (2011). Chronic pain: Symptoms, diagnosis, and treatment. *NIH Medline Plus, 6*(1), 5–6. Retrieved from https://medlineplus.gov/magazine/issues/spring11/toc.html

Navratilova, E., Atcherley, C. W., & Porreca, F. (2015). Brain circuits encoding reward from pain relief. *Trends in Neurosciences, 38*, 741–750.

Norton, P. J., & Asmundson, G. (2004). Anxiety sensitivity, fear, and avoidance behavior in headache pain. *Pain, 111*(1–2), 218–223.

Penzien, D. B., Irby, M. B., Smitherman, T. A., Rains, J. C., & Houle, T. T. (2015). Well-established and empirically supported behavioral treatments for migraine. *Current Pain and Headache Reports, 19*(7), 34.

Prince, P. B., Rapoport, A. M., Sheftell, F. D., Tepper, S. J., & Bigal, M. E. (2004). The effect of weather on headache. *Headache, 44*(6), 596–602.

Purves, D., Augustine, G. J., Fitzpatrick, D., Hall, W. C., LaMantia, A., & White, L. E. (2012). *Neurosciences* (5th ed.). Sunderland, MA: Sinauer Associates.

Shea, A., Walsh, C., MacMillan, H., & Steiner, M. (2004). Child maltreatment and HPA axis dysregulation: Relationship to major depressive disorder and posttraumatic stress disorder in females. *Psychoneuroendocrinology, 30*, 162–178.

Smith, J. C. (2007). The psychology of relaxation. In P. M. Lehrer, R. L. Woolfolk, & W. E. Sime (Eds.), *Principles and practice of stress management* (3rd ed., pp. 16–37). New York: Guilford Press.

Stetler, C., & Miller, G. E. (2011). Depression and hypothalamic-pituitary-adrenal activation: A quantitative summary of four decades of research. *Psychosomatic Medicine, 73*(2), 114–126.

Tietjen, G. E. (2016). Childhood maltreatment and headache disorders. *Current Pain and Headache Reports, 20*(4), 26.

Tietjen, G. E., Herial, N. A., Hardgrove, J., Utley, C., & White, L. (2007). Migraine comorbidity constellations. *Headache, 47*(6), 876–877.

Tietjen, G. E., Khubchandani, J., Ghosh, S., Bhattacharjee, S., & Kleinfelder, J. (2012). Headache symptoms and indoor environmental parameters: Results from the EPA BASE study. *Annals of Indian Academy of Neurology, 15*(Supp 1), 595–599.

Vachon-Presseau, E., Centeno, M. V., Ren, W., Berger, S. E., Tetreault, P., Ghantous, M., et al. (2016). The emotional brain as a predictor and amplifier of chronic pain. *Journal of Dental Research, 95*(6), 605–612.

Van Voorhees, E., & Scarpa, A. (2004). The effects of child maltreatment on the hypothalamic-pituitary-adrenal axis. *Trauma, Violence, & Abuse, 5*(4), 333–352.

Voscopoulos, C., & Lema, M. (2010). When does acute pain become chronic? *British Journal of Anaesthesia, 105(S1),* i69–i85.

Vreeburg, S. A., Hoogendijk, W. J., van Pelt, J., Derijk, R. H., Verhagen, J. C., van Dyck, R., et al. (2009). Major depressive disorder and hypothalamic-pituitary-adrenal axis activity. *Archives of General Psychiatry, 66*(6), 617–626.

Wittrock, D. A., & Foraker, S. L. (2001). Tension-type headache and stressful events: The role of selective memory in the reporting of stressors. *Headache, 41*, 482–493.

Woolf, C. J. (2011). Central sensitization: Implications for the diagnosis and treatment of pain. *Pain, 152*(3 Suppl), S2–S15.

Yaqub, F. (2015). Pain in the USA: States of suffering. *The Lancet, 386*(9996), 839.

Yu, S. P., & Hunter, D. J. (2015). Managing osteoarthritis. *Australian Prescriber, 38*(4), 115–119.

Chapter 7
A Pathways Approach to Mood Disorders

Abstract Mood disorders, particularly major depression is one of the most common mental illnesses, causing distress and impairing function. Genetic studies have confirmed an increased risk for depression in those with a positive family history, but environment, particularly chronic exposure to stressful events is a major contributor to etiology. Bipolar disorder has a lower prevalence in adults but a higher concordance. Difficulties in normal functioning in those with severe mood swings are striking in their intensity and effects on many areas of life. This chapter describes two cases of mood disorder, one of a patient with bipolar disorder and one with major depressive disorder. In both examples, the pathways model is applied to both symptom management and to elucidation of root psychological issues. The interventions were not curative but provided significant benefit to the individuals in the short term and assisted them in maintaining mood stability in the long term.

Keywords Major depressive disorder · Bipolar disorder

Bipolar Disorder; the case of Danielle

"Danielle had begun to behave erratically in the classroom and on the court. She reported racing thoughts "all in a jumble…""

"… the coach said that Danielle was playing out of control at times; last week at practice one of Danielle's teammates commented that Danielle was "acting crazy.""

The Case of Danielle Danielle was a 20-year-old college basketball player. She came to the counseling center at her university on the recommendation of her coach. Danielle had begun to behave erratically in the classroom and on the court. She reported racing thoughts "all in a jumble"; she had multiple school assignments partially done with deadlines approaching. She told the staff during the evaluation that all she wanted was to get out on the court and put all her

© Springer International Publishing AG, part of Springer Nature 2018

A. McGrady, D. Moss, *Integrative Pathways*,

https://doi.org/10.1007/978-3-319-89313-6_7

efforts into her sport. Unfortunately, the coach had reported that Danielle was playing out of control at times; last week at practice one of Danielle's teammates commented that Danielle was "acting crazy."

Most mood disorders are chronic illnesses, which are characterized by deviations from normal mood, either low or depressed mood, excessively positive mood (mania), or combinations of depression, mania, or hypomania. Exacerbations affect quality and function in all domains of life. Specific criteria are required for diagnosis (APA, 2013).

Bipolar disorder (BD) is a debilitating mental illness that causes distress to the individual and family members. Mood cycling presents particular challenges to normal life and to the providers caring for those patients, particularly medical professionals who must account for both expansive and depressed mood states. In bipolar disorder, successful management focuses on maintaining mood stability instead of labile and fluctuating moods. Medical management is described by many as the mainstay for the patient with this mood disorder. There are guidelines for medication management of bipolar disorder to include mood stabilizers, atypical antipsychotics, and antidepressants (Rapport et al., 2015). Despite years of experience with medication and the introduction of newer mood stabilizers, patients with BD may not respond or may relapse. Thus, psychotherapy and other non-pharmacological interventions are critical to assist patients with coping skills, day-to-day functioning, and stress management (Price & Marzani-Nissen, 2012).

Knowledge about the contribution of genetics to the emergence of a mood disorder, in particular bipolar disorder, can be discouraging to patients diagnosed with these conditions. They may assume that the appearance of behaviors or moods in themselves which caused them so much distress when they observed them in their parents is a foregone conclusion. So it is important to conduct an honest discussion, particularly with patients with bipolar disorder. It is true that additional risks, above those of the general population, are conferred with a family history of bipolar disorder and depression (Capuron et al., 2008; Craddock & Sklar, 2013). However, many other factors are also relevant to etiology, course, and outcome of intervention. Studies of relevant psychosocial factors highlight life stress, a history of abuse, alcohol use, and pain as affecting etiology (Hua et al., 2011; Larsson et al., 2013; Rapport et al., 2016). Adults who were abused as children may not be able to develop mature defense mechanisms nor the mainstays of coping behaviors. Research shows that the more severe the abuse, the more likely the person is to use emotional expression in coping (Daruy-Filho, Brietzke, Lafer, & Grassi-Oliveira, 2011). But many environmental or psychosocial factors can be modified or effectively treated, thus improving the probability of a positive outcome of treatment.

Bipolar disorder is associated with physiological disruptions in the sleep cycle, autonomic nervous system imbalance, and sometimes chronic pain, particularly headaches (Frank, Gonzalez, & Fagiolini, 2006; Leboyer et al., 2012). The relationship between mood and sleep may be bi-directional—irregular sleep may bring on a disturbance of mood and mood symptoms may make sleep irregular and nonrestorative (Gruber et al., 2011). Those individuals whose employment requires frequent travel across time zones will be at greater risk for mood swings and are more likely to experience disruptions in their normal functioning after travel to areas even with only 1 or 2 hours difference in time.

Danielle's History Danielle was diagnosed with bipolar disorder at age 15 in the midst of a manic episode during basketball season. She was unable to sleep for 48 hours and began talking about grandiose schemes involving leaving home, hiring a coach, and trying out for the Olympics. She described the feelings as "a high" and reported plans to take online classes so that she could graduate early from high school. She denied using any drugs or alcohol, and there was no observational report or serum evidence of drug use.

During grade school, Danielle was taller than her classmates and was very awkward. She would stumble or run into objects, providing entertainment for some classmates. But being different also drew the attention of a class bully. He made fun of her—called her "the gawker." At the end of middle school, her physical size and strength became an asset; she became a very good athlete. In high school, she played on the junior varsity as a freshman; as a sophomore, she began to play on the varsity team. She loved the workouts, being on the court; she was highly competitive, always willing to spend more time working on foul shots, and she was never disrespectful to upper classmen, girls from other teams or her coach. Altogether, Danielle was becoming a favorite of the coaches and potentially the star of the team.

Danielle's parents were at first disbelieving of the bipolar disorder diagnosis. They blamed Danielle's variable behavior and irritability on teen age defiance. "Now that she is playing varsity, she thinks that she is ALL THAT," said Roger, Danielle's dad. Although there was no physical abuse in the home of either Danielle or her younger brother, discipline was strict and criticism was frequent and sometimes caustic. Upon further questioning, it was revealed that there was a history of depression throughout mom's side of the family. Mom was not suffering depression at the time, but recalled months of sadness as a young child and her own mother's response of "get moving and you will feel better." The treating psychiatrist wanted to hospitalize Danielle, but her parents refused. All agreed to medical management with a mood stabilizer, to which Danielle responded well. She was adherent to the regimen although sometimes she reported missing that feeling of being able to do "everything fast."

Danielle was recruited to a Division I school in the Midwest to play basketball. During the recruitment interview, the coach was told about the bipolar disorder and its treatment and verbalized understanding. There were no episodes during her freshman year and she maintained a 3.0 grade point average. In her sophomore year, the courses became more challenging, and Danielle had trouble managing her time. She gave time and energy to all her required assignments and projects, but often gave a single task so much time that she did not complete the work in her other courses.

Danielle began having trouble concentrating in her classes so she decided to borrow a few tablets of Adderall from her roommate. Adderall is a combination of amphetamine and dextroamphetamine, frequently used to treat attention deficit disorders. The basketball season was just starting, and there was a lot of pressure to do well in order to be a starter, as well as to perform in the classroom. Danielle slept fewer hours and felt tired. So to improve her concentration, she started drinking caffeinated coffee, in addition to the Adderall. After 1 week, a manic episode was triggered.

Danielle showed up for practice and began warming up. She was unusually talkative and energetic, and soon the coach became concerned. Danielle was expending a lot of energy during the warm up instead of the slow increase in activity that the coach favored. This was going to be a "soft practice" because there was a game that night.

Recalling it later, the coach thought Danielle was overly excited about this particular game, which was against a team whose coach had snubbed her in recruitment. She had had a good week of practice so had been named a starter. Danielle couldn't stop talking about the upcoming game and began to suggest intricate plays that were not in the play book. At the end of practice, the coach asked Danielle to stay behind ostensibly to discuss the game but more so because she was more worried about how Danielle was acting. After another hour of restlessness, rapid speaking on topics ranging from playing time to term papers, making less and less sense, the coach walked Danielle to the counseling center and requested an immediate appointment. This was our first contact with Danielle and she was found to be in a manic state. Hospitalization was recommended and this time accepted in order to re-adjust medications. Inpatient services lasted 5 days and Danielle was released on the same mood stabilizer with an added atypical antipsychotic (*aripiprazole*, Abilify).

Both coach and athlete were hesitant about how to manage the rest of the season. Danielle felt that she had let down her coach and her teammates. She was supposed to start the game that night and instead was on the inpatient psychiatric unit when the game began. She felt sluggish as she adjusted to the new medication. She worried that her time in the hospital would result in her losing her place in the rotation. While in the hospital, she begged to go to the gym to work out. The hospital environment was far from ideal; there was some group therapy, short periods of individual therapy, a daily visit from the psychiatrist, but minimal physical activity. She was bored and scared. In addition, the coach was concerned that Danielle's natural enthusiasm and high energy, which made her potentially a great player, would be negatively affected by an additional medication.

Assessment and Treatment Plan After Hospitalization

Danielle was provided with a log book. The instructions were for Danielle to rate mood, energy, activity, and mental state. Mood charting is a common tool in the treatment of bipolar disorder so that relationships among life events, activities of daily living, and mood can be identified. She was willing to do this and brought her charts with her to her appointments. She was not to use caffeine in any form nor any other stimulants. Danielle again denied using alcohol or other recreational drugs.

She read up on the new medicine and found that many patients gain weight, some upward of 20 lb during this treatment, but this did not happen during the remainder of the season. Danielle played in most games and averaged 5–8 points per game. During the summer between junior and senior years, Danielle continued to work on her basketball skills and took two summer classes. She realized that she had gained 10 lb during the summer, so decreased her dosage of Abilify without medical supervision. Unfortunately, she had a relapse, becoming manic again. She told us that she would rather suffer the emotional turmoil of bipolar disorder than ruin her chances of a sports career by gaining more weight. The psychiatrist recommended going back to the original dosage, but this was refused. However, Danielle agreed to increase the frequency and the intensity of the non-pharmacological interventions.

Pathways Intervention Plan

Level One: Slow breathing, mindfulness, and cooling Danielle was instructed in mindful slow breathing and responded well. She found a breathing app on her phone that helped her focus. The recommended practice frequency was twice a day for 5 minutes of formal practice and shorter periods during the day if she felt that her thoughts were scattered.

Mindfulness training became an important part of Danielle's therapy, based on documented effectiveness for patients with bipolar disorder (Deckersbach et al., 2012; Haase et al., 2015; Ives-Deliperi, Howells, Stein, Meintjes, & Horn, 2013). This intervention can be used as a Level One strategy if it involves mindful breathing, or as a higher level intervention if it is coupled with cognitive therapy (Howells, Laurie Rauch, Ives-Deliperi, Horn, & Stein, 2014), as will be discussed later. Slow focused breathing was a challenge for Danielle since at rest her breath rate was 16 breaths a minute and her mind was easily distracted. The therapist conducted paced breathing with Danielle, a few minutes at a time. Suggestions of directing the breath through the body were easier for her; her breath slowed and her mind focused first on the lower body, then the central body and finally the upper body, including the head. The therapist spoke: "first direct your calming breath to your feet, lower and upper legs; the breath carries comfort and relaxation to the lower body…"; this process continued to the middle or central body and finally the neck and head. A phone app with phrasing similar to this was suggested and implemented by Danielle.

Danielle had the option of icing her muscles after rigorous practice sessions and she took advantage of it. Icing was soothing to her and she imagined that not only were her muscles cooling after exertion but also that she was cooling (calming) her mind. Icing helped her relax and slowly decrease the high energy levels summoned during a hard practice or after a game. We considered icing as a Level One self-care intervention.

Pathways Level Two: Passive relaxation Autogenic training was chosen as the relaxation option in Level Two (Davis, Eshelman, & McKay, 2008). Since mindful breathing in Level One consisted of directing the breath to three sections of the body, the autogenic phrases provided an ideal complement to mindful breathing in addition to providing the foundation for biofeedback which would come later. The autogenic phrases were taught and practiced in the same order. Suggestions of heaviness and warmth in the arms and legs and cooling of the face were made. Danielle described the sensations of heaviness as odd at first and questioned whether she would feel heavy when she was playing basketball which would not be a welcome sensation. The therapist carefully explained that heaviness associated with relaxation is appropriate, but that during physical activity, she would not experience this sensation; instead, the goal would be focused attention on the moment.

Pathways Level Three: Acceptance and Commitment therapy, thermal biofeedback, and health education   A series of thermal biofeedback sessions was implemented after the psychophysiological assessment revealed that Danielle usually had cool finger temperatures, ranging from 80° to 88°. This was unusual for an athlete whose performance depends on excellent circulation; in her case, we hypothesized that a cooler hand temperature than expected was evidence of over-arousal mediated by sympathetic/parasympathetic imbalance. Danielle mastered the passive relaxation technique and was able to warm her hands to 94° reliably. She appreciated the experience of being in control of her physiological reactions and accepted the feedback as "proof" of her progress in building self-efficacy and stabilizing her mood.

Acceptance and commitment therapy (ACT) was the mainstay of the Level Three interventions for Danielle. Danielle exhibited a tendency to perfectionism. When her performance in the classroom or particularly on the court fell short of her goals for that course or that game, she verbalized merciless self-criticism, reminiscent of her parents' verbal abuse, which then increased her anxiety and lowered her mood. She became depressed about her "failure," then anxious about the possibility of another failure in the next game (Stoeber & Janssen, 2011). Her ACT therapist guided Danielle to recognize that the poor performance was a disappointment, not a life-altering event, nor a condemnation of herself as a person. She learned to accept the reality of the poor performance, while realizing that her labels of "failure" were not realistic. Danielle believed in hard work and passion for what she chose to do; these values were emphasized in therapy and the anxiety associated with what was perceived as less than adequate performance was accepted, then redirected to a framework of personal growth (Orsillo, Roemer, Block Lerner, & Tull, 2011). Gradually, the "parental voices" (critical words and phrases that she had heard in childhood and adolescence) were quieted and mood became more stable.

Education about her bipolar disorder illness was also crucial in helping Danielle understand potential triggers for relapse and ways to decrease the impact of those stimuli (Lim, Nathan, O'Brien-Malone, & Williams, 2004; Mondimore, 2014). Health education—provided by a health educator, health coach, nurse, or counselor—can facilitate patients to more effectively manage their own illness, whether a chronic medical condition or mental health disorder.

Challenges

Prior to Danielle's senior year, a new basketball coach was hired who unfortunately had little understanding of psychiatric issues in student athletes and no appreciation for Danielle's struggles with mental illness. She did not understand why traveling across time zones was so difficult and actually suggested that if Danielle couldn't adjust to travel, maybe she should not undertake road games. This suggestion was devastating to Danielle. It is true that disruption in circadian rhythms and the resulting sleep deprivation is difficult for those with bipolar disorder and that good consistent sleep lowers the risk for mania (Frank et al., 2006; Gruber et al., 2011). However, staying behind from the road games was not an option in Danielle's mind. She proposed to the coach that she would utilize yoga and slow breathing at bedtime (White, 2014), but the coach was not persuaded.

Arrangements were made for the coach to speak with another psychiatrist at the medical center, who was not involved in Danielle's treatment. The physician provided an excellent explanation of bipolar disorder, asserting that Danielle's basic athletic ability was not affected by her illness and that she was working hard to maintain mood stability with medication and other non-pharmacologic interventions. The psychiatrist had treated many other student athletes and was able to thoughtfully reassure the coach that mood disorders may not be cured, but can often be effectively managed. She offered to remain in contact with the coach should there be additional concerns, but there were none after that occasion.

Follow-up: Continued Use of Pathways Skills to Manage Mood

Five years after graduation, Danielle was finished with her professional basketball career, which had occurred mostly overseas. During her playing years, there had been several relapses of her mood disorder, but each time Danielle was able to identify her triggers and the early signs of imbalance in mood. Residual symptoms are not uncommon in stable bipolar disorder; patients should be educated on this topic so that they can prevent worsening of symptoms which could require hospitalization (Miklowitz, 2011; Samalin et al., 2014). After her relapses, Danielle was able to recover a more stable mood state through medication adjustments, which remained the mainstay of treatment (Smith, Cornelius, Warnock, Bell, & Young, 2007). However, utilizing the nonpharmacological interventions daily was also critical to mood stability. No additional hospitalizations had been necessary at last contact.

Major Depressive Disorder: the case of Cherie

The Case of Cherie Cherie was a 58-year-old nurse at the local hospital. She came to the clinic because of a prolonged grief reaction to her husband's death. She had been on leave from her job to care for her husband, and had returned to work, but was not functioning well. She was missing work for various reasons. Some days, she could not drag herself out of bed; other days, she could not face another day of taking care of sick people. Her husband had died a year ago from an aggressive cancer. A close friend of Cherie's, another nurse at the hospital, finally confronted Cherie in a kind, concerned manner. The friend knew Cherie and her husband and had witnessed several conflicted interactions, so it didn't seem normal to her that Cherie remained grief stricken 1 year later. The friend accompanied Cherie to her first appointment at the clinic. During the evaluation, Cherie was tearful, talked slowly, and demonstrated psychomotor retardation. Her answers were quietly spoken and guarded. Her mental status exam showed deficits in immediate recall and recent past memory. There was no evidence of psychosis, and suicidal thoughts, plan or intent were denied. The diagnosis was complicated bereavement disorder and major depressive disorder.

Major depressive disorder is a very common mood disorder among adults which results in high disease burden, significant costs of care, and sometimes lifelong impairments. Similarly to treatment of bipolar disorder, psychopharmacology is an important part of management of recurrent major depression, but lifestyle changes and non-pharmacological interventions are vital to obtain remission and to maintain optimal functioning long term. Psychotherapy, social support, and medication adherence are associated with longer periods of remission and fewer episodes of depression (Altman et al., 2006).

Depression is characterized by low mood (sadness), loss of motivation, lack of interest, lethargy, and a pessimistic view of oneself, the environment, and the future (APA, 2013). Moderate or severe symptoms are often associated with thoughts of self-harm. Patients report suicidal ideations ranging from passive thoughts (such as being better off dead) to active cognitions, careful planning, and attempts to kill themselves. Depression interferes with all aspects of the person's life, from daily self-care to interactions with family and work performance. Depressed employees are pessimistic and lower in productivity due to fatigue and poor concentration. There is no correlation between age of illness onset and severity of impairment or number of affective episodes (Mehta et al., 2014). Persons with major depressive disorder are at greater risk of accidents at the workplace because of lower motivation and less concern about safety (McIntyre, Liauw, & Taylor, 2011). The global burden of disease from this mood disorder is increasing both from the specific effects of depression and the correlation between depression and cardiovascular disease (Topic et al., 2013). As discussed in subsequent chapters, there is significant comorbidity between depression and heart disease attributed in part to chronic inflammation.

"Depression interferes with all aspects of the person's life, from daily self-care to interactions with family and work performance. Depressed employees are pessimistic and lower in productivity due to fatigue and poor concentration. There is no correlation between age of illness onset and severity of impairment or number of affective episodes (Mehta, Mittal, & Swami, 2014)."

Multiple factors including genetic predisposition contribute to the emergence of symptoms. Those abused physically, emotionally, or sexually or neglected during childhood are at risk for recurrent and persistent depression (Nanni, Uher, & Danese, 2012). In comparison to bipolar disorder, milder impairments are associated with major depressive disorder, in terms of work productivity, interpersonal functioning, and cognitive impairment, but the experience of the patient who is depressed still involves intense suffering.

Depression affects the body as well as the person's cognitive and emotional states (Stapelberg, Neumann, Shum, McConnel, & Hamilton-Craig, 2015). Linkages among depression and hypertension, coronary heart disease, and Type 2 diabetes illustrate the concept that chronic stress and underlying inflammation may be common denominators (Howren, Lamkin & Suls, 2009; Miller, Maletic, & Raison, 2009). Recent meta-analyses confirmed the association between elevated levels of C-reactive protein, interleukins 1 and 6 and depression (Dowlati et al., 2010; Gimeno et al., 2009; Lopresti, Hood, & Drummond, 2013). Patients with low mood also manifest autonomic dysfunction, specifically low heart rate variability (Vasudev, Cha, & McIntyre, 2015). Frequent activation of the stress response system results in changes in neuroendocrine responses, such as cortisol dysregulation (Deshpande et al., 2014). For example, trait emotion (positive or negative) is related to cortisol levels at awakening and total output. Flattened cortisol curves are associated with increased sensitivity to stress and are also the result of frequent stress (Ong, Fuller-Rowell, Bonanno, & Almeida, 2011).

Losses that occur during life, such as jobs or financial downturns, are expected to produce short-term grief reactions, which usually resolve with time and support from others. More severe life-changing losses, such as spousal death, are expected to produce both more acute symptoms and longer lasting impairments. Although initial grief reactions are socially sanctioned, family and friends assume that grief will subside within 6 months and be significantly reduced in 1 year. Persistence of symptoms signals the development of persistent complex bereavement disorder (APA, 2013). There are several factors that impede resolution of the grief, such as guilt, the violent nature of the death, or questionable circumstances. Those with a history of recurrent depression are at greater risk for complicated bereavement.

Medical management is important in the treatment of depression and the selective serotonin reuptake inhibitors are commonly prescribed by primary care physicians. Unfortunately, patients often do not continue the medicine for a minimum of 4 weeks to determine efficacy. Changes are then made to the regimen and patients can remain frustrated at lack of progress (Kemp, Gordon, Rush, & Williams, 2008). Several types of psychotherapy are effective. For example, cognitive behavioral therapy in particular requires active patient engagement and frequent homework as patients learn and then practice countering negative thoughts and beliefs. Psychodynamic psychotherapy in contrast focuses on identifying areas of conflict, building mature defense mechanisms and exploring and resolving past traumatic memories.

Cherie's History: Chronic Recurrent Depression Cherie described struggles with low self-esteem since the early years of college. She found the subject material in the nursing major to be difficult and questioned her decision to be a nurse. But when the clinical training began, Cherie performed very well; she enjoyed taking care of patients. Her supervisors complimented her on her nursing and communication skills, which increased Cherie's confidence. Disruptions in mood occurred less frequently as she built her success history. Graduation brought a good job offer and Cherie began her nursing career at a large urban hospital.

Cherie met her husband Eric, a purchasing officer at the same hospital, at an employee event. They married 2 years later. Cherie experienced post-partum depression after the births of both of their children. Supportive therapy was recommended by her obstetrician, but each time Cherie discontinued after a few sessions, saying that her return to work would "bring me back to normal." Periods of low mood occurred at intervals, but each time, mood lifted within a few months. Eric was not supportive or patient during these times, criticizing Cherie when she was in her most vulnerable mindset. He complained that she didn't manage the household bills well enough, she didn't pay enough attention to the kids, or she wasn't promoted at her job, and he felt that he had too much of the financial responsibilities. One day, during an argument about family finances, Eric pushed Cherie to the wall and threatened her. She was devastated by this and began to think about leaving him. Around the same time, there were subtle changes at the hospital, producing an increasing malaise among the nurses who worked alongside Cherie. The atmosphere became more and more negative, raising doubts in her mind about the meaning of her work.

At the end of the evaluation session, Cherie was asked whether she would return and she agreed. Knowing her history with previous therapists, it was important to ask her for commitment to at least begin the process. She was already on an antidepressant, sertraline (Zoloft), prescribed by her family medicine physician. Cherie seemed disconnected from her job, which in the past had given her a sense of being part of something important and vital to the community of sick men and women. An exaggerated grief response was in evidence, and there was a need to explore and resolve this conflict before Cherie decided to leave therapy as she had in the past.

The Pathways model was implemented. However, the team felt that elements of Level One, Two, and Three should be intermingled and the path to Level Three accelerated. On the one hand, she needed the self-regulation activities of Level One so that she could begin to gain more of a sense of control. On the other hand, her depression was severe and suicidal risk a concern, so early professional intervention (Level Three) seemed time-urgent.

Pathways Intervention Plan

Pathways Levels One and Three: Mindful breathing, heart rate variability biofeedback, and interpersonal therapy The goal of Level One is to restore normal rhythms so mindful breathing training began. At the same time, Cherie's therapist began heart rate variability biofeedback (Level Three), which utilizes paced breathing to produce optimal heart rhythms and restore autonomic nervous system regulation. Heart rate variability biofeedback has also been demonstrated to assist depressed persons to lift mood, while enabling patients to take a more active role in their care (Katsamanis, 2016).

Cherie was fascinated by the biofeedback; first, seeing her highly maladaptive breathing pattern reflected her feelings—that she was depressed that and could not cope. Interestingly, Cherie said that low heart rate variability was "proof" that she was depressed and her body was demonstrating what she felt. Observing her pattern slowly improve with a guided breathing exercise gave her a feeling of self-control. "When I feel better mentally, that will show up in my breathing;" to which the therapist replied "when you breathe better you will feel better mentally also." Cherie practiced breathing daily with the aid of the app called Breath2Relax. Supportive therapy was utilized to maintain motivation, to build on the therapist-client relationship, and to slowly begin to bring depression-relevant issues into the conversation.

The choice of psychotherapy for Cherie was interpersonal therapy, which focuses on conflict between persons close to the patient, grief and loss, life stressors, and inadequate social supports (Constantino, Greenberg, & Laws, 2014). It was decided that cognitive behavioral therapy might be too confrontational and there were hints that the relationship with Eric had not been a happy one. As the weeks went on, a fuller story emerged. Cherie wanted to end the marriage and had met with an attorney when Eric came home with the news that he had cancer. The prognosis was not good, even with aggressive treatment. Cherie's guilt became overwhelming—"I couldn't leave him to die." Eric became more and more debilitated until chemotherapy treatment was stopped to give him some quality time before death.

Cherie took a leave of absence from work, feeling partially relieved to remove that stress from her life, but concurrently, missing her friends and her routine. Those days and weeks were excruciating. Cherie's conflicting feelings and thoughts continued—ranging from "I should have left him when I had the chance" to "he needs me—how can I be so cruel?" She felt closed in, isolated and depressed. In the last days before his death, Eric wanted to "be honest" and told her that he had not loved her for a long time. He said that he wanted her to be free after he was gone. He appreciated what she had done for him during his illness, but he wanted her to forget about him and go on with her life. This conversation led to a worsening of Cherie's depression and suicidal thoughts, as she rued past decisions to put up with Eric's abuse, and regretted wasting her life with him.

In the second month of weekly therapy, Cherie announced that she was glad that Eric was dead, and these thoughts automatically made her a terrible person in her own eyes. After all, he had not abused her for the entire marriage and he was a good father. She asked the therapist if she was better off "just killing myself." The weekly therapy sessions were supplemented by phone calls to assess for suicidal intent and to gauge the need for hospitalization. Gradually, these phone calls were no longer necessary and discontinued as Cherie came to terms with her thoughts and feelings about Eric and decided that she wanted to continue to live.

Level Two: Spiritual support Cherie consulted the minister at her church and talked to him about "feeling closed in" and needing to "open up." Cherie joined a prayer group where the other participants helped her to open up to the Lord with regular prayer and time spent listening to readings from the Bible and the messages therein. Quiet time within the group was used to listen for the Lord's voice in calm and peacefulness. She volunteered for church activities, first in the church's grief support group, but she found it "too closed." The instructional groups for people wanting to join the church were a much better fit for her; these people were full of hope, searching for meaning, and yearning for a spiritual connection. Cherie's faith was deepened as she taught the tenets of the faith to others and participated in their initiation into the church.

After almost a year of intensive psychotherapy, Cherie felt well enough to space out the appointments. She had gone back to work in a different setting and reported that the atmosphere in her new job was more positive than at the hospital where she had worked before. Her mood was significantly improved and suicidal thoughts were denied.

Level Three: Acupuncture Unbeknownst to the team, Cherie had consulted a physician acupuncturist. This was another Level Three intervention since it was provided by a professional. There are many evolving explanations for how acupuncture affects the body, including some based on scientific research (Kawakita & Okada, 2014), but the primary model in traditional Chinese medicine is that acupuncture frees the flow of Qi or life energy within the body. Cherie described her experience of acupuncture as "liberating," being the final piece in "opening up everything that was blocked, sad, and tight." Therapy with the Pathways team was terminated on mutual decision of Cherie and her treatment team.

Follow-up

Cherie returned 2 years later to request help with the grief over the death of her best friend, who had died from cancer 3 months ago. She had attended a support group but was concerned that her mood would spiral down into severe depression again so she made contact fairly early in the grief process. The team performed an evaluation and determined that although Cherie was actively mourning the death of her friend, she did not demonstrate symptoms of pathological bereavement. There was no guilt about not doing enough for her friend nor were there memories of past intense conflicts. Cherie and her friend had shared interests in theater and music. In the last weeks of life, her friend was in Hospice and they discussed all the wonderful times they had shared. Listening to music together had comforted them both. After 4 weeks of supportive therapy and resumption of the relaxation exercises, Cherie accepted that her grief was normal and there was very minimal risk of a severe depressive episode. However, she was encouraged to continue the support group and to contact us if necessary in the future.

References

Altman, S., Haeri, S., Cohen, L. J., Ten, A., Barron, E., Galynker, I. I., et al. (2006). Predictors of relapse in bipolar disorder: A review. *Journal of Psychiatric Practice, 12*(5), 269–282.

American Psychiatric Association. (2013). *Diagnostic and statistical manual of mental disorders* (5th ed.). Arlington, VA: American Psychiatric Association.

Capuron, L., Su, S., Miller, A. H., Bremner, J. D., Goldberg, J., Vogt, G. J., et al. (2008). Depressive symptoms and metabolic syndrome: Is inflammation the underlying link? *Biological Psychiatry, 64*(10), 896–900. https://doi.org/10.1016/j.biopsych.2008.05.019

Constantino, M. J., Greenberg, R. P., & Laws, H. B. (2014). To prevent depression recurrence, interpersonal psychotherapy is a first-line treatment with long-term benefits. *Current Psychiatry, 13*(4), 33–41.

Craddock, R., & Sklar, P. (2013). Genetics of bipolar disorder. *Lancet, 381*(9878), 1652–1662.

Daruy-Filho, L., Brietzke, E., Lafer, B., & Grassi-Oliveira, R. (2011). Childhood maltreatment and clinical outcomes of bipolar disorder. *Acta Psychiatrica Scandinavica, 124*(6), 427–434.

Davis, M., Eshelman, E. R., & McKay, M. (2008). *The relaxation & stress reduction workbook* (6th ed.). Oakland, CA: New Harbinger Publications, Inc..

Deckersbach, T., Hölzel, B. K., Eisner, L. R., Stange, J. P., Peckham, A. D., Dougherty, D. D., et al. (2012). Mindfulness-based cognitive therapy for nonremitted patients with bipolar disorder. *CNS Neuroscience & Therapeutics, 18*(2), 133–141.

Deshpande, S. S., Kalmegh, B., Patil, P. N., Ghate, M. R., Sarmukaddam, S., & Paralikar, V. P. (2014). Stresses and disability in depression across gender. *Depression Research and Treatment, 2014*, 735307. https://doi.org/10.1155/2014/735307

Dowlati, Y., Herrmann, N., Swardfager, W., Liu, H., Sham, L., Reim, E. K., et al. (2010). A meta-analysis of cytokines in major depression. *Biological Psychiatry, 67*(5), 446–457. https://doi.org/10.1016/j.biopsych.2009.09.033

Frank, E., Gonzalez, J. M., & Fagiolini, A. (2006). The importance of routine for preventing recurrence in bipolar disorder. *American Journal of Psychiatry, 163*(6), 981–985.

Gimeno, D., Kivimaki, M., Brunner, E. J., Elovainio, M., De Vogli, R., Steptoe, A., et al. (2009). Associations of C-reactive protein and interleukin-6 with cognitive symptoms of depression: A 12-year follow-up of the Whitehall II Study. *Psychological Medicine, 39*(3), 413–423. https://doi.org/10.1017/S0033291708003723

Gruber, J., Miklowitz, D. J., Harvey, A. G., Frank, E., Kupfer, D., Thase, M. E., et al. (2011). Sleep matters: Sleep functioning and course of illness in bipolar disorder. *Journal of Affective Disorders, 134*(1–3), 416–420. https://doi.org/10.1016/j.jad.2011.05.016

Haase, L., May, A. C., Falapour, M., Isakovic, S., Simmons, A. N., Hickman, S. D., et al. (2015). A pilot study investigating changes in neural processing after mindfulness training in elite athletes. *Frontiers in Behavioral Neuroscience, 9*, 229. https://doi.org/10.3389/fnbeh.2015.00229

Howells, F. M., Laurie Rauch, H. G., Ives-Deliperi, V. L., Horn, N. R., & Stein, D. J. (2014). Mindfulness based cognitive therapy may improve emotional processing in bipolar disorder: Pilot ERP and HRV study. *Metabolic Brain Disease, 29*(2), 367–375.

Howren, M. B., Lamkin, D. M. & Suls, J. (2009). Associations of depression with C-reactive protein, IL-1 and IL-6: A metanalysis. Psychosomatic Medicine 71 (2) 171–186.

Hua, L. L., Wilens, T. E., Martelon, M., Wong, P., Wozniak, J., & Biederman, J. (2011). Psychosocial functioning, familiarity and psychiatric comorbidity in bipolar youth with and without psychotic features. *Journal of Clinical Psychiatry, 72*(3), 397–405.

Ives-Deliperi, V. L., Howells, F., Stein, D. J., Meintjes, E. M., & Horn, N. (2013). The effects of mindfulness-based cognitive therapy in patients with bipolar disorder: A controlled functional MRI investigation. *Journal of Affective Disorders, 150*(3), 1152–1157.

Katsamanis, M. (2016). Heart rate variability biofeedback for major depression. In D. Moss & F. Shaffer (Eds.), *Foundations of heart rate variability biofeedback: A book of readings* (pp. 73–75). Wheat Ridge, CO: Association for Applied Psychophysiology and Biofeedback.

Kawakita, K., & Okada, K. (2014). Acupuncture therapy: Mechanism of action, efficacy, and safety: a potential intervention for psychogenic disorders? *Biopsychosocial Medicine, 8*(4), 1–4. https://doi.org/10.1186/1751-0759-8-4

Kemp, A. H., Gordon, E., Rush, A. J., & Williams, L. M. (2008). Improving the prediction of treatment response in depression: Integration of clinical, cognitive, psychophysiological, neuroimaging, and genetic measures. *CNS Spectrums, 13*(12), 1066–1086.

Larsson, S., Aas, M., Klungsoyr, O., Agartz, I., Mork, E., Steen, N. E., et al. (2013). Patterns of childhood adverse events are associated with clinical characteristics of bipolar disorder. *BMC Psychiatry, 13*, 97. https://doi.org/10.1186/1471-244X-13-97

Leboyer, M., Soreca, I., Scott, J., Frye, M., Henry, C., Tamouza, R., et al. (2012). Can bipolar disorder be viewed as a multi-system inflammatory disease? *Journal of Affective Disorders, 141*, 1–10.

Lim, L., Nathan, P., O'Brien-Malone, A., & Williams, S. (2004). A qualitative approach to identifying psychosocial issues faced by bipolar patients. *Journal of Nervous and Mental Disease, 192*(12), 810–817.

Lopresti, A. L., Hood, S. D., & Drummond, P. D. (2013). A review of lifestyle factors that contribute to important pathways associated with major depression: Diet, sleep and exercise. *Journal of Affective Disorders, 148*, 12–27.

McIntyre, R. S., Liauw, S., & Taylor, V. H. (2011). Depression in the workforce: The intermediary effect of medical comorbidity. *Journal of Affective Disorders, 128S1*, S29–S36.

Mehta, S., Mittal, P. K., & Swami, M. K. (2014). Psychosocial functioning in depressive patients: A comparative study between major depressive disorder and bipolar affective disorder. *Depression Research and Treatment, 2014* (Article ID 302741), 6 pages. http://dx.doe.org/10.1155/2014/302741

Miklowitz, D. J. (2011). Functional impairment, stress, and psychosocial intervention in bipolar disorder. *Current Psychiatry Reports, 13*(6), 504–512.

Miller, A. H., Maletic, V., & Raison, C. L. (2009). Inflammation and its discontents: The role of cytokines in the pathophysiology of major depression. *Biological Psychiatry, 65*(9), 732–741.

Mondimore, F. M. (2014). *Bipolar disorder: A guide for patients and families* (3rd ed.). Baltimore, MD: John Hopkins University Press.

Nanni, V., Uher, R., & Danese, A. (2012). Childhood maltreatment predicts unfavorable course of illness and treatment outcome in depression: A meta-analysis. *American Journal of Psychiatry, 169*(2), 141–151.

Ong, A. D., Fuller-Rowell, T. E., Bonanno, G. A., & Almeida, D. M. (2011). Spousal loss predicts alterations in diurnal cortisol activity through prospective changes in positive emotion. *Health Psychology, 30*(2), 220–227.

Orsillo, S. M., Roemer, L., Block Lerner, J., & Tull, M. T. (2011). Acceptance, mindfulness and cognitive-behavioral therapy. In S. C. Hayes, V. M. Follette, & M. M. Linehan (Eds.), *Mindfulness and acceptance expanding the cognitive-behavioral tradition* (pp. 66–95). New York: The Guilford Press.

Price, A., & Marzani-Nissen, G. (2012). Bipolar disorders: A review. *American Family Physician, 85*(5), 483–493.

Rapport, D., Kaplish, D., McGrady, A., McGinnis, R., Whearty, K., Fine, T., et al. (2015). A descriptive analysis of factors leading to or failing to lead to a clinically meaningful recovery in bipolar disorder. *Journal of Psychiatric Practice, 21*(5), 351–358.

Rapport, D., Lynch, D., McGrady, A., Kaplish, D., McGinnis, R., & Whearty, K. (2016). Psychosocial factors and comorbidity associated with recovery in bipolar disorder. *Journal of Depression and Therapy, 1*, 11–17. https://doi.org/10.14302/issn.2476-1710.JDT-15-762

Samalin, L., Bellivier, F., Giordana, B., Yon, L., Milhiet, V., El-Hage, W., et al. (2014). Patients' perspectives on residual symptoms in bipolar disorder. *The Journal of Nervous and Mental Disease, 202*(7), 550–555.

Smith, L. A., Cornelius, V., Warnock, A., Bell, A., & Young, A. H. (2007). Effectiveness of mood stabilizers and antipsychotics in the maintenance phase of bipolar disorder: A systematic review of randomized controlled trials. *Bipolar Disorders, 9*(4), 394–412.

Stapelberg, N. J. C., Neumann, D. L., Shum, D. H. K., McConnel, H., & Hamilton-Craig, I. (2015). From physiome to pathome: A systems biology model of major depressive disorder and the psycho-immune-neuroendocrine network. *Current Psychiatry Reviews, 11*(1), 32–62.

Stoeber, J., & Janssen, D. P. (2011). Perfectionism and coping with daily failures: Positive reframing helps achieve satisfaction at the end of the day. *Anxiety, Stress, and Coping, 24*(5), 477–497. https://doi.org/10.1080/10615806.2011.562977

Topic, R., Milicic, D., Stimac, Z., Loncar, M., Velagic, V., Marcinko, D., et al. (2013). Somatic comorbidity, metabolic syndrome, cardiovascular risk, and CRP in patients with recurrent depressive disorders. *Croatian Medical Journal, 23*(12), 1672–1686.

Vasudev, A., Cha, D. S., & McIntyre, R. S. (2015). Autonomic dysfunction and depression: A biomarker of MDD across the life span. *Current Psychiatry, 11*, 1–7.

White, R. C. (2014). *Preventing bipolar relapse*. Oakland, CA: New Harbinger Inc.

Chapter 8
Pathways Approaches for Post-traumatic Stress Disorders

Abstract Post-traumatic stress disorder is a psychophysiological disorder, characterized by chronic sympathetic nervous system activation; persisting perceptual/sensory vigilance for threats; recurrent distressing memories of the event, including intrusive memories, flashbacks lived as if in the present moment, and nightmares; and a persisting negative emotional state including fear and shame. The psychophysiological basis for this disorder calls for psychophysiologically based interventions. This chapter presents the case narrative of a 29-year-old national guardsman, exposed to combat trauma, and later to civilian trauma in public safety work. His treatment followed the Pathways model, comprised of multi-modal interventions, beginning with self-directed behavioral changes, then the acquisition of skills (including self-hypnosis), and finally professional treatment including clinical hypnosis and EMDR.

Keywords Post-traumatic stress disorder · Psychophysiological · Hypnosis · Neurofeedback · EMDR

Introduction: Trauma is a Psychophysiological Phenomenon

> "During World War II an American psychiatrist, Abram Kardiner, called the disorder affecting soldiers after combat a physioneurosis, meaning that it is at the same time physiological and a nervous condition."

During World War II, Abram Kardiner, called the disorder affecting soldiers after combat trauma a "physioneurosis," meaning that it is at the same time physiological and a nervous condition (Kardiner, 1941). Traumatic experiences impact mind and body and full-fledged post-traumatic stress disorder is a psychophysiological illness, with measurable changes in

This chapter is adapted with the permission of Taylor and Francis from a previous version which appeared as: D. Moss (2017), *The frustrated and helpless healer*: Pathways approaches to post-traumatic stress disorders. *International Journal of Clinical and Experimental Hypnosis, 65*(3), 336–352. doi.org/10.1080/00207144.2017.1314744.

physiology and a wide spectrum of mental and emotional effects. Today's traumatized soldiers show the same five markers that Kardiner described 75 years ago: a persistent startle response and irritability, preoccupation with the trauma, explosiveness and aggressive outbursts, nightmares, and interpersonal and social constriction.

One of today's leading spokespersons on traumatic experiences and PTSD, Bessel van der Kolk, has emphasized that trauma causes serious problems in affect regulation and impulse control. Many of the therapies favored today for the treatment of PTSD, such as cognitive behavioral therapy and "exposure therapy," require that patients must manage intense emotions and keep their attention focused to a degree not possible for many traumatized individuals. Van der Kolk advocates for a variety of mind-body-based therapies as first level interventions for trauma, including yoga, physical exercise, and EMDR (this therapy, eye movement desensitization and reprocessing, will be discussed later) (van der Kolk, 2014; van der Kolk et al., 2014).

This chapter applies a Pathways intervention program (McGrady & Moss, 2013) for a combat veteran with PTSD and utilizes a variety of mind-body skills and strategies in addressing the individual's traumatic memories and post-traumatic symptoms. These psychophysiological interventions are delivered within the context of an integrative multi-modal program of behavioral and lifestyle change.

The patient was a 29-year-old National Guardsman who served in Iraq until injured by an improvised explosive device (IED). His post-traumatic symptoms were noticeable, and he received some treatment at a veterans' medical facility, but his condition remained manageable until he began service as a local public safety officer, cross-trained in both police and fire service, and encountered a series of traumatic incidents.

Introducing Francesco

Francesco was the first born of two sons in an Italian-American family. He grew up in a close knit Catholic family, in an urban neighborhood in the Midwest. His father was a former Marine and a police officer and his mother was a dispatcher. Francesco played baseball in high school and earned a B+/A− grade point. He earned a partial scholarship to a large Midwestern university for baseball and gained admittance to the criminal justice program. He found that he couldn't play sports and keep up his grades, so he gave up his scholarship, reduced his course load, and worked two jobs to pay expenses.

Francesco entered the National Guard while in college to further defray college costs. He was proud of serving and declared his willingness to be assigned to Iraq or Afghanistan if called to active duty. He qualified as an emergency medical technician (EMT) while in college. He graduated in June 2005, and was activated in August 2005, to serve for 1 year in Iraq, but his mobilization to Iraq was prolonged due to strain on active duty units at that time. During his 17th month in Iraq, the armored personnel carrier in which he was riding hit an IED (improvized explosive device) and exploded. Francesco watched one National Guardsman friend bleed to death in the wreckage of the carrier, while he himself was pinned into the side of the vehicle, and unable to assist. Francesco suffered bruises and lacerations over much of his body, and two fractures in his left arm, but remained conscious. He survived and rehabilitated without any significant physical disability.

Symptoms of acute stress disorder Francesco suffered nightmares, occasional flashbacks, and periods of heightened anxiety after the incident, and after 3 weeks, he was diagnosed with acute stress disorder (ASD). ASD is the diagnosis applied to affected individuals who show significant post-traumatic symptoms, in the immediate period after the traumatic event, before they qualify for the diagnosis of post-traumatic stress disorder (PTSD). Many individuals diagnosed with ASD later qualify for the PTSD diagnosis (APA, 2013).

Initial treatment Francesco participated in a veterans administration (VA) sponsored group therapy for veterans with combat trauma-based disorders. He grew frustrated with the group conversations, which triggered his flashbacks and anxiety, but did not alleviate his symptoms, so he discontinued the VA-sponsored services. He used willpower and running to manage his symptoms, which remained present for the next several years, but at a moderate level. Most noticeable were chronic heightened alertness and anxiety and occasional nightmares in which he re-lived the explosion. He decided to use his veteran status and his bachelor's degree in criminal justice to seek employment in either fire safety or police work. (Most police and fire service agencies give preferential status to job applicants who are veterans).

Employment as Public Safety Officer

Francesco was hired by a small municipal fire department. He learned rapidly, came to love fire service work, and upgraded his EMT certifications to strengthen his role as a first responder. After Francesco completed 2 years of service in fire safety, his municipality required all police and fire personnel to cross-train, so they were assigned to wherever there was a staffing need. Francesco enjoyed responding to medical emergencies and police crises, but came to strongly dislike road patrol, jail duty, and assignments to transport prisoners.

Trauma on the job Over the next 2 years, Francesco faced a series of traumatic incidents in the course of duty. He was called to an early morning car fire on the shoulder of an interstate, and risked his own life to pull the driver from the fire, only to discover that the driver was a shooting victim, probably dead before the fire was started. He suffered burns on his arms but also an exacerbation of his nightmares. The Iraq incident and the roadside incident became confused in his nightmares, and he dreamed of being trapped in a truck watching his guardsman friend shot and burned. Several weeks later, he was on a late-night road patrol and was called to the scene of a two-car accident. As he assisted another police officer in lifting a barely breathing adolescent victim off the pavement, he realized that it was his niece. He initially began to shake uncontrollably, but managed to get the girl into an ambulance, before he broke down sobbing.

Initial referral Francesco was referred for counseling by the Department of Public Safety, because, from his supervisor's point of view, he had "let his emotions interfere with performing his responsibilities." Francesco was referred to a group of psychologists who regularly provided critical incident debriefing for public safety officers. His assigned psychologist diagnosed post-traumatic stress disorder, based on a mixture of symptoms related to both the original Iraq incident and the two recent traumatic incidents. His psychologist encouraged Francesco to continue his running, and arranged to make Public Safety Department funds available for use of a gym facility with an indoor track, because it was hard for Francesco to keep up his running through the Midwestern winter.

Francesco was then offered a course of 10–12 sessions of eye movement desensitization and reprocessing (EMDR), which is frequently utilized for trauma. EMDR involves the therapist using hand motions to guide the patient's eyes back and forth laterally, while the patient mentally visualizes the trauma (Shapiro, 2001). In many cases, there is a lessening of subjective anxiety and a diminution of physiological activation over the course of several sessions (Sack, Lempa, Steinmetz, Lamprecht, & Hofmann, 2008). The International Society for Traumatic Stress Studies has categorized EMDR among the first rank interventions for PTSD (DeAngelis, 2008). Van der Kolk et al. (2007) found that brief EMDR reduced both PTSD and depression symptoms in most victims of adult-onset trauma. Shapiro (2014), the psychologist who developed the EMDR intervention, reviewed 24 randomized controlled trials of EMDR for treating emotional trauma and other adverse life experiences. She reported that 12 studies of the 24 showed a rapid decrease in negative emotion and/or in vividness of traumatic images. She also cited eight additional studies reporting other beneficial effects.

Francesco underwent five sessions of EMDR and reported significant lessening of nightmares and anxiety. He mentioned his improvement to his shift supervisor, which resulted in the Department canceling further sessions, explaining that from their point of view he was "sufficiently improved." Because he had been referred under a self-funded Employee Assistance Program, the employer had the right to terminate the services.

Francesco continued his running regimen and sustained improved sleep and better managed anxiety for several months, but continued to experience intrusive daytime traumatic memories as well as nightmares. He was exposed to two additional traumatic incidents in the line of duty over the next year. First, he was on road patrol and was the first to arrive at a traffic accident. The accident involved a young female patrol officer with whom he had worked closely; she had been hit head on by a drunk driver and lost her life. Two weeks later, he was summoned to a worksite accident. A utility worker in his twenties was working in a raised bucket with a chain saw, attempting to cut away fallen tree limbs following a straight-line windstorm. One of the tree limbs collapsed on the worker and his bucket, pushing the chain saw into his leg and crashing the worker and the bucket to the ground. Francesco called for backup, applied a tourniquet to the leg gashed by the saw, and held the utility worker while he died.

Francesco began to suffer daily flashbacks, more frequent nightmares, shortened sleep and increased anxiety. He found it difficult to concentrate on his work, with current events triggering flashbacks to the point that he was confused between present events and flashbacks. He asked for some days off, and this time his supervisor placed him on indefinite disability leave, and renewed the referral for psychological services. The supervisor called ahead of the initial appointment, asked to speak with the scheduled therapist, and stated his opinion that the psychological services should include "counseling this maladjusted individual out of public safety work." The supervisor stated that Francesco should never have been hired and had long-term psychological disturbances that made him unsuited for public safety work. The supervisor also stated that he hoped that psychological services could be wrapped up within a month, with a termination of employment.

The clinic director was able to intervene and arrange coverage by Francesco's health insurance program, so that the treatment course would be independent of the Department of Public Safety. This action protected his access to longer term psychological treatment, but left his public safety job in jeopardy.

Pathways Intervention

Pathways Assessment

Psychosocial and lifestyle Francesco was active socially and athletically in college. He was engaged to be married when he was mobilized, but his fiancée ended the engagement when his Iraq mobilization was extended beyond 12 months. He had a number of close friendships in the National Guard, both in his home state of Michigan and in Iraq. He sustained an exceptionally close relationship with his younger brother, Antonio, speaking with him twice a week by SKYPE™ from Iraq. He initially made friends at the Department of Public Safety, played basketball after work with other public safety officers, and dated one of the dispatchers. Although he could not clearly describe the sequence of events, he knew that something changed in him during the time period of the initial traumatic incidents in his public safety work. He found himself not answering phone calls, even from his brother and the girlfriend. He felt strangely detached in his relationships and found himself snapping at and arguing with co-workers over trivial matters. Both the friendships and his dating relationship faded away without any discussion or resolution. Looking back, Francesco could see that his self-isolation began after the second work-related trauma incident (finding his niece on the pavement), but became more severe after the later incidents (the death of his female co-worker and of the young utility worker).

Francesco continued his running schedule and felt less tense after each run. But he no longer played basketball with his co-workers and avoided break and lunch times with them. He rarely left his apartment except for work and runs and spent most evenings watching television. Both detachment in relationships and emotional constriction are symptoms of PTSD (APA, 2013, pp. 271–277).

Psychodiagnostic assessment Francesco showed sufficient signs and symptoms to meet the DSM-V diagnosis for post-traumatic stress disorder, with dissociative symptoms (DSM-V Code 309.81). He suffered significant impairment from his symptoms for over 1 month. He reported the following symptoms/diagnostic markers for PTSD:

- Direct experience of a life-threatening event, fatal to a significant other
- Recurrent distressing memories of the event, including intrusive memories, flashbacks lived as if present moment, and nightmares
- Persisting emotional state including fear and shame
- Loss of interest in once regular activities
- Marked detachment from others
- Hypervigilance
- Unprovoked irritability
- Sleep disturbance
- Moderate levels of dissociation, feeling as if he were watching life without being engaged in it

Readiness for change Francesco appeared to be strongly motivated for change and ready to implement change. He rated himself at the 8–9 level on the Stages of Change Ruler, and behaviorally showed signs of being solidly in the Preparation for Change stage, with some indications of moving into the action stage (DeSalle & Agley, 2015). He had persisted in running throughout the time period of his worsening PTSD symptoms. He initiated the request for psychological services, and in his first interview he asked whether there was a way that he could continue in treatment if his employer again attempted to terminate the services. The pathways treatment team viewed these actions as indications of his high readiness for change. Francesco readily agreed to work with both a health coach and a psychologist on the Pathways team to facilitate his recovery.

Pathways Interventions

Level One Pathways Activities

Level One in the Pathways Model consists of self-directed behavior and lifestyle changes, with the goal of restoring biological rhythms, re-establishing psychosocial supports, and eliminating/moderating any health risk factors.

Level One Pathways activity: Running The choice of Level One activities was discussed at length with Francesco. Because Francesco was already a runner, he asked if he could continue running and "get credit for this" as a Pathways Level One activity. In general, persons with PTSD, especially those with heightened autonomic nervous system arousal, are physically less active compared to healthy normal persons (Vancamfort et al., 2016). Research has shown that physical exercise can moderate depression, anxiety, and PTSD symptoms (Manger & Motta, 2005; Smith, 2015). Francesco committed to running for at least 30 minutes 4 days a week, a slight increase over his average frequency at the time of initial evaluation.

Level One Pathways activity: Breathing   Breath training and the regular practice of paced diaphragmatic breathing are effective tools to reduce anxiety, including the anxiety accompanying PTSD. Scotland-Coogan and Davis (2016) proposed combining breath training with mindfulness training, yoga, and meditation, as a supplement to psychotherapy for PTSD. A study in the Netherlands showed that adding biofeedback-assisted breath training to trauma focused cognitive behavioral therapy (TF-CBT) produced a quicker reduction in PTSD symptoms in an adult sample than treatment with TF-CBT alone (Rosaura Polak, Witteveen, Denys, & Olff, 2015).[1]

Francesco's health coach taught him to do a simple mindful breathing exercise, with an emphasis on breathing slowly, evenly, gently, smoothly, and mindfully, at a rate of approximately six breaths per minute. Francesco learned to follow a breath training "app" on his iPhone called Breathing Zone, which guides one to breathe with the expansion and contraction of a lotus blossom, and the waxing and waning of a sound track, at a breathing rate set by the trainee. (The "app" provides a variety of audio and image choices so each user can customize the display).

Level One activity: Communicate   Because of his extreme isolation, Francesco's Pathways health coach asked him to consider whether there was anyone he would feel comfortable making contact with on some regular basis. He hesitated and then decided that he was ready to resume phone calls and possibly SKYPE calls with his brother two or more times a week. He also set the goal of phoning a friend from the National Guard, Brad, who was at the same base in Iraq at the time of Francesco's injuries. He set a goal of calling Brad once, before he would consider commiting to a more challenging goal.

Level One Progress

Francesco reported some initial feelings of resistance to running, now that it was "prescribed" by someone else. He was able to remind himself that he had personally requested this goal, and this recognition reduced his resistance. He ran in late afternoons or early evening and found himself calmer both during and after his runs. He was able to sit quietly and practice his paced diaphragmatic breathing after his runs.

Francesco found the paced breathing soothing. Initially, he practiced only when he was already calm, so he could concentrate on his breathing more easily. After the first week, however, he began to use paced breathing to calm himself whenever he became anxious and whenever he recognized some sensory cue for his traumatic memories. He found that his everyday anxieties calmed and when he experienced a memory related to his injuries in Iraq or any of his police/fire service traumas, he could accept the memory and allow it to emerge, but with greater calmness.

---

[1] TF-CBT is a form of psychotherapy, which is empirically supported by extensive outcome research (Seidler & Wagner, 2006).

Throughout the first 2 weeks, Francesco made excuses to himself not to call his brother or his National Guard friend, Brad. As his 2-week appointment with his Pathways health coach approached, he felt a sense of pressure to prove that he was serious about change, and called his brother Antonio at midnight on the evening before the appointment. They talked for 3 hours. He felt a tremendous release as he poured out to his brother the events of the last 2 years, and especially when his brother voiced his acceptance and support. Francesco promised Antonio to call him regularly and visit soon, and Antonio promised to pursue him if he broke contact again. Francesco reported feeling less alone with his trauma and recommitted to contact with Antonio and his friend Brad.

Level Two Pathways Activities

Level Two in the Pathways model consists of the acquisition of self-regulation, coping skills, and wellness practices, aided by educational materials (smart phone "apps," YouTube videos, educational CDs, handouts) as well as community-based resources.

Level Two activity: Self-hypnosis One of the effects of traumatic experiences is a chronic state of perceptual/sensory vigilance and physiological hyperarousal. The individual experiences an immediate sense of danger as though the traumatic event were still present. Clinical hypnosis has long been recognized as a powerful tool to facilitate muscular relaxation, moderate autonomic nervous system activation, reduce chronic perceptual/sensory vigilance, and conduct therapeutic affective abreaction following trauma (Barabasz & Barabasz, 2013; Spiegel & Cardena, 1990), and two recent meta-analyses supported its effectiveness as a treatment for PTSD (O'Toole, Solomon, & Bergdahl, 2016; Rotaru & Rusu, 2015).

Francesco inquired about using hypnosis as a coping strategy and after discussion he requested to include self-hypnosis as a Level Two coping strategy. Francesco's Pathways psychologist conducted a hypnotic session with him, including the Elkins Hypnotizability Scale (Elkins, 2014; Kekecs, Bowers, Johnson, Kendrick, & Elkins, 2016). Francesco's score was 8, placing him in the high range of hypnotic ability, and suggesting that hypnosis would be an effective intervention for his post-traumatic stress symptoms. Francesco's psychologist carried out two self-hypnosis scripts with him in the remainder of that single hypnotic session, and provided him with handouts with instructions for these and two additional auto-hypnosis techniques. His instructions were to begin practicing these hypnotic scripts on his own at home, remaining with each script for a full week.

Script One. Eye fixation and breathing, with staircase imagery Initially, the therapist invited Francesco to breathe slowly while staring at the wall across from him. He then was instructed to allow his eyes to drift upward (keeping the head stationary while the eyes moved) until some place on the wall, above eye level, drew his attention. Then, he was to remain focused on that spot and notice the deepening heaviness and fatigue in his eyelids until he began to blink and eventually could no longer resist eye closure. Once his eyes closed, he was invited to visualize himself at the top of a staircase of 20 steps leading downward into a profoundly safe and tranquil place. He was instructed to count downward from 20 as he descended the stairs and notice the deepening safety and calm enveloping him as he descended each step. Once in the tranquil and secure hall, "deep within his own mind," he was invited to experience himself cherishing the peacefulness of this sanctuary, repeating the words "safe" and "relax" to himself, savoring the comfort and tranquility, and "saving up" the experience for moments when it might be helpful. Finally, he was instructed to slowly ascend, counting his way back up to 20, and retain the experience to be recalled whenever he repeated the words "safe" and "relax," and whenever he pictured himself descending the staircase.

Script Two. Eye roll with soothing breath The second script was designated for Francesco to use after a week of practice with Script One. Script Two was recommended whenever he felt anxiety but lacked the privacy or the time for the first script. Francesco was taught to sit comfortably in his chair, and on the count of one, two, three to:

- Roll his eyes up and back into his skull, as far as was comfortable
- Take a long gentle in-breath and hold that breath while he continued to hold his eyes up and back in his head
- Release his breath slowly and allow his eyes to close

Francesco showed a dramatic amount of sclera (white area) in the eyes during the eye roll, believed by some to be another positive indication of hypnotic ability (Spiegel & Spiegel, 2004). He was encouraged to practice these self-hypnotic inductions whenever he had a free moment, and especially to practice when he felt acute anxiety coming on, or the beginnings of a flashback or traumatic memory.

Scripts Three and Four Once Francesco had practiced the first two scripts to the point of complete automaticity, he was encouraged to begin experimenting with Scripts Three and Four, which used muscle relaxation (Script Three) and imagery of a peaceful scene (Script Four) to induce trance and relaxation.

Level Two activity: Yoga classes A leading expert on trauma treatment, Bessel Van der Kolk, has promoted yoga as a beneficial practice for patients with trauma histories (Interlandi, 2014; van der Kolk, 2014). Francesco's Pathways health coach suggested yoga, and Francesco recalled a positive experience with a yoga class during his college years. He selected a twice-weekly Hatha yoga class at a nearby yoga center as a Level Two activity, and began attending. He also purchased an educational CD with demonstrations and instructions for conducting hatha yoga at home.

Level Two Progress

Francesco found self-hypnosis a useful tool for calming his anxieties and diminishing his sensitivity to trauma-related cues. Initially, he favored long sessions of self-hypnosis using eye fixation and the staircase image. He said he often felt like Jello®, with almost no tension anywhere in his mind or body after a session. This was a breakthrough for him after years of vigilant nervous activation. Over time he learned that he could induce a moderate trance by means of a quick eye roll, with a long inhalation and exhalation, or a combination of slow paced breathing and soothing images. In this way, he could deal with anxiety or re-experiencing of traumatic memories, in the moment, wherever he was in his everyday world.

> "The psychotherapist guided Francesco through a series of hypnotic inductions and deepening steps, to elicit progressively deeper trance states. He was guided to experience a lessening of his chronic vigilance and baseline tensions, and a deepened sense of safety."

Francesco found yoga satisfying and compared it to running. He felt more settled in his body when posing in a yoga asana, and felt calmer at the end, especially after the brief period of yogic breathing at the end of each class. Occasionally, he experienced flashbacks—upsurges of traumatic memories, experienced as vivid present-moment experiences—during yoga class and even during yoga practice at home. His Pathways coach encouraged him to use his new self-hypnosis skills to calm himself whenever traumatic memories occurred. He was somewhat anxious about doing yoga when it first began to trigger traumatic memories, but when he learned that the memories lost their intensity with repetition and with his self-hypnosis, he felt more confident in continuing yoga. The onset of traumatic memories themselves became less intimidating.

Level Three Pathways Treatment

Level Three activities in the Pathways Model consist of professional interventions by psychologists, physicians, and other health professionals. The patient is encouraged to continue the Level One and Two Pathways activities during the Level Three treatment programs and to continue them as elements in their new lifestyle after treatment ends.

Level Three intervention: Hypnotically assisted psychotherapy Francesco's Level Three treatment began with hypnotically assisted psychotherapy, with the goals of reducing baseline autonomic activation, desensitizing traumatic memories, and ameliorating chronic anxiety and negative affect. The psychotherapist guided Francesco through a series of hypnotic inductions and deepening steps to elicit progressively deeper trance states. The suggestions were to experience a lessening of his chronic vigilance and persisting everyday tensions. He was given several cues to add to his daily self-hypnosis to deepen his sense of safety.

Next, the therapist used a series of dissociative images while Francesco remained in a profoundly relaxed trance state, viewing past traumatic events on a film screen, viewing them through clouded windows, and viewing them at a comfortable distance. Then, he was guided to enter the memories, navigate through them, while sustaining a state of trance and safety. The purpose was to de-sensitize the memories and assist him in recovering a sense of mastery in trauma-related situations.

Level Three intervention: EMDR Francesco reported a positive response to the first trial of EMDR, for trauma in the line of public safety work, until his department chief terminated his therapy abruptly. He asked his Pathways team if he could have another course of EMDR to supplement the positive therapeutic effects he was having in hypnosis. The team psychologist agreed to alternate sessions of hypnosis and EMDR, and as Francesco once again became familiar with the process of EMDR, the psychologist began to integrate hypnosis and EMDR into the same sessions.

"The time-regressions used a staircase to deepen trance, and then introduced images of a long hallway with doors to the left and right. All of the doors on the left led to 'soothing rooms,' rooms of comforting images, and each door on the right led to a specific traumatic incident."

As mentioned above, in an EMDR session, the client selects a painful or traumatic memory as a starting point and calls this event to mind. The therapist begins to move his/her hand laterally, from left to right and back again, as the client's eyes follow from left to right and back. Typically, the client experiences a vivifying or intensifying of the remembered experience, frequently with abreactions of intense emotion. With repetition, the eye movement frequently produces a lessening of the accompanying affect. However, in many instances clients, especially those with complex and multiple trauma histories, find it difficult to persist in extended sessions because of the intensity of the emotional experience.

Integrating hypnosis and EMDR Francesco chose to begin EMDR with images and memories from his original Iraq experiences in the armored personnel carrier. However, the imagery spontaneously shifted at times from moments of helplessness while trapped in that vehicle to experiences of helplessness in his police work. The desire to reach out and save his trapped National Guardsman friend and to rescue the injured utility worker intermingled as Francesco participated in the eye movement process. He spontaneously asked on multiple occasions whether he could use self-hypnosis to moderate the intensity of his emotion, and then stated his readiness to resume eye movement.

Level Three: Hypnotic time-regressions Later in his therapy, the psychologist guided Francesco into hypnotic time-regressions to actively revisit both the Iraq incident and his later police service traumatic scenes. The time-regressions used a staircase to deepen trance and then introduced images of a long hallway, with doors to the left and right. All of the doors on the left led to "soothing rooms," rooms of comforting images, and each door on the right led to a specific traumatic incident. Francesco was encouraged to enter the soothing rooms first and use hypnotic soothing to create a calm and sense of safety, then to enter a door on the right, leading to a traumatic memory or situation. He was invited to first observe the trauma through a colored glass window in the door, and then to enter the trauma room, but sit initially on an elevated chair close to the door, observing the scene from above. Eventually, he was encouraged to enter the scene and experience it along with his previous self. However, Francesco was also permitted to leave the trauma room at any time to seek respite in the soothing rooms.

Level Three Progress

> "The IED explosion in Iraq forced Francesco to watch helplessly as his comrade bled. He was 'a frustrated and helpless healer'—a medic who could not stop his companion's slow death."

Francesco reported a gradual decrease in his sense of tension and apprehensiveness in everyday life, as both his hypnosis and EMDR sessions continued. He began watching television shows with police trauma and occasional combat-focused films, which he could not do before. Each time he viewed traumatic scenes he found himself apprehensive, holding his breath, and tensing his musculature. Using his breath exercises and self-hypnosis, he was able to persist in watching, reduce his physiological activation, resume a relaxed breathing, and experience a sense of relief whenever some resolution was achieved on screen.

Hypnosis and psychotherapy Francesco's hypnosis was delivered in the course of ongoing psychotherapy. He became aware and articulated a new understanding of himself and his trauma, through the series of trance exposures to traumatic memories and the time-regression experiences. He came to recognize that serving as a healer or helper for persons in distress, in Iraq, in his public safety work, and in his everyday relationships was appealing to him. The IED explosion in Iraq forced Francesco to watch helplessly as his comrade bled. He was "a frustrated and helpless healer"—a medic who could not stop his companion's slow death. He re-experienced this helplessness repeatedly in the traumatic experiences during his public safety work, most acutely as he held the dying utility worker. He remembered that often in childhood, he had protected or rescued his baby brother on the playground and from neighborhood bullies. He reported a deep sense of worthlessness and uselessness, when he could no longer seem to help others. Francesco slowly accepted that his "baby brother" could now serve and help Francesco, the older brother, and that this was a natural transition in their adult relationships. Francesco's renewed sense of closeness with his brother, and his brother's expression of sadness at the lost time between them, encouraged Francesco in reaching out to other acquaintances, including co-workers.

Discussion: The Future

Francesco continued to incorporate several of his Level One and Two activities as regular parts of his lifestyle. He utilized his paced relaxed breathing and self-hypnosis several times a week to sustain a more relaxed physiology, and soothe himself emotionally. He ran regularly and almost always felt calmer afterwards. Francesco continued in his yoga class, once a week, and often practiced yoga *asanas* before his runs. He reported that he was less jumpy though he still felt a surge of reaction when he faced sensory cues eliciting traumatic memories. For example, his breath always caught when he glimpsed a bucket truck on the side of the road.

Francesco's weekly psychotherapy continued for 6 months. Thereafter, he utilized sessions of verbal therapy, hypnosis, and EMDR occasionally, about every 6–8 weeks. He continued to ask for both hypnosis and EMDR to de-sensitize residues of traumatic reactivity.

Human beings who have experienced cumulative trauma, and especially those who have developed full blown PTSD as a disorder, continue to be at a higher risk than the general population for new trauma-related symptoms. One of the key questions for Francesco was whether he should return to emergency public safety work, with the high likelihood of facing new traumatic events in his work. Francesco loved many aspects of his public safety work. The everyday positive experiences of helping others, providing emergency medical attention, and resolving community crises gratified him. Yet he recognized the cumulative load of the many traumatic situations he had experienced. He also understood that the supervisory team did not welcome his return. Research has documented that non-supportive work environments are a factor increasing the incidence of PTSD symptoms, in police work and in other settings (Maguen et al. (2009).

After several months of psychotherapy and hypnosis, Francesco elected to take a partial disability retirement from his department and sought work as a medical technician in a primary care office where the burden of traumatic events was significantly lower.

References

American Psychiatric Association. (2013). *Diagnostic and statistical manual of mental disorders* (5th ed.). Washington, DC: Author.

Barabasz, A., & Barabasz, M. (2013). Hypnosis for PTSD: Evidence-based placebo controlled studies. *Journal of Trauma and Treatment, S4*, 006. https://doi.org/10.4172/2167-1222.S4-006

DeAngelis, T. (2008). PTSD treatments grow in evidence, effectiveness. *Monitor on Psychology, 39*(1), 40.

DeSalle, M., & Agley, J. (2015, September 15). SBIRT: Identifying and managing risky substance abuse. *Counseling Today.* Tag Archives: Substance Abuse and Addictions. Retrieved from https://ct.counseling.org/tag/substance-abuse-addictions/

Elkins, G. (2014). *Hypnotic relaxation therapy: Principles and applications.* New York: Springer.

Interlandi, J. (2014, May 22). A revolutionary approach to treating PTSD. *The New York Times Magazine.* Retrieved from https://www.nytimes.com/2014/05/25/magazine/a-revolutionary-approach-to-treating-ptsd.html?_r=0

Kardiner, A. (1941). *The traumatic neuroses of war. Psychosomatic Medicine Monograph II-III.* Washington, DC: National Research Council.

Kekecs, Z., Bowers, J., Johnson, A., Kendrick, C., & Elkins, G. (2016). The Elkins Hypnotizability Scale. *International Journal of Clinical and Experimental Hypnosis, 64*(3), 285–304. https://doi.org/10.1080/00207144.2016.1171089

Maguen, S., Metzler, T. J., Moccasin, S. E., Inslicht, S. S., Henn-Hase, C., Neylan, T. C., et al. (2009). Routine work environment stress and PTSD symptoms in police. *Journal of Nervous and Mental Disease, 197*(10), 754–760.

Manger, T. A., & Motta, R. W. (2005). The impact of an exercise program on posttraumatic stress disorder, anxiety, and depression. *International Journal of Emergency Mental Health, 7*(1), 49–57.

McGrady, A., & Moss, D. (2013). *Pathways to illness, pathways to health.* New York: Springer.

Moss, D. (2017). The frustrated and helpless healer: Pathways approaches to post-traumatic stress disorders. *International Journal of Clinical and Experimental Hypnosis, 65*(3), 336–352. https://doi.org/10.1080/00207144.2017.1314744

O'Toole, S. K., Solomon, S. L., & Bergdahl, S. A. (2016). A meta-analysis of hypnotherapeutic techniques in the treatment of PTSD symptoms. *Journal of Traumatic Stress, 29*(1), 97–100. https://doi.org/10.1002/jts.22077

Rosaura Polak, A., Witteveen, A. B., Denys, D., & Olff, M. (2015). Breathing biofeedback as an adjunct to exposure in cognitive behavioral therapy hastens the reduction of PTSD symptoms: A pilot study. *Applied Psychophysiology and Biofeedback, 40*(1), 25–31. https://doi.org/10.1007/s10484-015-9268-y

Rotaru, T.-S., & Rusu, A. (2015). Meta-analysis of the efficacy of hypnotherapy for alleviating PTSD symptoms. *International Journal of Clinical and Experimental Hypnosis, 64*(1), 116–136.

Sack, M., Lempa, W., Steinmetz, A., Lamprecht, F., & Hofmann, A. (2008). Alterations in autonomic tone during trauma exposure using eye movement desensitization and reprocessing (EMDR)—Results of a preliminary investigation. *Journal of Anxiety Disorders, 22*(7), 1264–1271. https://doi.org/10.1016/j.janxdis.2008.01.007

Scotland-Coogan, D., & Davis, E. (2016). Relaxation techniques for trauma. *Journal of Evidence-Informed Social Work, 13*(5), 434–441. https://doi.org/10.1080/23761407.2016.1166845

Seidler, G. H., & Wagner, F. E. (2006). Comparing the efficacy of EMDR and trauma-focused cognitive-behavioral therapy in the treatment of PTSD: A meta-analytic study. *Psychological Medicine, 36*(11), 1515–1522.

Shapiro, F. (2001). *Eye movement desensitization and reprocessing* (2nd ed.). New York: Guilford.

Shapiro, F. (2014). The role of eye movement desensitization and reprocessing (EMDR) therapy in medicine: Addressing the psychological and physical symptoms stemming from adverse life experiences. *The Permanente Journal, 18*(1), 71–77. https://doi.org/10.7812/TPP/13-098.

Smith, J. (2015). Cognitive behavioral therapy and aerobic exercise for survivors of sexual violence with posttraumatic stress disorder: A feasibility study. *Journal of Traumatic Stress Disorders and Treatment, 4*(1), 1–6. https://doi.org/10.4172/2324-8947.1000136

Spiegel, D., & Cardena, E. (1990). New uses of hypnosis in the treatment of posttraumatic stress disorder. *Journal of Clinical Psychiatry, 51*(Suppl), 39–46.

Spiegel, H., & Spiegel, D. (2004). *Trance and treatment: Clinical uses of hypnosis* (2nd ed.). Arlington, VA: American Psychiatric Association.

van der Kolk, B. (2014). *The body keeps the score: Brain, body, and mind in the healing of trauma.* New York: Viking.

Van der Kolk, B., Spinazzola, J., Blaustein, M. E., Hopper, J. W., Hopper, E. K., Korn, D. L., et al. (2007). A randomized clinical trial of eye movement desensitization and reprocessing (EMDR), fluoxetine, and pill placebo in the treatment of posttraumatic stress disorder: Treatment effects and long-term maintenance. *Journal of Clinical Psychiatry, 68*(1), 37–46.

van der Kolk, B. A., Stone, L., West, J., Rhodes, A., Emerson, D., Suvak, M., et al. (2014). Yoga as an adjunctive treatment for posttraumatic stress disorder. *Journal of Clinical Psychiatry, 75*(6), e559–e565. https://doi.org/10.4088/JCP.13m08561

Vancamfort, D., Richards, J., Stubbs, B., Akello, G., Gbiri, C. A., Ward, P. B., et al. (2016, May). Physical activity in people with PTSD: A systematic review of correlates. *Journal of Physical Activity and Health, 13*(8), 910–918.

Chapter 9
A Pathways Approach for an Anxiety Disorder

Abstract Caregiver stress is a growing problem with an aging population; many spouses are cast in the caregiver role for extended periods. Pre-existing anxiety disorders commonly recur in the face of caregiver stress. This chapter narrates the case of a 71-year-old retired professional woman, serving as caregiver for a husband with dementia. The stress of the caregiver role served to trigger a recurrence of a previously treated anxiety disorder. The case narrative illustrates the value of breath training and heart rate variability biofeedback for the anxiety disorder, as well as an effort to instill sustainable self-regulation skills and lifestyle changes for greater resilience in this long-term situation.

Keywords Caregiver stress · Anxiety disorder · Lifestyle medicine · Heart rate variability · Mindfulness · Acceptance and commitment therapy

Introduction

Anxiety is a normal dimension of human experience. Anxiety, fear, and worry are experienced by most human beings when major life transitions emerge and when threatening or unmanageable situations occur (Moss, 2016b). Anxiety becomes an anxiety disorder when it becomes persistent (generally at least 6 months in duration), significantly impairs everyday life functioning, and meets the diagnostic criteria in the DSM-V or ICD-10.

Once present, anxiety disorders are often chronic, with a relapsing and remitting pattern in the life cycle. An 8-year American longitudinal study showed varying rates of recurrence of anxiety disorders, for a variety of anxiety disorders, as high as

This chapter is adapted with permission of the Association for Applied Psychophysiology and Biofeedback from a previous version that appeared as: D. Moss (2016a), The house is crashing down on me: Integrating mindfulness, breath training, and heart rate variability biofeedback for an anxiety disorder in a 71-year old caregiver. Biofeedback, 44(3), 160-167. doi: 10.5298/1081-5937-44.3.02.

64% for women with panic disorder (Yonkers, Bruce, Dyck, & Keller, 2003). Dutch researchers recently documented that recurrence rates are consistently higher if we look beyond the artificial confines of DSM-V diagnoses. When they limited their measurements only to the recurrence of anxiety disorders with the same diagnosis, recurrence rates were approximately 24% overall, but when other anxiety disorders were included, the recurrence rate was approximately 55%, and in populations with comorbid anxiety and depressive disorders the recurrence rate was 66% (Scholten et al., 2016).

When life stress is more severe, the symptoms of anxiety proliferate and the anxiety disorder intensifies. The anxiety disorders in the DSM-V include panic disorder, agoraphobia, specific phobia, generalized anxiety disorder, social anxiety disorder, separation anxiety disorder, and selective mutism (American Psychiatric Association, 2013).

Introducing Judy

At the time Judy was referred for evaluation, she was a 71-year-old retired social worker, and wife of a retired dentist with debilitating Alzheimer's disease. She was also a mother of four adult children and grandmother of six. Judy was embarrassed to ask for professional help. She had experienced anxiety of varying severity intermittently throughout her adult years, commencing in college years. However, she had completed several periods of counseling for her anxiety and thought that her accumulated coping skills should be more effective now. She also had prided herself in helping anxious clients herself in her decades as a clinical social worker. She apologized repeatedly for taking up the psychologist's time and assured the clinic staff that she probably would not need lengthy services.

History

Initial Course of Illness

Judy grew up in a professional family, with a physician mother and an attorney father. She was a gifted child both academically and musically, and aspired in adolescent years to a career as a concert pianist. Her father was a cellist, and he nurtured her interests in music with special summer institutes and family travel to attend major orchestral performances. She attended a private liberal arts college and was encouraged in her musical dreams by the music faculty.

Initial onset of anxiety disorder In the fall of her sophomore year, her father died suddenly of a heart attack, and Judy felt that her world was coming apart. She flew home from college for her father's funeral. When severe turbulence affected the flight, she developed a panic attack with fears of the plane crashing. The panic per-

"Judy began shaking physically during this initial conversation, and experienced her worst panic attack yet, with rapid breathing, rapid heart rate, and a physical sense of *the house crashing down on her body.*"

sisted throughout the flight. She experienced a recurrence of the panic when viewing her father's body and again at the funeral. She was able to return to college although she arranged for a cousin to drive her back to campus to avoid another flight. She experienced intermittent panic around thoughts of her father's absence from her life, yet managed to complete her fall semester courses.

When Judy returned home for Christmas vacation, her mother discussed a need for Judy to interrupt her studies at the private college. The family's finances were devastated by the deceased father's law firm debts. Both the father and his business partner had taken on substantial loans to expand the firm, signing to personally guarantee the loans, and his sudden death left the firm and the family in crisis. Judy's mother asked her to leave the private college for at least the spring semester and to consider enrolling at a nearby community college. Judy began shaking physically during this conversation, and experienced her worst panic attack yet, with rapid breathing, rapid heart rate, and a physical sense of *the house crashing down on her body.*

Previous management of disorder Judy sought out counseling in the months after returning to the family home. Her initial counselor was warm and encouraging, but non-directive and inexperienced with anxiety disorders. Judy's family physician, a close friend of her mother, intervened and arranged for her to work with a female clinical psychologist who used cognitive behavioral therapy and was able to help Judy manage the panic episodes in 3 months of psychotherapy. With the psychologist's guidance, she used self-talk and a process of systematic desensitization, facing and coping with progressively more frightening situations in her life.

Judy resumed college studies the following summer, completed a two-year degree at a nearby community college, and then earned a bachelor's degree in music at a nearby state college. She added sociology and psychology courses to her curriculum in her junior and senior years and determined to become a social worker instead of a professional musician. Judy had been deeply impressed with her psychologist's compassion and skill, with both Judy and her mother. She was confident that she could be satisfied by putting music into second place in her life, as her father had done, while pursuing a career as a helping professional.

Judy earned an MSW in clinical social work and developed a clinical practice with a group of mental health professionals in her home community. She met and married her husband David at the age of 26, while he was still in dental school. Together they raised three daughters and one son, and Judy took an active role in community service.

Judy experienced intermittent generalized anxiety and worry through graduate school and in the years of her young adulthood. She suffered a series of panic episodes at the time her youngest daughter (her youngest child) left home for college. David was encouraging and insisted that she get professional help for the panic. Again she worked with a female psychotherapist and used cognitive strategies to manage her anxiety. Looking back, she believes that she was more secure about her life overall at that time, with financial security and a comfortable supportive marriage. She experienced a loss of purpose and sense of loss with the daughter's departure from home, but it lacked the catastrophic feeling she experienced with her father's death.

In her 50s and 60s, Judy managed life with intermittent but manageable anxiety. Her social work career was satisfying, and she developed long-term friendships with several colleagues in mental health professions. She maintained her passion for piano and music, performing occasional solo performances at area churches, accompanying vocalists at a nearby University music school, and became a fixture leading sing alongs at parties. She played improvizational "bluesy-jazz" when alone and found that the music freed her thoughts and settled her emotions.

Judy's marriage survived times of distance and strain and became a comfortable and rewarding companionship. Her husband retired from his dental practice at 63, after which they traveled and enjoyed long hours walking and bicycling, alone and with friends. Judy continued her social work practice part time until she was 68. That year David's occasional forgetfulness progressed to a frightening and more pervasive cognitive decline. Increasingly, he struggled to find the words to express himself, could not recall information which she provided repeatedly, and failed to recognize longtime friends.

A thorough neurological evaluation resulted in a diagnosis of Alzheimer's disease. Increasingly, Judy found herself acting as a nurse and caregiver, on a 24/7 basis. After David wandered around the neighborhood on two occasions, lost, confused, and crying, she stopped leaving him home alone even briefly. Her younger sister began to provide an occasional afternoon of respite care.

Recurrence of anxiety disorder Two weeks after Judy's 71st birthday, she noticed David staring blankly at her and realized that he did not recognize her. She experienced her heart racing and found herself overwhelmed with panic. She felt terribly alone, and felt a resurgence of the experience she had at age 19, after her father's death. She felt as if *the house was crashing down on her.*

In the next few months, her husband showed only occasional moments of not knowing her. He was still manageable and on many days a good companion. Her episodes of panic, however, increased in frequency until she realized she needed help.

The initial triggers for Judy's anxiety were episodes of David not recognizing her or one of their children. Increasingly, however, the anxiety generalized and was set off by thoughts of a future alone and apprehensions that an attack might be coming on. This *anticipatory anxiety* frequently plays a part in the escalation of anxiety. Physical sensations she associated with the panic began to serve as triggers for anxiety. Whenever she noticed her heart beating faster or her face flushing, Judy became fearful of another episode, and this increasing fear seemed to trigger the very episode she feared.

Judy's daughter accompanied her to her primary care physician, and the daughter and physician insisted with Judy that she accept help for herself. The physician referred her to a team of integrative mental health professionals, who provide counseling, biofeedback, hypnosis, and other mind-body practices, integrated into a program of behavioral and lifestyle change.

Pathways Assessment

Diagnostic assessment Judy met the DSM-V diagnostic criteria for a panic disorder with agoraphobia. She reported severe episodes at least twice weekly of an overwhelming experience of anxiety, with attacks persisting over 6 months, from their recurrence shortly after her 71st birthday (American Psychiatric Association, 2013). She reported racing and pounding heart beat, rapid and shallow breathing, facial flushing, and profuse sweating. She experienced fears of her life crashing in on her, of being alone in the world, and of dying. Increasingly, she stayed home and avoided public places. In part she was needed at home to watch and care for David, but increasingly she stayed home because she feared having an attack in public and not being able to manage the anxiety.

Judy completed some behavior checklists and a physiological assessment. On the Beck Depression Inventory, she scored 23, indicating moderate depression. On the Beck Anxiety Inventory, she scored 38, indicating severe anxiety. A 10-minutes sample of heart rate variability data was gathered, along with a sample of respiration. Her SDNN, a statistical index of heart rate variability, was 39, suggesting compromised health and well-being (a ten minute sample of heart rate variability data is less reliable than a 24-hours monitor in categorizing health and well-being). Her baseline breathing indicated a respiration rate of 21, in the hyperventilation range, with periods of breath holding in the sample as well.

Judy's family history suggested a genetic predisposition to anxiety disorders; her mother suffered a lifelong anxiety disorder, requiring long-term treatment. Judy's own anxiety disorder was present for approximately five decades, with exacerbations in times of transition in her life. The current episode was triggered by the progressive loss of her spouse as a support and companion, and the stress of the caregiver role. The parallels to the circumstances in her life when her father died appeared to be the dynamic trigger for the recurrence of the frightening experience that *the house is coming down on her.*

Judy's anxiety was disruptive of daily life functioning. Judy still provided daily care for her husband and managed their household and finances, but frequently felt that her coping and functioning were slipping. She feared losing her own cognitive capacities. Her sleep was disturbed and she found it difficult to concentrate on bookkeeping and paying her household bills.

Caregiver stress Judy is not unique or alone in her challenges. The 2015 study sponsored by AARP and the National Alliance for Caregiving, *Caregiving in the US*, provides a number of informative statistics (AARP/NAC, 2015, pp. 6–7). 43.5 million adults had provided unpaid care to an adult or child in the previous 12 months. Approximately 16.6% of adult Americans are in the caregiver role. Seven percent of caregivers themselves are 75 years or older, and older caregivers tend to receive less unpaid help than younger caregivers. Those persons giving more hours of care to someone each week have been in that role on average for 10 years or longer.

The longer the caregiving situation continues, the more likely the caregiver is to report deterioration in his/her own health. Persons caring for a spouse or parent report more emotional stress and about half of those caring for someone with a mental health problem or Alzheimer's report emotional stress (AARP/NAC, 2015, pp. 9–10).

Lifestyle assessment Judy reported poor sleep many nights, with long delays in sleep onset and an anxious vigilance about her husband, with her anxiety often persisting through the night. She awoke frequently in the night, apprehensive about sounds and movement in the bedroom. She associated her poor concentration with sleep deprivation. On the few nights when she slept through the night, she felt mentally sharper and more able to think and make decisions.

As a mental health professional, Judy believed in the benefits of coping skills, relaxation techniques, social supports, physical exercise, and healthy lifestyles to buffer the effects of stressful situations. She was embarrassed that the caregiver role had come to eat up so many hours in her day and that her life was empty of all of these useful health and wellness supporting activities. She reported almost no physical exercise, little social contact with friends and extended family, and no use of the various coping skills she previously had taught her patients.

She also reported that with the demands of caregiving she was relying more and more on pre-packaged meals with high sodium content and very few fresh vegetables or fruits. She had prided herself on the family's positive nutritional choices in past years, with minimal fast food or box meals, but she found herself so exhausted from care for David, dressing him, washing him, soothing him, laundering his soiled clothing, that the idea of going to the kitchen and making a meal from fresh market ingredients sounded overwhelming. She rarely had any appetite and had lost 18 pounds since the of David's dementia diagnosis.

Pathways Intervention Plan

Judy was enthusiastic when her therapist discussed the Pathways Model, and a plan to make wellness-oriented lifestyle changes on multiple levels. The therapist explained that during the first two phases of implementing the Pathways Model he would act more as a health coach, not undertaking formal psychotherapy. He would act as a coach facilitator/wellness educator, help her identify options, encourage her to set goals, and assist her in assessing her progress and modifying her Pathways plan as needed. Judy expressed a desire to increase her activity, resume contact with her sister and friends, but broke down in tears at the impossibility of leaving David alone in the house, or even of going into the next room to exercise or practice some form of relaxation or self-care.

Community-based respite care Judy's therapist/coach discussed the cumulative erosion of well-being with prolonged caregiver stress. She accepted this warning, as she was already experiencing anxiety, cognitive lapses, and worries that she might have early signs of dementia. Her therapist discussed available forms of respite care for David, as well as self-care skills that she might be able to practice without leaving her husband's side. A consultation with her physician about the health risks of continuing her current level of 24/7 care reduced her resistance. Judy reluctantly agreed to begin a trial of respite day care with a local church affiliated programs for adults with dementia. David's physician had already recommended a long-term Alzheimer's unit placement, and respite seemed a more tolerable compromise to her. She welcomed a social worker on the respite team to her home to evaluate David and consider him as a candidate for the program. David was assessed to be able to tolerate all of the current activity programs in the respite day program. Judy elected a trial period of two afternoons of respite care weekly, with a plan to increase further if David responded positively.

Level One Plan

In the Pathways Model, intervention begins with Level One activities, which consist of self-directed behavioral and lifestyle changes. Judy dialogued for 2 weeks with her therapist about which self-care activities to choose for her Level One plan. She already felt a boost from experiencing two afternoons a week that were her own, for any activity she might choose. She finally chose three initial Level One activities.

Level One activities: Mindful breathing Judy's therapist/coach recommended she consider breath training, emphasizing that mindful, paced diaphragmatic breathing is a useful skill in managing anxiety symptoms. The therapist also proposed that Judy could practice breathing exercises while in the room with David, which might serve to calm David as well as herself.

Judy recognized that rapid and shallow breathing were a significant part of her anxiety experience and decided to select mindful breathing as her first Level One activity. Judy practiced the mechanics of mindful, paced breathing with her therapist, monitoring her breathing with one hand on her chest and one on her abdomen, to follow the process of her breathing. She learned to breathe in through her nostrils and out through "pursed lips" (making a small circle with her lips), which increased her awareness of her out breath.

Judy's therapist emphasized a mindfulness component in her breathing practices. She learned to mindfully absorb her awareness fully into the breathing process, following the flow of air in through her nostrils, through her airways, into her lungs and back out again through her mouth. Judy's therapist cautioned her that some wandering thoughts are normal, and encouraged her to notice, observe, and accept distractions and wandering thoughts without any self-judgment, and then to bring her attention back to her breathing.

Next Judy and her therapist practiced breathing at a slower rate. They breathed together following a breath pacer that she downloaded to her smart phone, called Breathing Zone, which uses an expanding and shrinking lotus blossom accompanied by one of several sounds. As the lotus expanded she filled her lungs, and as it shrank she exhaled and emptied her lungs. She initially set the breath pacer at nine breaths per minute, which felt very slow but tolerable for her. Judy committed to practice mindful diaphragmatic breathing twice a day, for 15 minutes, and to use the same mindful breathing exercises whenever she experienced the onset of anxiety. She was also instructed to gradually lower her breathing rate until she could breathe comfortably at six breaths per minute, a relaxation-promoting breathing rate for most persons.

Level One activities: Nutrition Judy had attended many professional workshops on nutrition, diet, and wellness, and was embarrassed to disclose the full decline of her diet since the caregiving role had fully worn down her energies. She was knowledgeable about meal planning, the use of fresh market ingredients, and the advantages of a high fiber, low-fat diet with lots of garden vegetables and fruit. It was the stress and exhaustion of being a caregiver, and not ignorance, that had led her to surrender her past role as careful planner of highly nutritional meals. After the first 3 weeks of her husband's participation in respite care, she felt able to set some Level One nutritional goals.

The local farmer's market operated on Wednesdays, one of the days her husband participated in respite care. Judy had not used the farmer's market since her husband's dementia was diagnosed. She decided to begin buying enough vegetables, fruit, and fresh poultry for three to four dinners a week, and set herself the goal of preparing two to four healthy dinners each week.

Judy's therapist stepped in during this planning session and encouraged her to also consider accepting lunches from the local community's senior center meals program, at least on the days that David was in the home. Initially that seemed like a sacrilege to Judy, but the therapist reminded her that the meals program actually provided fairly high quality healthy fare, and also reminded her that the strain of preparing meals, when she was also watching David every moment, had led to the fast food/box meals regimen of the past year.

Judy decided to try the senior lunch meals 3 days a week—the 2 weekdays David was home and Saturdays when he was again home.

Level One activity: Sleep hygiene Sleep hygiene includes attention to optimizing the sleep environment and examining personal habits that might disrupt sleep readiness. Judy's initial observation was that her anxiety and vigilance about the husband's occasional nocturnal wandering was the single greatest factor disrupting her sleep. She had awakened to find him missing on repeated occasions. On two occasions, he had urinated into a closet which produced more work for her, but on one other occasion she found him wandering in the street three blocks from home. With her therapist's guidance, she purchased a motion sensor alarm for the hallway outside the bedroom. If the husband remained in the bedroom or master bath, the alarm was silent, but whenever he wandered further, she was awakened by an electronic chime.

Judy was also instructed to use her mindful breathing exercises herself, and to include David whenever possible, at bedtime to reduce physiological arousal and prepare herself neurophysiologically for sleep.

Level One Progress

After 10 weeks, Judy met with her therapist/coach and reviewed her progress in each of the Level One activities:

Progress: Mindful breathing Judy experienced a calming and inward absorption as she practiced the breathing exercises. By the 3-week point, she was breathing at six breaths per minute, for at least 20–30 minutes a day. She found that she could pace her breathing at about six breaths per minute quite well now, without the pacer.

Judy felt that when she paced her breathing, the world slowed down around her. When upsetting things happened, she felt she was watching them in slower motion. By week six, she reported using the paced mindful breathing several times a week in moments of increasing anxiety, noticing that in many cases the physical symptoms of anxiety moderated from severe to mild within 10 minutes of mindful breathing.

She also began to sit with David when she practiced her breathing. He couldn't seem to comprehend the breath pacer or her instructions, but she sat close and breathed audibly, sometimes stroking up his arm as she inhaled and down his arm as she exhaled. His breathing was not even, but slowed, resembling hers, and the process seemed to calm him. She began to use her breathing practices, whenever he was agitated, simply holding him and breathing and saying aloud, "Peace David, peace."

Judy committed to continuing her breathing practices indefinitely and placed yellow dots and sticky notes on the bathroom mirror, on the refrigerator, and on her dashboard, to remind herself to slow her breathing, and to wrap her awareness around the breathing, whenever she felt anxious, whenever she feared an attack, and whenever she had a few moments free.

Progress: Nutrition Initially, the senior meals program was the most successful part of Judy's nutritional change program. Judy and David had always preferred a simple breakfast of oatmeal, honey, and nuts, with an occasional boiled egg. Now they also enjoyed regular lunches, delivered to their door and ready to serve. She soon set up a 6-day meal schedule, with a luncheon meal for herself when David was in respite. She supplemented the delivered meals with salads and fruit from the farmer's market. She felt her body responding with more appetite to regular tasty foods, and now could feel a lightness and energy in her movements many days.

The presence of respite care helped Judy with the second portion of her nutritional goals. She began to spend some of her time online reviewing recipes, especially exploring new uses for foods from the farmer's market. She took pride in using all of the purchases from the market by the weekend and made occasional trips to the Saturday market. She began to buy grains that she had never used before (quinoa, bulgur wheat, and wheat berries) and added these to her menu.

David never commented on the meals, but his appetite increased, and he made no objections to any of her experiments in *nouveau cuisine*. She noticed that both of them were filling out their clothes better. She regained eight pounds in the 10 weeks she spent on Level One.

Progress: Sleep hygiene   The use of the motion sensor reduced Judy's nighttime vigilance and frequent awakening. She still was awakened several times a week when he wandered beyond the master suite, but she now could fall asleep with confidence that she would be awakened before the husband could engage in anything harmful. Her use of mindful breathing also helped in sleep onset, with greatly reduced sleep latency. When she occasionally awakened in the night and could not sleep, she began to play her keyboard with a headset, and found she could usually get back to sleep within 20–30 minutes.

Level One Summary

Judy experienced perhaps the largest benefit from the new use of respite care. By the end of 10 weeks, David was participating in 3 days of respite care. The reduction in stress for her was substantial, and the available time enabled her to engage in the beneficial self-care activities she had chosen for Level One. She was encouraged at her engagement and progress with all three Level One activities and felt ready to start Level Two. She embraced mindful breathing as her best tool in reducing physiological tensions and coping with anxiety, and determined not to let go of her regular practice. She also embraced continuation of the two components in her nutritional goals. Her sleep continued to be challenged, but she felt enough benefit in improved cognitive function that she expressed determination to further improve her sleep.

Level Two Plan

In the Pathways Model, Level Two involves the individual using educational materials and community resources to acquire additional self-care and self-regulation skills. Patients utilize self-help workbooks, educational CDs and DVDs, or classes and training programs in their community. Judy deliberated thoughtfully about her options in Level Two, just as she had in Level One.

Level Two: Mindfulness training and mindful meditation   Judy loved the sensation of her life slowing down around her as she performed her mindful breathing. She especially liked the process of mindfully accepting distractions. She had previously engaged in a lot of self-criticism and perfectionism, and she enjoyed the idea of accepting without judgment whatever happened during her breathing practices. She asked for more mindfulness at Level Two. Initially, Judy read Jon Kabat-Zinn's *Full Catastrophe Living* (Kabat-Zinn, 1990). Then, she began listening three times a week to two Jon Kabat-Zinn audio-CD programs (Kabat-Zinn, 2005, 2006). The CD programs provided instructions on how to pay attention to life in a particular way, attending to whatever unfolds in this moment, with acceptance and heightened awareness, and without judgment or self-critical commentary. Her therapist sought out a mindfulness class for her as well, but none was available in that time period.

Level Two activities: Emotional journaling Judy kept a journal in college years, especially after her father's death, and found the process of journaling soothing at that time. Her therapist introduced James Pennebaker's research on journaling. Pennebaker is a research psychologist who studied self-disclosure in several forms, including the use of an emotional journal. His extensive research showed that expressing negative emotions and experiences in a journal can have many positive therapeutic effects, including improved mood, reduced anxiety and fearfulness, enhanced immune function, reduced blood pressure and other effects (Klapow et al., 2001; Pennebaker, 1997).

Judy's therapist gave her a copy of Pennebaker's most recent workbook, *Expressive Writing, Words that Heal,* designed to guide individuals through the journaling process (Pennebaker & Evans, 2014). Her therapist instructed Judy as follows:

- Dedicate a relatively short time period (15–20 minutes) each day to writing.
- Use that time to write about your deepest and most intense emotions, especially emotions about painful and traumatic times in your life.
- Allow yourself to express yourself freely, without concern about handwriting, grammar, or literary concerns.
- Remind yourself that this writing is for you—you alone. No one else will ever read it unless you decide to share it.
- Once you have reached the 15 or 20 minutes point, close the journal, place it in a drawer, and go on about your day.

Her therapist also repeated the Pennebaker and Evans guidance from the workbook: openly acknowledge emotion, work to construct a story about the event, switch perspectives within your journal entry, and find your own voice (Pennebaker & Evans, 2014, pp. 17–18). He offered to read any journal entry she wished to share, but also encouraged her to burn, shred, or just hold back anything she felt uncomfortable sharing. Judy purchased a beautiful leather bound blank book and committed to write in the journal for about 15–20 minutes, at least four times per week.

Level Two activities: Pastoral care After the first week of respite care for David, Judy began to feel extreme guilt at sending him away from the home. He cried as she dropped him off the first day, and when a bus with two caregivers arrived to transport him for the second day, he crumpled on the floor and clung to her, while crying softly. The caregiving staff assured her at the end of each day that David had enjoyed several activities, and they showed her a smartphone video of a smiling David pushing a beach ball toward other participants in the program. She intermittently considered cancelling the respite care and dropping out of her treatment program.

Judy's parents were devout Lutherans, and she had remained active in a Lutheran church throughout her adult life. She joked with her therapist about Lutherans really knowing how to experience guilt, but she still found herself thinking that God must be judging her for not living up to her marriage vows. The words "for better, for worse, in sickness and in health" ran through her mind, and she felt that she was not living up to her nuptial commitment.

Her therapist initially discussed with Judy a balance between self-care and devotion to others, giving her the example, that every airplane safety talk reminds the passengers to place their own oxygen masks over their own mouths before trying to help others. Cognitively, Judy could understand that a burned out caregiver isn't much help, yet the sense of God judging her, of not being a loving wife troubled her. In spite of seeing the benefit for herself of reclaiming parts of her life, with John now in three full days of respite each week, Judy continued to struggle with ruminations on guilt and sin.

Judy decided that one of her Level Two activities should be weekly pastoral sessions with her senior pastor, a biblical scholar who seemed to convey acceptance.

Level Two Progress

Progress: Mindfulness training and mindfulness meditation Judy was enthusiastic over her mindfulness experiences. She had enjoyed the mindful acceptance of stray thoughts during her Level One mindful breathing. Now the readings and exercises in mindfulness enabled her to more fully embrace a mindful awareness toward her life and her anxieties. Judy began to set goals for herself each morning, about certain times of day and certain situations that she wished to enter and experience mindfully. She also began to meditate for the first time in her life, on days when her spouse was in respite care. She practiced quiet sitting, with paced breathing, and a deliberate mindful attention to each sensation, thought, and urge entering her awareness. The combination of meditating several days a week and practicing mindful acceptance of events and thoughts through the day increased her sense of calm in daily life, even when her husband had a disturbing day.

Progress: Emotional journaling Judy began journaling the day of her initial evaluation. The journaling gripped her strongly, and she found herself making time to write almost every day of the week. Initially, she journaled about changes in her husband David, and about her own fears for the future. She found herself crying over images of her husband in a nursing home, or images of his funeral. Writing about her husband dying took her back to the experience of her father's death.

Her journaling quickly led her to experience the similarities in her circumstances around the father's death and around David's decline. The sense of her life-as-it-had-been being shattered, and the tangible physical experience of the *house crashing down on her* were like the same experience all over again. She continued to cry as she journaled although the heaviness moderated as she continued to journal into the second week.

By the fourth week, Judy reported being able to write about her experiences without tears and began describing in her journal joyful memories of past travel with David and also with her father. She found herself realizing that in many positive ways, more than she had recognized, her husband's place in her life resembled her father's place in her childhood. He had been a steady support, encouraging her talents, especially her music, seeking out avenues for her to receive support for her piano performance.

Judy remembered a phrase she frequently utilized in her years as a therapist and found herself repeating this phrase to herself as she journaled: "I have this one, I have it." This conveyed a sense that she felt a confidence to handle a problem or a situation. Frequently, she repeated to herself, "I have this," about David's dementia and the changes it wrought in her life.

Level Two Progress: Pastoral care Judy's participation in pastoral care sessions was as emotional and intense initially as her first weeks of journaling. Initially, she cried about David's diagnosis, his wandering in the neighborhood, his blank stares when she spoke to him. Then she shifted to expressing her sense of burden and duty to be a good caregiver for him now. She had a sense of owing him so much for their years together and felt intense guilt for placing him in respite.

Her pastor had no quick answers for her suffering and her sense of guilt. She had feared he might quote scriptures and platitudes at her, but he did not. Initially, he read a Psalm to her each week, choosing Psalms about suffering and "tribulation," and then listened and acknowledged the depth of her challenge. The words of Psalm 88 stayed with her:

> I am overwhelmed with troubles
> and my life draws near to death.
> I am counted among those who go down to the pit;
> I am like one without strength…
> I call to you, LORD, every day;
> I spread out my hands to you.
> (Psalm 88, v. 1–4, 9. New International Version, 2015)

When she condemned herself for placing David in respite care, he asked how much longer she thought she would have been able to continue as she had been doing, without a breakdown. He also asked what she as a professional social worker thought about her self-condemnations. She laughed and accused him of tricking her, but realized she would without fail have counseled self-forgiveness and self-care for any of her clinical patients.

The pastor confronted Judy's occasional image of a judging God sitting in a sky-high tribunal watching her moments of self-pity and punishing her with additional suffering. He suggested that by asking for spiritual grace, she might find moments of strength, new purpose, and peace, within this "season of suffering" in her life.

The pastor also encouraged her new mindfulness meditation practices and affirmed the positive contributions of Buddhist traditions to bringing a contemplative/meditative dimension back into the stressful pace of Western life. This acceptance by an ordained Lutheran pastor relieved a nagging concern that she had been experiencing about using non-Christian spiritual practices.

Setback

In the sixth week of Judy's Level Two activities, David fell in the bathtub at home, while she was helping him bathe. She had been supporting him as he stepped into the tub, and he seemed to startle and break from her supporting hold. He fractured his proximal right femur. David was given an analgesic for acute pain, and he became more confused on the analgesic. The hospital team performed a surgical fixation of the femur, and then treated him for infection and loss of blood flow in the hip joint. The team recommended an extended rehabilitation placement with occupational therapy. In hospital, David needed help even getting up from a chair, showed confusion about where he was, and persisted in trying to climb out of his hospital bed risking further injury. He was placed in restraints which produced episodes of crying and additional confusion.

Judy accepted the accident and felt relief not having to manage David in his further diminished state. She decided to suspend her weekly Pathways clinic sessions temporarily, in order to be able to participate fully in David's rehabilitation treatments, to help him recover. Her Pathways therapist encouraged her to continue her mindfulness exercises and journaling, at least 3 days a week, to continue her mindful paced breathing, and to continue her progress in managing anxiety. She accepted this suggestion and also agreed to keep appointments with her Pathways therapist and with her pastor every 3 weeks, with the hopes of resuming her own full Pathways program relatively soon.

The rehabilitation team was able to reduce David's analgesic medication after 3 weeks, and he showed some improvement in orientation, but remained affected cognitively. He began to adjust to the rehabilitation setting, and physical therapy (PT) began work with him in his fourth week, to recover strength. David initially improved with PT, and then his cognitive status deteriorated further. After 8 weeks, David's rehabilitation team recommended placement in an Alzheimer's unit adjacent to the rehabilitation unit, with plans for intermittent PT and long-term custodial care. Judy reported increased sadness and anxiety as David deteriorated. Yet she could see his decline objectively and agreed to the suggested placement.

Level Two Progress and Decisions

After David's move to the Alzheimer's unit, Judy resumed more frequent Pathways appointments and resumed all of her Level One and Two activities. She felt again that she "had this," that is, that she was able to face and manage her transitions. She asked to begin her Level Three professional services and expressed that some professional counseling might assist her now to make some life decisions that were on her mind.

Level Three Plan

In the Pathways Model, Level Three consists of professional services and treatment interventions, ranging from biofeedback to psychotherapy to acupuncture. Judy asked for more help with anxiety and more mindfulness.

Level Three intervention: Heart rate variability (HRV) biofeedback Judy agreed to begin her Level Three interventions with HRV training because it has been shown to benefit patients with anxiety (Moss, 2016a, 2016b) and is understood to improve autonomic nervous system regulation (Moss & Shaffer, 2016). The HRV training was also a natural extension of Judy's extensive use of mindful, paced, diaphragmatic breathing. Initially, she spent one session watching the biofeedback display—a multiple line graph showing her breathing and the fluctuations in her heart rate. Next, she learned to further smooth the process of her breathing and watched the corresponding smoothing of the heart rate line graph on the screen. Judy's therapist asked her to call to mind disturbing events of the past 6 months, and she saw the smooth hills and valleys of breathing and heart rate deteriorate into jagged and more irregular activity. She also practiced breathing with the pacer on the screen, which duplicated her practice at home with the Breathing Zone pacer.

Next, the therapist guided Judy through breathing at various breath rates, between 7.5 and 5 breaths per minute. Through this process, the therapist identified her resonance frequency as 7.0 breaths per minute. This is the breathing rate that produced the best phase synchrony between breathing and heart rate. At seven breaths per minute, her highest HR came just as she shifted from inhalation to exhalation, and the lowest HR came almost exactly where she shifted from exhalation to inhalation. This was also the breathing rate producing the largest oscillations in HR and the highest SDNN (the SDNN is a statistical index for the variability of the time in milliseconds between heart beats).

Level Three intervention: Acceptance and commitment therapy Judy specifically wanted counseling as one of her Level Three activities. She also asked for a kind of counseling that would parallel her self-guided mindfulness practices. Acceptance and commitment therapy (ACT) is a form of psychotherapy developed by Stephen Hayes (Hayes, Strosahl, & Wilson, 2003), which integrates the approach of mindful acceptance of all events, including negative emotions. Through ACT, patients learn to "just notice," accept, and even embrace their moment to moment experiences, especially those they have previously avoided.

Judy was excited at this emphasis on acceptance and found herself increasingly integrating her pastor's idea of discovering strength and purpose within her season of suffering.

Level Two: Meditation (continued) Judy continued her meditation practice during David's treatment, rehabilitation, and long-term placement. She experienced a recurrent image of a circle, first an image of a geometric circle and then an image of a circular path. That image took on meaning for her, and she explained that her father's death had taken her away from her original dream of a music career, and now David's decline was calling her back around the circle to music. She declared that the mental health and mind-body aspects of her Pathways treatment were sufficient and chose musical instruction as her final Level Three intervention.

Level Three intervention: Master class in piano Judy announced that she was taking 2 weeks to attend a piano master class in Germany. She asked her oldest daughter to stay at Judy's home and visit David several times a week, while Judy got away and immersed herself in music. She explained that she did not imagine a concert career at her age, but wanted to allow music to reclaim her, regardless of what form that might take.

Level Three Progress

Judy continued in her HRV biofeedback for eight sessions and continued in the ACT psychotherapy for 12 sessions.

HRV biofeedback: Progress Judy was able to produce smooth, synchronized oscillations of heart rate and respiration quite consistently after five sessions of HRV training. She continued to practice her breath exercises at home, with the pacer now set at her resonance frequency of 7 breaths per minute. During the week of her sixth HRV session, her husband had another fall at his Alzheimer's unit and was badly bruised with aggravation of pain in his hip. She experienced increased sadness and anxiety, initially, but by the eighth HRV session she was again producing high-level HRV with over 90% of her HRV in the target range during most of her session.

Subjectively, the primary effects of her HRV training were a strengthening of her management of anxiety and a reduction in negative emotional states. She reminded her therapist of the "I have this" experience that came to her during emotional journaling. She explained that now she had gone from "I have this" to "bring it on." She expressed that the HRV practice was making her into the "Dirty Harry of anxiety" who would take on any adversary and keep her body calm and self-regulated. She didn't really want more adversity, but felt a surprising level of confidence that she could deal with whatever life was bringing.

Acceptance and commitment therapy: Progress Judy reported that acceptance of events and acceptance of her thoughts was producing a kind of ability to experience her life in slow motion. She embraced the ACT model as more suited to herself than her past efforts to dispute or restructure her anxious thoughts. She had decided to identify a future training for either ACT or a mindfulness-based therapy as part of her ongoing social work continuing education activity.

Master class: Progress Judy waited until her HRV and ACT treatments were complete and left for the 2-week piano class. She sent postcards to the Pathways treatment team and proclaimed a sense of ecstasy at spending 12 hours each day in studying, playing, and listening to music. She enrolled in classical and improvizational piano and stayed on three extra days to participate in a special improvizational music festival.

Post-Treatment Assessment

By the time she returned from her piano class, Judy felt no need for further treatment. She assessed herself as having achieved a sustainable program for managing the stress of her life. In fact, she reported that joy and enthusiasm now outweighed any negative emotion most days. She committed to maintain her seven breaths a minute exercises, along with her regular meditation practices. She continued to journal although less often. She felt an overall breakthrough in using mindful acceptance for anything new emerging in her life.

Judy agreed to participate in a formal assessment session and completed the Beck Depression and Anxiety Inventories again, as well as a final psychophysiological recording. She subjectively described herself as only occasionally anxious or depressed in response to setbacks in her husband's condition. On the BDI, she scored a 14 indicating only mild depression. On the BAI she scored a 9, indicating minimal, normal range anxiety. Her psychophysiological sample showed an SDNN of 88, indicating that she was much closer to the "good health" range, and her breath rate while sitting and reading a magazine was 12 breaths per minute, with no evidence of breath holding.

Judy announced several life decisions at her assessment session. She had decided to sell the large family home and purchase a condominium near several girlfriends. She said that she would enjoy walking away from the house that she felt was "crashing down on her." She asked her children to help with disposing of decades of belongings. She also persuaded the rehabilitation system where David had been placed to take her on for 15 hours a week, initially, as a medical social worker/music therapist. She intended to blend breath training, meditation, and piano in group sessions, and in patient rooms for those who were bed-bound. She purchased a cart on wheels for her keyboard and was excited at the image of becoming an iterant performer around the rehabilitation system.

Anxiety disorders are chronic remitting and relapsing conditions (Scholten et al., 2016), recurring under stress, during life transitions, and sometimes without apparent provocation. Judy had already experienced five decades of intermittent anxiety episodes. She was assured by her treatment team, that it would be normal for anxiety to recur in some future time of loss, stress, or ill health, but also assured that the self-care skills she was currently utilizing would serve her well in managing any recurrence. She was also assured that she would be welcome to return for Pathways refresher sessions as needed or as desired in the future.

Judy's story is a reminder that impactful therapeutic transformation is not confined within the services of the mental health and health care profession. Educational pursuits, volunteer service, and expressive arts activities all frequently impart powerful life-transformative effects. In her case, both her piano master's class and her activities as a volunteer mind-body-spirit-music therapist in the rehabilitation setting were significant components in re-directing her life and health.

References

AARP/NAC. (2015). *Caregiving in the US. 2015.* Washington, DC: AARP and National Alliance for Caregiving.

American Psychiatric Association. (2013). *Diagnostic and statistical manual of mental disorders* (5th ed.). Washington, DC: Author.

Hayes, S. C., Strosahl, K. D., & Wilson, K. G. (2003). *Acceptance and commitment therapy: An experiential approach to behavior change.* New York: Guilford.

Kabat-Zinn, J. (1990). *Full catastrophe living: Using the wisdom of your body and mind to face stress, pain and illness.* New York: Delacorte.

Kabat-Zinn, J. (2005). *Guided mindfulness meditation: A complete guided mindfulness program from Jon Kabat-Zinn* (Educational CD). Louisville, CO: Sounds True.

Kabat-Zinn, J. (2006). *Mindfulness for beginners: Reclaiming the present moment* (Educational CD). Louisville, CO: Sounds True.

Klapow, J. C., Schmidt, S. M., Taylor, L. A., Roller, P., Li, Q., Calhoun, J. W., et al. (2001). Symptom management in older primary care patients: Feasibility of an experimental, written self-disclosure protocol. *Annals of Internal Medicine, 134*(9 Pt 2), 905–911.

Moss, D. (2016a). *The house is crashing down on me:* Integrating mindfulness, breath training, and heart rate variability biofeedback for an anxiety disorder in a 71 year-old caregiver. *Biofeedback, 44*(3), 160–167.

Moss, D. (2016b). Anxiety and anxiety disorders. In G. Tan, F. Shaffer, R. Lyle, & I. Teo (Eds.), *Evidence-based treatment in biofeedback and neurofeedback* (3rd ed., pp. 27–31). Wheat Ridge, CO: Association for Applied Psychophysiology and Biofeedback.

Moss, D., & Shaffer, F. (Eds.). (2016). *Foundations of heart rate variability.* Wheat Ridge, CO: Association for Applied Psychophysiology and Biofeedback.

Pennebaker, J. (1997). *Opening up: The healing power of expressing emotions* (revised edition). New York: Guilford.

Pennebaker, J., & Evans, J. (2014). *Expressive writing: Words that heal.* Enumclaw, WA: Idyll Arbor.

Scholten, W. D., Batelaan, N. M., Penninx, B. W., Balkom, A. J., Smit, J. H., Schoevers, R. A., et al. (2016). Diagnostic instability of recurrence and the impact on recurrence rates in depressive and anxiety disorders. *Journal of Affective Disorders, 195*, 185–190. https://doi.org/10.1016/j.jad.2016.02.025

Yonkers, K. A., Bruce, S. E., Dyck, I. R., & Keller, M. B. (2003). Chronicity, relapse, and illness-course of panic disorder, social phobia, and generalized anxiety disorder: Findings in men and women from 8 years of follow-up. *Depression and Anxiety, 17*(3), 173–179.

Chapter 10
A Pathways Approach to the Metabolic Syndrome

Abstract Psychosocial factors interact with genetics, environment, and lifestyle to increase risk for the metabolic syndrome (essential hypertension, Type 2 diabetes, hyperlipidemia, and obesity). Patients with the metabolic syndrome often suffer from anxious and depressive symptoms, negatively affecting motivation for self-management. A biopsychosocial approach is important in the care of patients such as Carmella, the case described in this chapter. Treatment of this multifaceted chronic disorder is complex and is best coordinated among multiple specialists and in addition requires the active participation of the patient. Based on the Pathways Model, the mental health provider's role is to empower the patient in effective self-management. Psychophysiological therapies offer the opportunity for regulation of physiological stress responses, engaging the relaxation response. Patients learn to make daily decisions which benefit their short- and long-term health. The psychotherapies, particularly cognitive behavioral therapy are consistent with the theme of self-awareness, patient choices, and significant changes in behavior. One of the complementary therapies, Reiki is also utilized by Carmella to achieve her goal of better metabolic control.

Keywords Metabolic syndrome · Diabetes · Hypertension · Hyperlipidemia · Obesity · Pathways Model

Metabolic Syndrome: Definition

"The *metabolic syndrome* comprises Type 2 diabetes mellitus, essential hypertension, hyperlipidemia, and obesity. The prevalence of the metabolic syndrome has been steadily increasing both during the past decade and in younger people ..."

The *metabolic syndrome* comprises Type 2 diabetes mellitus, essential hypertension, hyperlipidemia, and obesity. The prevalence of the metabolic syndrome has been steadily increasing both during the past decade and in younger people (Aguilar, Bhuket, Torres, Liu, & Wong, 2015; Ogden et al., 2006). Type 2 diabetes is defined as hyperglycemia (elevated blood glucose) and insulin resistance.

© Springer International Publishing AG, part of Springer Nature 2018   181
A. McGrady, D. Moss, *Integrative Pathways*,
https://doi.org/10.1007/978-3-319-89313-6_10

The person may produce sufficient insulin, but the cell membrane impedes instead of facilitates the entry of glucose into the cells. Diagnosis is made based on strict criteria developed by the American Diabetes Association (ADA, 2015a). Initial treatment consists of oral hypoglycemic agents, diet, and exercise which may provide sustained control of blood glucose for years; however, endocrinologists who care for patients with Type 2 diabetes guide their patients toward an insulin regimen if optimal control is not achieved after initial therapy (ADA, 2015b).

Essential hypertension is defined as chronically elevated blood pressure. Usually both systolic and diastolic blood pressures are higher than normal, but occasionally a person has either systolic or diastolic blood pressure elevations without the other (High Blood Pressure, 2016). The cutoff values for diagnosis have decreased, and treatment is initiated at lower levels of blood pressure; antihypertensive medication, diet, and exercise are recommended therapies (James et al., 2014). A recent scientific statement from the American Heart Association reviewed other approaches to lowering blood pressure, including exercise, relaxation, and biofeedback (Brook et al., 2013). Most of the behavioral or psychological non-drug therapies were rated as low risk, low to medium efficacy, while the exercise-based protocols had stronger, more consistently positive effects.

Central obesity, that is, an accumulation of fat around the mid-section, is another hallmark of the metabolic syndrome. Hyperlipidemia consists of increased blood levels of triglycerides, cholesterol, and low density lipoproteins. Medical treatment for hyperlipidemia comprises the class of medications called statins coupled with recommendations for improved diet and increasing activity (Catapano et al., 2016).

Risk Factors for the Metabolic Syndrome

The components of the metabolic syndrome share risk factors from the genetic, environmental, and psychosocial domains. The genetic predisposition to develop obesity, high blood pressure, and insulin resistance is shared among these disorders. Behavior is an important risk factor for metabolic syndrome, specifically overeating and unhealthy food choices leading to obesity in addition to a sedentary lifestyle (Healthy Lifestyles, 2016). Psychosocial factors, such as depression, anger, and anxiety, contribute to risk, onset, maintenance, and worsening of the metabolic syndrome (Goldbacher & Matthews, 2007). The impact of some of these variables in Type 2 diabetes and in essential hypertension is reviewed by Linden and McGrady (2016) and McGrady and Lakia (2016), respectively. However, the effects of depression and anxiety must be detailed further as they are most relevant to the case contained in this chapter.

Cumulative distress has a negative impact on glycemic control both acutely and long term (Aikens, 2012). In particular, clinical depression is well known to be linked to Type 2 diabetes. But a diagnosis of major depressive disorder or dysthymia is not necessary to observe an effect on blood glucose; even subclinical depressive symptoms influence adherence to a prescribed regimen (Gonzalez et al., 2008). The association between depression and diabetes is thought to be mediated by inflammatory processes that decrease cell membrane insulin sensitivity (Capuron et al., 2008;

McIntyre et al., 2007). Low mood also affects motivation and therefore adherence to the demanding daily regimen for diabetes control. For example, physical activity is less likely and caloric intake is usually higher during times of stress or when depressed mood predominates (Gonzalez, Shreck, Psaros, & Safren, 2015; Simon et al., 2008).

Chronic stress produces a burden on the patient's adaptive resources, making the coping demands more and more difficult to meet (Chandola, Brunner, & Marmot, 2006; Kim, Bursac, DiLillo, White, & West, 2009). Several mechanisms may account for the failure to adapt: poor recovery, lack of habituation, hypo-reactivity, or over-responsiveness to minor stimuli. Each of these maladaptive reactions is associated with emotional and physiological responses. Over time, repeated sympathoadrenal medullary disruptions increase blood pressure, blood glucose, and often body weight (Branth et al., 2007). Behavioral reactions to chronic stress—overeating of foods with poor nutritional value and withdrawal into an inactive lifestyle—may precede, co-exist with, or follow the diagnosis of metabolic syndrome.

The provider has a major effect on patients' perception of their own role in maintaining control of blood pressure, blood glucose, and blood lipids. Perceived personal control and a solid sense of self-efficacy are associated with better adherence (McSharry, Moss-Morris, & Kendrick, 2011) as exemplified by the mentality of "what I do makes a difference in my health." A provider skilled in motivational interviewing will facilitate change talk, elicit patients' motivation for change, and increase their sense of personal control (Lundahl & Burke, 2009).

Early life adversity[1] affects the risk for cardiovascular disease, as it does for many physical and emotional disorders. As detailed in the first chapter of this volume, negative life events lay the foundation for later illness, including diabetes and heart disease (Wickrama, O'Neal, Lee, & Wickrama, 2015). Dysfunction in the autonomic nervous system can be mediated by serotonin levels, the release of cytokines, and an accumulation of platelets; each of these factors comprises a biological risk (Davies, Hood, Christmas, & Nutt, 2008). Sociological factors also influence biology. Low socioeconomic status (SES, captured by educational level, income, and occupation) is correlated with the etiology and worsening of the metabolic syndrome (Maty, Lynch, Raghunathan, & Kaplan, 2008). Patients' perception of current SES and appraisal of their future (positive or negative) link with overall physical health (Matthews & Gallo, 2011).

Hormones related to metabolism exhibit variations during the day/night that are controlled by the central timing neurons in the brain, specifically the master clock (Froy, 2010). Circadian rhythms of cortisol, catecholamines, insulin, ghrelin, and leptin orchestrate metabolism and determine the timing of appetite, subsequently providing feedback to the master clock. People with disrupted sleep schedules are prone to demonstrate alterations in metabolic balance that eventually increase the risk for Type 2 diabetes. Eating during night time hours, sleeping during the daylight hours, and too few hours of sleep all have the potential to interfere with normal regulation of body weight (Knutson & Van Cauter, 2008; Patel, 2009). The major

---

[1] In health care research, this factor of early adversity is operationalized as *adverse childhood experiences* (ACE) and recognized as a significant contributor to negative adult physical and mental health outcomes (American Academy of Pediatrics, 2014).

long-term regulatory factor for feeding and stable body weight is leptin, which is a chemical released by fat cells and then distributed through the blood stream to the feeding control center in the hypothalamus. The adherence of leptin to the receptors in the hypothalamus produces a signal to decrease appetite and stop food intake. Other hormones such as cortisol, neuropeptide Y, and ghrelin are appetite stimulants. A relatively constant body weight can be maintained via communication among receptors in peripheral energy stores, the gastrointestinal nervous system, and the hypothalamus. Disruption in any component of the feedback loop may have one or more sequelae in the cardiovascular or endocrine systems (Kyrou, Chrousos, & Tsigos, 2006).

In contrast, positive affect, infrequent or minor distress, and few adverse life events provide a counterpoint to the effects of negative events and high distress. Positive psychology emphasizes a positive attitude and positive beliefs about the self, the environment, and the future. It is possible to feel more satisfied, to be more engaged with life, find more meaning, have higher hopes and laugh or smile more, regardless of what is going on at the time. Creating enjoyment in life can counter the effects of negative stress in patients with diabetes (Moskowitz, Epel, & Acree, 2008; Steptoe, O'Donnell, Marmot, & Wardle, 2008). Physical exercise, particularly of the aerobic type, not only conditions the body but is also associated with mental health benefits, increased sense of accomplishment, and more consistent positive affect (Carnethon & Craft, 2008).

In each of the disorders that constitute the metabolic syndrome, motivation may be affected by delay discounting, and the tendency to prefer smaller, quicker rewards to larger, long-term reinforcement. For most patients, the rewards for adherence to a regimen that comprises daily monitoring (blood glucose, blood pressure, body weight), exercise, nutrition, and medication are perceived as being far in the future. There is little if any immediate gratification in following the regimen compared to eating favorite foods, and being sedentary while watching television or communicating online (Dixon, Lik, Green, & Myerson, 2013; Petry et al., 2013).

Case of Carmella

Carmella was a 55-year-old Hispanic woman who was referred for therapy by her internal medicine physician because of low motivation, apparent lack of interest in improving blood glucose levels, and reported feelings of being overwhelmed by multiple responsibilities. At the time of the interview, she was highly anxious about her multiple diagnoses, her family history, and reported major stressors in her current life. There was a strong family history of Type 2 diabetes and heart disease; her grandfather had died at age 50 from a stroke; an uncle on her dad's side had a foot amputated because of diabetes.

Carmella was 5 ft, 6 in. and weighed 175 lb; her BMI was 28.3, which placed her in the overweight range. At age 40 her blood pressure started to increase and she was medicated with an antihypertensive at age 41. Later that same year, increased cholesterol and triglycerides necessitated medication with a statin. Four years later, Carmella was diagnosed with Type 2 diabetes; fasting blood glucose levels were 130 and 2-hours postprandial values were 180 mg/dL. Her glycohemoglobin A1C was 7.5%, indicating abnormally high blood glucose. She was prescribed Metformin, which kept her hemoglobin A1C under reasonable control for 5 years. Then her weight increased as she became more and more sedentary. Her physician began to talk about starting insulin and that is when she described her feelings of being overwhelmed. She told her physician that she couldn't do any more, "not one more thing." He responded that he could approve an FMLA (family medical leave act), so she could take time off work. Instead of this offer producing the intended relief, Carmella refused it immediately, saying that she could never go to her boss with this request.

Carmella was employed as an administrative secretary for a local school system. Her duties included setting the superintendent's schedule, taking minutes at meetings, and interacting with parents, members of the school board, and teachers. Her schedule was very busy during the academic year, somewhat less so in the summer months. The school system had received poorer ratings in the past year from the state board so mood around the office was often tense. She saw ways that the functioning of the office could be improved, but she had no energy and was reluctant to make any suggestions for fear of being told: "go ahead and do it."

Carmella's husband Bobby was 58 years old and of non-Hispanic origin. He worked as a nurse in the pediatric unit of the hospital; his work days changed each week but his hours were constant at three 12 hours shifts per week. His health was generally good although he had times of low back pain. Carmella and Bobby met after college and had been married for 27 years. Their three adult children were college graduates. Two lived on their own, one in the same city as Carmella and Bobby and one in a large city 4 hours away; their 21-year-old son lived at home.

The psychosocial evaluation revealed significant stressors at home and at work, but the major stress was identified as her medical illnesses and the burden of meeting what she saw as her physician's expectations. She met diagnostic criteria for generalized anxiety disorder, but not for major depression, although she endorsed three of the required five criteria for major depression (APA, 2013). Physically, she was often tired, had trouble getting to sleep at night, and woke up fatigued in the morning. A few times a month, she woke up with a mild headache and pain in the jaw area of her face. She had diffuse body pain several times a week; but her main physical complaint was sensations of tingling and burning in her feet. These unpleasant sensations were most noticeable at night when she tried to fall sleep, during times of hot weather, or when she had been on her feet for several hours.

Pathways Model of Intervention

Pathways Level One: Breathe, Feed, and Sleep Carmella expressed reluctance to begin active therapy; she could not imagine taking on "one more thing" and answering to a mental health team, besides "having excuses for her physician." She refused to schedule 1-hour appointments after the evaluation; instead agreeing to 30 minutes every other week. The team did not endorse this plan but accepted it, fearing that additional demands would drive the patient away with no benefit.

> "After 2 weeks, Carmella reported that she practiced mindful breathing daily and at bedtime, and felt some sense of quieting her mind as her breathing slowed ..."

Mindful breathing was explained as a low time commitment practice with potential high yield (Baer, 2003; Davis, Eshelman, & McKay, 2008). Her breathing rate at rest was 16 breaths per minute so the recommendation was to focus on slowing the breath first to 12, then to 10 breaths per minute. Training sessions were short and emphasized her gaining control, first over her breathing and later other physiological responses. She accepted the recommendation that she practice mindful breathing during the day and at bedtime. The team offered text messaging and phone apps as reminders, but these were refused. Carmella said that we should take her word that she would do the breathing practice and she would be back in 2 weeks.

Complaints about non-restorative sleep were part of the clinical presentation; specifically, Carmella did not sleep well and was always tired. She wondered if her low motivation for change was related to insufficient sleep. Her physician had prescribed Lunesta but she did not want to start it, "not another medicine!" Sleep hygiene recommendations were kept very simple; the entire list was not given to the client; only two suggestions were made, one of which also related to eating behavior (Ho et al., 2015).

Carmella often waited until her husband got home from work to eat her largest meal of the day, delaying the meal until after 8 p.m. The new plan was to prepare the meal at 6 p.m.; Carmella would eat alone or with her son and later would share a hot beverage and fruit while her husband ate his meal. She reported that this worked well, since in the past, she was very hungry earlier than 8 p.m. and snacked on high fat, high salt foods. The other sleep hygiene recommendation was to limit her nap to 15 minutes after getting home from work. Sometimes Carmella was so fatigued after work that she slept for more than an hour and then felt groggy and irritable the rest of the evening.

Progress on Pathways Level One activities   After 2 weeks, Carmella reported that she practiced mindful breathing daily and at bedtime and felt some sense of quieting her mind as her breathing slowed (Black, O'Reilly, Olmstead, Breen, & Irwin, 2015). She said that eating earlier had made a big difference in how she felt at bedtime. She thought she was falling asleep sooner and staying asleep longer. The fatigue was still there, but she was not "exhausted" at the end of the work day. A total of four sessions (8 weeks' time) focused on her Level One interventions. Although the team wanted to build the program a little faster, Carmella resisted these attempts, telling us that she would keep her appointments, but she couldn't do any more and needed time to adjust to the new ways.

Pathways Level Two The Level Two interventions were progressive relaxation, imagery, and increasing activity. Progressive relaxation was demonstrated and practiced within the session (Davis et al., 2008), but at first, only upper body, neck, and face instructions were given. Carmella liked this experience and accepted the concept that this exercise gave her more control over her physical tension. It was suggested that she practice on awakening and at bedtime; these instructions were given with different hoped for outcomes. On awakening, progressive relaxation can increase blood flow to muscles and provide a sense of movement and energy, thus facilitating the waking state. At bedtime, the emphasis was placed on relaxation; the instructions were to utilize shorter periods of tension and longer times of relaxation, while she breathed slowly and mindfully.

Imagery of a pleasant scene was integrated into the breathing exercise and Carmella was able to recreate an image of a beach vacation that she and her husband had taken years ago. She found this easy to do and enjoyed re-experiencing that time. At this point in therapy, the topic of increasing activity was mentioned. This was met with immediate resistance and repeated statements of this being "one more thing." The team was concerned about a lapse in motivation for the entire program, so once again no additional recommendations for activity were made. Carmella was encouraged to continue with breathing and imagery until the next session and was told that the Pathways Model was flexible and could accommodate a faster or slower pace. Acknowledgment of the difficulties that she was experiencing with making changes in behavior was frequently mentioned along with strong positive reinforcement for the changes already in place.

"... she had borrowed a step counter from a friend and was shocked at the relatively few steps that she took. She considered herself an active person, but seemingly had confused 'busy' with 'active,' two different concepts. She committed to increasing her step count to 5000."

Progress on Pathways Level Two activity As it happened, the next session did not occur for 4 weeks because of scheduling issues. On her return, Carmella offered an apology for her reaction to our suggestion for increasing physical activity. She said that in the past month, she had borrowed a step counter from a friend and was shocked at the relatively few steps that she took each day. She considered herself an active person, but seemingly had confused "busy" with "active," two different concepts. She committed to increasing her step count to 5000, which was encouraged by the team so specific suggestions were made to slowly increase aerobic activity. After a stressful day, Carmella was advised to do a short period of exercise, which was intended to buffer the anticipated increased blood pressure and recovery failure associated with the stress response of the day, potentially damaging to a person with essential hypertension (Hamer, Taylor, & Steptoe, 2006).

Pathways Level Three   The Level Three interventions were thermal and heart rate variability (HRV) biofeedback, psychotherapy, and Reiki (Rice, 2007). Biofeedback was explained as a way of reducing the feelings of being overwhelmed by gaining control over physiological reactions to stress (McGinnis, McGrady, Cox, & Grower-Dowling, 2005). Carmella understood the concept of heart rate variability, but achieving resonance frequency breathing took multiple sessions. Her responses after a few minutes were either giving up: "too hard—can't do it" or "don't have time to give to this." Thermal feedback for hand warming seemed easier to grasp and to implement and within five sessions, she was able to reliably warm her hands to above 90°. The usual next step, warming the feet, presented a theoretical and practice challenge. Carmella did not complain of cold feet as she did her cold hands, but experienced sensations of burning, possible indicators of diabetic neuropathy.

> "Carmella nodded her head and told us that she felt at peace and experienced a sense of connectedness within herself; there was no pain in her feet and no burning."

In response to these concerns, the team designed a guided imagery intervention that would focus on mental pictures of healthy warmth of the feet. Relaxation was induced through mindful breathing, then an image of a pleasant scene was suggested; instead of the ocean, an image of clear lake water was suggested. She was guided in imagining her burning feet in flowing water of changing colors. She started describing the colors to the therapist as she saw them, starting with orange/yellow colors (associated with the burning sensation), then yellow/green, followed by green/blue and bluish white. The first time this intervention was attempted, Carmella's breathing slowed and was counted at 8 breaths per minute. When she opened her eyes, tears streaked her cheeks. Carmella nodded her head and told us that she felt at peace and experienced a sense of connectedness within herself; there was no pain in her feet and no burning. She talked for several minutes, telling us that for the first time, she believed in the therapy and in her own ability to improve.

Factors relevant to the psychotherapy were learning to cope with her responsibilities at work and the perceived demands placed on her by her parents and adult children. Her parents were in their late 70s and independent, but both were retired and engaged in few activities, so they waited for Carmella and her siblings to come over and visit, which her brother and sister did infrequently. Carmella said: "I got into the habit of going over there 2–3 times a week and now they expect it and make me feel guilty if I don't see them." "We grew up in a close family and my mother took care of her mother which is expected in our Hispanic culture." My husband doesn't understand this, as his grandmother went into assisted living after her husband died and seemed happy there with activities, new friends and no responsibilities." That conversation led into a discussion of their adult children. She and Bobby believed they raised their kids to be independent and self-sufficient, but they didn't act like it.

I was hoping for an adult relationship at least with my daughter but it isn't. She calls me daily, sometimes twice a day and I hate to admit it but it drives me crazy. My son tells me all these details about his relationship with his girlfriend and asks me what to do about issues. One of my friends told me her son calls twice a month and she envies me!! I wanted to tell her—NO—this is TOO MUCH. I am so involved with my family that I don't see friends much anymore; between my husband's schedule at the hospital and my family, Bobby and I are not together much, sex is infrequent. *Facebook* is not a substitute for seeing a friend face to face.

Cognitive behavioral therapy (CBT) focused on reframing her overwhelming sense of responsibility for her parents, her adult children, and her job, and setting clearer boundaries. After the guided imagery sessions, Carmella was at the same time, calm, focused, and empowered, and more willing to brainstorm some solutions. Later that week, she talked to her sister who agreed readily to go over and visit their parents once a week, surprising Carmella. In fact, as she found out later, Carmella's sister, husband, and son showed up at the parents' home several times a week around dinner time, which pleased her parents as mom still liked to cook; this arrangement also seemed helpful to her sister who did not like to prepare daily meals.

Carmella gently suggested to her daughter and sons that she had to devote time to her health and couldn't talk to them every day because she was meditating or working on increasing her activity. These conversations did not go well; Carmella was disappointed that her children could not see the importance of their mother devoting time to care for herself. Further, her daughter reminded Carmella that other parents would be thrilled to have frequent phone contact with their adult children. After discussion with Bobby, Carmella suggested a weekly family dinner night where the in-town children would come over and eat with her and Bobby; this would give them a chance to prepare and share a meal and stay current with each other's activities. The out-of-town son could participate via Skype although he would miss the actual food. This weekly dinner became a treasured ritual, as Bobby made it a point to come home on time, Carmella planned the meal the previous weekend, and the kids sometimes brought over dessert or salad. When their son came for a visit, the family made sure to schedule a family meal. Gradually, the daily phone calls decreased to once or twice a week, but the family dinners were rarely missed.

Carmella's workplace was a larger challenge, but timing was in her favor, since the school year was ending soon and summer break was beginning. After teachers and students left for the summer, the administrative staff continued to work, but the atmosphere was much less stressful and deadline pressures were rare. Carmella talked to her boss at length, being truthful with him. She began the conversation by admitting that the past 2 years had not been her best and she appreciated his tolerance and understanding. Her boss said that he saw the fatigue in her expression and the suffering in her eyes when she was slow to complete tasks. He also told her that he observed in meetings that she "*almost* said things, seemed to have something to say, then said nothing." Carmella ruefully agreed; she did have ideas of how some tasks could be made more efficient, but didn't dare offer anything because she was afraid she would not be able to carry out what she herself suggested. At the end of the meeting, there was agreement that Carmella would have time during the summer to work on two of her ideas and present them to the superintendent by early August. Implementation would then be discussed. Carmella worked on one of the projects during the summer and felt more intellectually challenged than she had been in a long time. As her ideas grew into concrete proposals and implementation strategies Carmella felt validated. She told the team: "I thought my ideas were good, but my fatigue and depression made me question everything and minimize my contributions." In August of that year, Carmella presented a detailed plan which was accepted and formulated into an action plan. Carmella's boss encouraged her to begin to speak up at meetings during the next school year and promised that she would not be assigned multiple new tasks. In fact, she would be allowed to allocate time to her "baby," the computerized student attendance tracking system.

Complementary medicine intervention Eighteen months into treatment, Carmella mentioned the topic of complementary medicine, specifically Reiki and supplements, which had been discussed among the staff at school. She did not want to explore supplements or herbals, but the concept of energy medicine was intriguing for her. Reiki is a complementary health approach in which practitioners place their hands lightly on or just above a person, with the goal of facilitating the person's own healing response. Emerging research has shown that Reiki may benefit patients with diabetes (Gillespie, Gillespie, & Stevens, 2007; NCCAM, 2015). The team helped Carmella to locate a local provider who had been affiliated with the hospital at one time but who was in private practice now. Several weeks later, Carmella reported that the feelings that she experienced during Reiki were similar to those of the relaxation exercises. In contrast to her active participation with our team, Reiki was passive, and Carmella enjoyed sitting quietly while the Reiki practitioner moved his hands a few inches from her body. She decided that monthly sessions with the Reiki provider would supplement what she was doing on her own and in our therapy sessions. The use of Reiki for its effects on pain and anxiety (Thrane & Cohen, 2014) is consistent with the Pathways Model.

Session frequency decreased during year two of treatment to monthly 50-minutes appointments, and this schedule continued for another year. Carmella lost 25 lb in 3 years, which resulted in a significant decrease in blood glucose. The improvement in fasting and postprandial blood glucose was reflected in her glycohemoglobin of 6.5%, eliminating the "threat" of insulin injections. Medication for essential hypertension and hyperlipidemia remained the same. Carmella shared the details of the Pathways program with her physician; he said that she was doing extremely well and encouraged her to continue using the skills that she had learned. He would manage the medicines and she would be in charge of every other part of diabetes care. Carmella continued daily practice of mindful breathing, relaxation, and imagery. When her feet burned, she practiced the specifically designed imagery exercise and achieved relief.

Termination of her treatment program was mutually agreed upon at the end of 3 years. Carmella expressed gratitude to the team, ruefully commenting: "I guess I was a challenge in the beginning, but I am so glad you stuck with me; the changes were huge to me at that time and all I could think about was "One More Thing." "Thanks for your patience."

Summary

The metabolic syndrome is a chronic illness for which cure is not a reasonable expectation. However, patients can achieve decreases in blood glucose, blood pressure, and lose weight, by following established medically based protocols supplemented by psychophysiological interventions. Motivation for change and self-management is a key to improvement (West, DiLillo, Bursac, Gore, & Greene, 2007), but a therapeutic relationship with the health care team is essential to support the patient's efforts. Carmella reported no history of trauma or abuse during early development or in her relationship with her husband. Conversely, ethnicity, family history, sedentary lifestyle, anxiety, and burdensome responsibilities at home and at work increased the risk for the metabolic syndrome and led to its gradual emergence during middle adulthood.

As Carmella continued in the Pathways program, her growing sense of empowerment facilitated reframing suggestions not as evidence of failure or burdens, but as encouragement to continue and expand good health practices. Medical management was not much different at the end compared to the beginning of treatment, but the mental regimen was dramatically different. Carmella's care presented particular challenges: she needed to feel in control, refused the usual timing of sessions, and initially actively resisted suggestions for increased activity. Her reaction to certain components of the treatment plan necessitated adapting the biofeedback protocol to her specific needs. The addition of Reiki, initiated by Carmella provided a good complement to self-guided practice of relaxation. CBT provided new, flexible frameworks for rethinking work responsibilities and eliciting creative potential. Since the Pathways Model allows for flexibility and elasticity in scheduling and choice of interventions, it is particularly useful for clients such as Carmella.

References

Aguilar, M., Bhuket, T., Torres, S., Liu, B., & Wong, R. J. (2015). Prevalence of the metabolic syndrome in the United States, 2003-2012. *Journal of the American Medical Association, 313*(19), 1973–1974.

Aikens, J. E. (2012). Prospective associations between emotional distress and poor outcomes in type 2 diabetes. *Diabetes Care, 35*(12), 2472–2478. https://doi.org/10.2337/dc12-0181

American Diabetes Association (ADA). (2015a). Diagnosis and classification of diabetes mellitus. *Diabetes Care, 38*(Suppl. 1), S8–S16.

American Diabetes Association (ADA). (2015b). Standards of medical care in diabetes. *Diabetes Care, 38*(Suppl. 1), S1–S93.

American Psychiatric Association. (2013). *Diagnostic and statistical manual of mental disorders* (5th ed.). Arlington, VA: American Psychiatric Publishing.

American Academy of Pediatrics (2014). Adverse childhood experiences and the lifelong consequences of trauma. https://www.aap.org/en-us/Documents/ttb_aces_consequences.pdf.

Baer, R. A. (2003). Mindfulness training as a clinical intervention: A conceptual and empirical review. *Clinical Psychological Science Practicum, 10*(2), 125–143.

Black, D., O'Reilly, G., Olmstead, R., Breen, E., & Irwin, M. (2015). Mindfulness meditation and improvement in sleep quality and daytime impairment among older adults with sleep disturbances: A randomized clinical trial. *JAMA Internal Medicine, 175*(4), 494–501.

Branth, S., Ronquist, G., Stridsberg, M., Hambraeus, L., Kindgren, E., Olsson, R., et al. (2007). Development of abdominal fat and incipient metabolic syndrome in young healthy men exposed to long-term stress. *Nutrition, Metabolism, and Cardiovascular Diseases, 17*, 427–435.

Brook, R. D., Appel, L. J., Rubenfire, M., Ogedegbe, G., Bisognano, J. D., Elliott, W. J., et al. (2013). Beyond medications and diet: Alternative approaches to lowering blood pressure. *Hypertension, 61*(6), 1360–1383.

Capuron, L., Su, S., Miller, A. H., Bremner, J. D., Goldbery, J., Vogt, G. J., et al. (2008). Depressive symptoms and metabolic syndrome: Is inflammation the underlying link? *Biological Psychiatry, 64*(10), 896–900.

Carnethon, M., & Craft, L. (2008). Autonomic regulation of the association between exercise and diabetes. *Exercise and Sport Sciences Reviews, 36*(1), 12–18.

Catapano, A. L., Graham, I., De Backer, G., Wiklund, O., Chapman, M. J., Drexel, H., et al. (2016). 2016 ESC/EAS guidelines for the management of dyslipidaemias: The Task Force for the Management of Dyslipidaemias of the European Society of Cardiology (ESC) and European Atherosclerosis Society (EAS) developed with the special contribution of the European Association for Cardiovascular Prevention & Rehabilitation (EACPR). *Atherosclerosis, 253*, 281–344. https://doi.org/10.1016/j.atherosclerosis.2016.08.018

Chandola, T., Brunner, E., & Marmot, M. (2006). Chronic stress at work and the metabolic syndrome: Prospective study. *British Medical Journal, 332*, 521–525.

Davies, S. J. C., Hood, S. D., Christmas, D., & Nutt, D. J. (2008). Psychiatric disorders and cardiovascular disease anxiety, depression and hypertension. In L. Sher (Ed.), *Psychological factors and cardiovascular disorders: The role of psychiatric pathology and maladaptive personality features* (pp. 69–96). Hauppauge, NY: Nova Scotia Publishers Inc..

Davis, M., Eshelman, E., & McKay, M. (2008). *The relaxation & stress reduction workbook* (6th ed.). Oakland, CA: New Harbinger.

Dixon, M. R., Lik, N. M. K., Green, L., & Myerson, J. (2013). Delay discounting of hypothetical and real money: The effect of holding reinforcement rate constant. *Journal of Applied Behavior Analysis, 46*(2), 512–517.

Froy, O. (2010). Metabolism and circadian rhythms—Implications for body weight. *The Open Neuroendocrinology Journal, 3*, 28–37.

Gillespie, E., Gillespie, B. W., & Stevens, M. J. (2007). Painful diabetic neuropathy: Impact of an alternative approach. *Diabetes Care, 30*(4), 999–1001. https://doi.org/10.2337/dc06-1475

Goldbacher, E. M., & Matthews, K. A. (2007). Are psychological characteristics related to risk of the metabolic syndrome?: A review of the literature. *Annals of Behavioral Medicine, 34*(3), 240–252.

Gonzalez, J. S., Peyrot, M., McCarl, L. A., Collins, E. M., Serpa, L., Mimiaga, M. J., et al. (2008). Depression and diabetes treatment nonadherence: A meta-analysis. *Diabetes Care, 31*(12), 2398–2403. https://doi.org/10.2337/dc08-1341

Gonzalez, J. S., Shreck, E., Psaros, C., & Safren, S. A. (2015). Distress and Type-2 diabetes-treatment adherence: A mediating role for perceived control. *Health Psychology, 34*(5), 505–513.

Hamer, M., Taylor, A., & Steptoe, A. (2006). The effect of acute aerobic exercise on stress related blood pressure responses: A systematic review and meta-analysis. *Biological Psychology, 71*(2), 183–190.

Healthy Lifestyles. (2016, January). 6th. Retrieved from https://www.icsi.org/guidelines__more/catalog_guidelines_and_more/catalog_guidelines/catalog_prevention__screening_guidelines/healthy_lifestyles/

High Blood Pressure (Hypertension): Tests and Diagnosis. (2016, September 9). Retrieved from http://www.mayoclinic.org/diseases-conditions/high-blood-pressure/basics/tests-diagnosis/con-20019580

Ho, F. Y. Y., Chung, K. F., Yeung, W. F., Ng, T. H., Kwan, K. S., Yung, K. P., et al. (2015). Self-help cognitive-behavioral therapy for insomnia: A meta-analysis of randomized controlled trials. *Sleep Medicine Reviews, 19*, 17–28.

James, P. A., Oparil, S., Carter, B. L., Cushman, W. C., Dennison-Himmelfarb, C., Handler, J., et al. (2014). 2014 evidence-based guideline for the management of high blood pressure in adults: Report from the panel members appointed to the eighth Joint National Committee (JNC 8). *JAMA, 311*(5), 507–520.

Kim, K. H. C., Bursac, Z., DiLillo, V., White, D. B., & West, D. S. (2009). Stress, race, and body weight. *Health Psychology, 28*(1), 131–135.

Knutson, K., & Van Cauter, E. (2008). Associations between sleep loss and increased risk of obesity and diabetes. *Annals of the New York Academy of Sciences, 1129*, 287–304.

Kyrou, I., Chrousos, G. P., & Tsigos, C. (2006). Stress, visceral obesity, and metabolic complications. In G. P. Chrousos & C. Tsigos (Eds.), *Stress, obesity, and metabolic syndrome: Annals of the New York Academy of Sciences* (Vol. 1083, pp. 77–110). Boston, MA: Wiley-Blackwell.

Linden, W., & McGrady, A. V. (2016). Essential hypertension. In M. S. Schwartz & F. Andrasik (Eds.), *Biofeedback: A practitioner's guide* (pp. 383–399). New York: The Guilford Press.

Lundahl, B., & Burke, B. L. (2009). The effectiveness and applicability of motivational interviewing: A practice-friendly review of four meta-analyses. *Journal of Clinical Psychology, 65*(11), 1232–1245.

Matthews, K. A., & Gallo, L. C. (2011). Psychological perspectives on pathways linking socioeconomic status and physical health. *Annual Review of Psychology, 62*, 501–530. https://doi.org/10.1146/annurev.psych.031809.130711

Maty, S. C., Lynch, J. W., Raghunathan, T. E., & Kaplan, G. A. (2008). Childhood socioeconomic position, gender, adult body mass index, and incidence of type 2 diabetes mellitus over 34 years in the Alameda County Study. *American Journal of Public Health, 98*(8), 1486–1494.

McGinnis, R. A., McGrady, A., Cox, S. A., & Grower-Dowling, K. A. (2005). Biofeedback-assisted relaxation in type 2 diabetes. *Diabetes Care, 28*(9), 2145–2149.

McGrady, A., & Lakia, D. (2016). Diabetes mellitus. In M. S. Schwartz & F. Andrasik (Eds.), *Biofeedback: A practitioner's guide* (4th ed., pp. 400–421). New York: The Guilford Press.

McIntyre, R. S., Soczynski, J. K., Konarski, J. Z., Woldeyohannes, H. O., Law, C. W. Y., Miranda, A., et al. (2007). Should depressive syndromes be reclassified as "metabolic syndrome type II?". *Annals of Clinical Psychiatry, 19*(4), 257–264.

McSharry, J., Moss-Morris, R., & Kendrick, T. (2011). Illness perceptions and glycaemic control in diabetes: A systematic review with meta-analysis. *Diabetic Medicine, 28*, 1300–1310. https://doi.org/10.1111/j.1464-5491.2011.03298.x

Moskowitz, J. T., Epel, E. S., & Acree, M. (2008). Positive affect uniquely predicts lower risk of mortality in people with diabetes. *Health Psychology, 27*(1 Suppl), S73–S82.

National Center for Complementary and Alternative Medicine. (2015). *Reiki: An introduction.* Retrieved from http://nccam.nih.gov/health/reiki/introduction.htm

Ogden, C. L., Carroll, M. D., Curin, L. R., McDowell, M. A., Tabak, C. J., & Flegal, K. M. (2006). Prevalence of overweight and obesity in the United States, 1999-2004. *Journal of the American Medical Association, 295*, 1549–1555.

Patel, S. R. (2009). Reduced sleep as an obesity risk factor. *Obesity Reviews, 2*(10), 61–68.

Petry, N. M., Cengiz, E., Wagner, J. A., Hood, K. K., Carria, L., & Tamborlane, W. V. (2013). Incentivizing behavior change to improve diabetes care. *Diabetes, Obesity, and Metabolism, 15*(12), 1071–1076.

Rice, B. I. (2007). Clinical benefits of training patients to voluntarily increase peripheral blood flow. *Diabetes Educator, 33*(3), 442–454.

Simon, G. E., Ludman, E. J., Linde, J. A., Operskalski, B. H., Ichikawa, L., Rohde, P., et al. (2008). Association between obesity and depression in middle-aged women. *General Hospital Psychiatry, 30*, 32–39.

Steptoe, A., O'Donnell, K., Marmot, M., & Wardle, J. (2008). Positive affect and psychosocial processes related to health. *British Journal of Psychology, 99*, 211–227. https://doi.org/10.1348/000712607X218295

Thrane, S., & Cohen, S. M. (2014). Effect of Reiki therapy on pain and anxiety in adults: An in-depth literature review of randomized trials with effect size calculations. *Pain Management Nursing, 15*(4), 897–908. https://doi.org/10.1016/j.pmn.2013.07.008

West, D. S., DiLillo, V., Bursac, Z., Gore, S. A., & Greene, P. G. (2007). Motivational interviewing improves weight loss in women with type 2 diabetes. *Diabetes Care, 30*, 1081–1087.

Wickrama, K., O'Neal, C. W., Lee, T. K., & Wickrama, T. (2015). Early socioeconomic adversity, youth positive development, and young adults' cardio-metabolic disease risk. *Health Psychology, 34*(9), 905–914.

Chapter 11
Pathways Approach to Cardiovascular Disorders

Abstract Cardiovascular diseases are the most common chronic illnesses and a major cause of morbidity and mortality. Comorbidity among the physical illnesses in this category and mood and anxiety disorders is very high. Management of symptoms of shortness of breath, rapid heart rate, fatigue, or a sense of malaise are signals requiring attention first by the patient experiencing the symptoms; then the patient must have the ability to decide whether emergency medical attention is necessary. Interference by low mood or high anxiety in the decision-making process can have serious consequences. This chapter considers cardiovascular disorders from the Pathways perspective. The first case is that of a middle-aged physician who struggles to adjust to his diagnosis of congestive heart failure. The second case describes a traumatic reaction to heart surgery, necessitating treatment for post-traumatic stress disorder. In each case, the Pathways Model organizes, step-wise interventions facilitating active involvement of the individual in his/her own health care. The effects of mood and anxiety on symptom management, response to treatment and outcome are explored. Both individuals achieve enhanced well-being in spite of the presence of a chronic cardiovascular condition.

Keywords Cardiovascular disorders · Congestive heart failure · Cardiac rehabilitation · PTSD · Pathways Model

The Case of Eduardo

"Eduardo was one of the angriest people the team had seen... He was furious at his body for letting him down."

Eduardo was a 50-year-old Hispanic physician, who was referred by his cardiologist friend and colleague. He noticed that his colleague was anxious, irritable, and displaying excessive anger. Eduardo was an emergency room physician with an excellent reputation as a caring and highly skilled caregiver. During the past 8 months, Eduardo became aware that he was more fatigued than usual. On two occasions while rushing into an exam room

© Springer International Publishing AG, part of Springer Nature 2018 195
A. McGrady, D. Moss, *Integrative Pathways*,
https://doi.org/10.1007/978-3-319-89313-6_11

during a code yellow (multiple victims coming to the emergency room), he was short of breath and had to slow his pace. The first time he attributed this to his rapid run down the hallway; the second time, his usually normal quick pace caused him to experience chest pain and difficulty taking a deep breath. He knew that the combination of shortness of breath, fatigue, and chest pain could indicate congestive heart failure.

Eduardo was one of the angriest people the team had seen. Despite his medical knowledge and extensive experience in the ER, he rebelled against his diagnosis and resisted psychological intervention. He was furious at his body for letting him down. Unfortunately, the young cardiologist, who conducted the preliminary workup before the full medical battery of testing was completed, suggested that Eduardo would have to cut back on his work hours, which caused immediate resistance and further outrage. The referral to the mental health team was finally accepted by Eduardo when the interventions were described as "helping patients gain control over their illness."

Congestive Heart Failure

Congestive heart failure (CHF) is a chronic cardiovascular condition characterized by the inability of the heart muscle to pump enough blood throughout the body. The damage to the heart can develop due to viral infections of the heart muscle, diseases of the valves, heart attack, or untreated hypertension, among other causes. The severity of symptoms and prognosis are related to the etiology. No matter what the cause, CHF is a stressful life experience because of its chronicity, the debilitating symptoms themselves, and the common comorbid mood symptoms (Yu, 2008). Non-surgical interventions include medication, primarily diuretics, ACE inhibitors (angiotension converting enzyme blockers), and nitrates. Successful surgical treatment depends on identifying the cause of heart failure accurately. For example, a pacemaker can be placed in the chest if patients have arrhythmias, while a ventricular assist device helps to prevent dangerously low heart rate (bradycardia). Heart valve surgery repairs or replaces a valve(s), usually the mitral valve.

Self-awareness, monitoring, and self- regulation are important, and it is fair to say even critical components to management of chronic cardiovascular disorders. Day-to-day decisions require effective problem-solving skills. The patient should be able to identify when a symptom is stable and when there has been a change. Potentially harmful variations necessitate the ability to devise a plan to prevent worsening and then re-stabilize the condition (Bosworth, Powers, & Oddone, 2010).

Multiple physical and psychological factors affect the progression of cardiac failure and (what is termed) "event-free length." For example, sleep disruption of any type, such as insomnia, multiple awakenings, or non-restorative sleep may upset normal endocrine or autonomic balance in addition to worsening mood (Krietsch, Mason, & Sbarra, 2014). Time spent awake during the night was shown in one study to increase sympathetic activity and interfere with the cortisol feedback ystem (Motivala, 2011). The malaise that accompanies sleep deprivation can mimic ickness behavior or depressed mood. Patients with heart failure often grieve their oss of cardiac health. Anxiety is a common experience as patients attempt to adjust heir physical activity, their work schedule, and family responsibilities (Gallagher & 3rimaldi, 2012). Similarly, to other chronic illnesses, management of cardiac failure requires a partnership among the patient and providers. Self-awareness and self-care strategies, based on realistic understanding of the illness, are keys to maintaining unction (Li & Shun, 2015).

Initial Psychological Evaluation of Eduardo

3duardo spent his early years in Puerto Rico. He was an only child, a happy boy who enjoyed activity and to his uneducated mother and father seemed to have a superior intellect. At age 8, Eduardo became seriously ill and his parents first tried 1ome remedies and consulted family members about his symptoms. Weeks later, hey took him to the local doctor. Rheumatic fever was suspected, but not diagnosed. Subsequently, Eduardo was treated with a short course of antibiotics. He recovered and resumed his active life; no one thought any more about it. When 3duardo was 10 years old, the family emigrated from Puerto Rico to Florida. 3duardo's parents improved their English and strived to assimilate into the American culture. Throughout their years in Miami and a later period in Tallahassee, Florida, 1is parents believed that education was the key to success in America. So they promoted school attendance, encouraged completion of homework, and fostered dreams of college. Eduardo completed college and then to his parents' great joy, he applied and was accepted into medical school. He was a good enough student in the basic sciences, but outstanding in his clinical work. He matched into emergency medicine, completed residency with superior grades, and entered a group practice. He married Carla, a nurse at the hospital, and they had three healthy children. Their marriage was stable and his children, now in college or working were a great source of pride for both Eduardo and Carla.

Carla came with Eduardo to the evaluation, offering to provide support in any way necessary. The couple was very close. Both had been shocked by the diagnosis and the recommendation that Eduardo would have to cut back on the work that gave 1is life so much meaning. Eduardo voiced his opinion that the young cardiologist had insulted him and judged him to be "unable" to continue his work schedule. "Nothing has happened to my mind!! I have many more years of experience than he has and he can't tell me what to do". Carla diverted the conversation away from the topic of what Eduardo would and would not be able to do, stating: "Let's hear more about the Pathways Model." The team provided an explanation of the Model, emphasizing the active collaboration between provider and patient, the logical progression of the steps in the model, and patient empowerment. Carla had rarely seen her husband as angry as he was during these weeks since the diagnosis and she was very concerned that the over-arousal would complicate the CHF. She encouraged her husband to try the Pathways interventions at least for a few weeks, as it could do no harm. Eduardo was on a short-term medical leave and did not have enough activity to fill his time, so he reluctantly agreed.

Pathways Interventions

> "The Pathways Model provided a return to normal rhythms (Level one), skill building (Level two), and advanced psychophysiological interventions (Level three) to help Eduardo regain emotional balance and improved physical health."

Pathways Level One Level One interventions were explained as restoring normal bodily rhythms, which had been disrupted by the illness and Eduardo's reaction to the diagnosis. The first Level One intervention was slow mindful breathing. We emphasized being in the moment with the breath, not seeing the breath as his enemy. He was instructed to practice several times a day for a few minutes, gradually increasing to 5 minutes, three times a day. A second Level One intervention, Soothing, was explained as the beginnings of self-care. Eduardo was to sit in his rocking chair and instead of reading a book, which he often did, to focus on the rhythm of the rocker and let himself relax. He reported that he found it difficult to "do nothing" while he was rocking, so he began to pray during this time, which was effective in soothing his mind and his spirit. He was pleased by the therapist's validation of his habit of prayer as another way to decrease sympathetic activity and improve autonomic regulation (Bernston, Norman, Hawkley, & Cacioppo, 2008).

Pathways Level Two The Level Two interventions were described as the necessary skills to cope with symptoms, make good decisions, and advance self-care. Emphasis was again placed on empowerment and building self-efficacy. Eduardo was taught progressive muscle relaxation as his first Level Two intervention and encouraged to add this exercise to his daily mindful breathing and soothing practices. After 2 weeks, he reported an increased sense of control over the tension in his body. He recognized that since the diagnosis of CHF, he had been so angry and tense, that he was gritting his teeth and tightening the muscles in his shoulders and back, feeling pain in those areas by the end of the day.

The "Pause" intervention was suggested as a strategy for moments when Eduardo started feeling angry, before letting his anger take control of him. He had "done everything right," worked hard in the ER, dealt with difficult patients more effectively than some of his colleagues, and had never had an ethical violation or a malpractice suit. He ate a healthy diet and walked on the track at the hospital facility several times a week. He felt punished for a transgression that he had not committed. Eduardo's accurate sense of himself as an astute clinician coupled with the discovery he had been at risk for heart failure for the previous 40 years since his childhood illness was almost more than he could bear.

Some of his expressed anger had actually begun to worry Eduardo—he had never been physically violent to another person and was usually slow to anger. Now, he directed his anger toward himself. He felt that he was a faker—advising patients to know their medical history and practice self-care, while all along he was a time bomb. The team realized that a mismatch between perception and reality can be the spark to instigate angry responses, which can become violent, and that anger can be a critical factor in heart failure (Brennan, 2011; Kucharska-Newton et al., 2014). An introductory anger management intervention was implemented in Level Two, with the plan to expand it in Level Three. Basically, the "pause" suggestion was a kind of "time out," to be implemented whenever Eduardo recognized physiological arousal and feelings of frustration or irritability. The sequence was as follows: become aware, pause, breathe mindfully until arousal decreases, and then re-engage with the situation, the memory, or the person eliciting the angry reaction and work to resolve it.

During this phase of treatment, the Eduardo sought a second full cardiac workup from a major medical center. When the physician discussed the results with him, it became clear that the episode of rheumatic fever when he was 8 years old had started the weakening of his heart valves, which were now damaged. The team of physicians credited Eduardo for his commitment to a healthy lifestyle, which "certainly" had delayed the damage to the valves until now. Hearing this acknowledgment of his efforts to stay healthy defused some of his anger toward himself and toward the illness. He was a candidate for valve replacement and had an excellent prognosis for recovery. Eduardo readily agreed to the surgical procedure, which was done at the major medical center. He would be followed closely locally and return for checkups if needed at the center. Surgery and recovery produced a hiatus in our work with this patient. When he returned to treatment, his attitude was much improved and his anger had decreased, but he still over-reacted to minor irritations and displayed physiological and emotional over-arousal. He realized that the first two levels in the Pathways Model had helped him get through a very difficult period in his life and he wanted to continue.

Pathways Level Three The Level Three interventions consisted of cognitive behavioral therapy (CBT), biofeedback, and advanced anger management. The team chose CBT as the first type of psychotherapy, since Eduardo resisted exploration of feelings, but could accept working on his thoughts. He was still recovering from surgery, often felt weak, and fatigued easily. His medical leave was extended for another 6 weeks. His return to normal physical activity was slow and he mercilessly called himself "disabled" and "pathetic." CBT is particularly effective in decreasing irrational beliefs related to illness. Cognitive restructuring taught Eduardo to challenge his thoughts of disability, worthlessness, and hopelessness about the future. Return to medical practice was realistic but it was still unclear if he could work a full schedule (Gallagher & Grimaldi, 2012).

Heart rate variability (HRV) biofeedback was offered to help Eduardo gain confidence in his ability to slow his breathing, also to understand the relationships among mood, anger, and breathing. When angry and self-critical, his breathing was shallow and asynchronous with heart rate. When he paused, mentally stepped back, and focused on breathing, he achieved resonance. The information (feedback) provided by HRV biofeedback gave Eduardo a sense of mastery over his physiological responses to stress. His adherence to home practice was excellent and he reported feeling more relaxed and more in control of his breathing and his mood. Often, patients with heart disease and particularly congestive heart failure report feelings of hopelessness and negative views of their future. However, research has shown therapeutic effects of achieving self-mastery on morbidity and mortality (Roepke & Grant, 2011; Surtees, Wainwright, Luben, Khaw, & Day, 2006).

Advanced anger management consisted of adapting standard techniques used when clients are angry or violent toward others to Eduardo's rage at himself and to an extent at his parents. The provider helped Eduardo identify his self-critical verbiage, his frequent "should" statements in the context of his current diagnosis. Slowly, Eduardo forgave himself for being ignorant about the effects of his early illness. He recalled his parents' worried faces when he was sick as a child and accepted that they did the best that they could with available medical resources. During this process, emotions became intense, and Eduardo worked on coping with these emotions. Later, a more problem-focused coping approach was introduced and integrated into treatment (Li & Shun, 2015).

The integrative approach to Eduardo's heart failure was crucial to successful resolution and a return to functionality for him (Kemper, Carmin, Mehta, & Binkley, 2016). A comprehensive medical workup provided an explanation for his symptoms, which he could understand and accept. Fortunately, surgery was available and the valve replacement surgery had a positive outcome. The Pathways Model provided a return to normal rhythms (Level one), skill building (Level two), and advanced psychophysiological interventions (Level three) to help Eduardo regain emotional balance and improved physical health. He returned to work after 6 months of medical leave, voluntarily decreasing his work hours by one quarter, but reporting that his colleagues and the staff were happy to have him back at any percentage of time. He told the team that he wanted more time with Carla and his kids and time to pursue other interests, that is, to enjoy the life that he had feared would be lost because of CHF.

The Case of Vanessa

Vanessa was a 51-year-old woman who was a patient in a cardiac rehabilitation program following a heart attack and surgical stent placement. The Pathways team was called in because Vanessa had dropped out of rehab after 1 week of structured exercise. After multiple attempts, contact was successful. Vanessa agreed to come in, but only if she was seen in a different location from the hospital and rehab facility. Vanessa came to the appointment with her daughter and provided a personal history of sporadic chest pain for several years prior to the heart attack and high blood pressure treated with an antihypertensive medication. There was a strong family history of heart disease on her mother's side of the family although the biological father's history was unknown.

Two months prior to the assessment by the Pathways team, Vanessa sustained a severe heart attack and was hospitalized. Stent placement to open two blocked arteries was recommended, but Vanessa resisted at first, telling the surgeon and her family that she knew that she was going to die during surgery. A psychiatric consult was scheduled and Vanessa told the psychiatrist that it probably didn't matter if she had the surgery or not. She had a strong feeling of dread and believed that she would not survive to see her grandchildren grow up. Eventually, Vanessa's daughter persuaded her mother to sign the consent form. Stent placement was successful and physical recovery uneventful. However, both mood and anxiety seemed to worsen, particularly when she drove by the hospital or had appointments in cardiac rehabilitation. The team recommended that the Pathways Model be implemented in the Department of Psychiatry on the opposite side of campus from the hospital.

Cardiovascular disease, according to recent literature, is responsible for about one-third of all deaths and is the leading cause of morbidity and mortality in the United States (Ruiz & Brondolo, 2016).The severity of the illness and outcomes are influenced to a great extent by gender, race, socioeconomic status, and psychological health or ill health. Specifically, depression and anxiety were shown to be predictors of recurrent myocardial infarction or worsening heart disease (Roest, Heideveld, Martens, de Jonge, & Denollet, 2014). Multiple hypotheses have been advanced to explain the mechanisms linking mood and anxiety with cardiovascular disease; the most widely studied are chronic inflammation, autonomic imbalance (sympathetic nervous system dominance), platelet aggregation, hyperactivity of the stress response system, and allostatic load. Behavioral and socioeconomic pathways for poor outcomes include sedentary lifestyle, unhealthy eating, and living in noisy, dangerous, low-income neighborhoods (Stewart, Janicki, & Kamarck, 2006; Wulsin, 2012). Nonetheless, these negative effects are not necessarily permanent and their impact can be lessened when the person acquires coping skills, builds a support network, and learns to modify the negative effects of stress (Kiviruusu, Huurre, Haukkala, & Aro, 2013).

Recommended treatment following a myocardial infarction (heart attack) includes medical management and cardiac rehabilitation. Completion of rehab is associated with attenuation of risk factors (Redfern, Briffa, Ellis, & Freedman, 2008), fewer re-hospitalizations, and lower mortality rates (Martin et al., 2012). Unfortunately, mood disturbances prevent some patients from finishing the required number of rehab sessions, the treatment with proven success (Huffman et al., 2008). Specifically, depression and anxiety are predictors of lower attendance and reduced completion of cardiac rehabilitation (McGrady, McGinnis, Badenhop, Bentle, & Rajput, 2009; McGrady, Burkes, Badenhop, & McGinnis, 2014) although the linking variables between psychological state and drop out have not been fully explored.

Initial Evaluation of Vanessa Vanessa had experienced multiple stressors in her early life which changed in nature over time but continued into adulthood. She grew up in a single parent household; her mother worked full time and Vanessa had responsibilities for her younger siblings by the age of 10. She was a marginal student, graduating from high school with a C average and no thoughts of college, but she had learned computer skills and found a part-time job at an auto dealership. She became pregnant by her boyfriend of 2 years and they lived together but never married. There were financial stressors, since her young partner, also with only a high school education, worked at minimum wage jobs. The relationship lasted 4 years and Vanessa was left with a young daughter to take care of with minimal support. She placed her daughter in federally funded day care and found a new job as a secretary at her church. With assistance, she paid her bills. The pattern continued. Vanessa's daughter become pregnant during high school, dropped out, and at the time of Vanessa's heart attack had two young children, but was not married. Vanessa was babysitting on the days that she did not work at the church. She loved many aspects of her job, particularly the interaction with the pastors, the friendliness of the members of the church, and her participation in church activities. However, the relationship with her daughter was sometimes conflicted. She loved her grandchildren and wanted the best for them, but she sometimes felt used by her daughter who always said she was looking for work, but somehow never found a stable position.

The Pathways Model was explained to Vanessa as a program to help her reduce her stress and regain her health so that she could go back to work at the church.

Pathways Interventions

Pathways Level One Since there were multiple Level 1 needs, the following were implemented: mindful breathing, feeding, sleep, and movement. Vanessa learned slow mindful breathing and practiced it in our presence with little difficulty. She agreed to slowly increase her activity from sedentary (since she stopped rehab) to taking a 10-minutes walk every day. With regard to her diet, she began to increase consumption of fruits and vegetables. She recalled frequently eating fruit when she was growing up in her mother's home and rekindled the enjoyment of the texture and taste of fruit. However, Vanessa's sleep did not improve. Her doctor had prescribed a sleep aid that was somewhat effective, but left Vanessa with a "hangover" the next morning. It was decided to move to Level Two interventions to address the sleep problem and to attempt to return Vanessa to the cardiac rehab program.

"The team comforted Vanessa, as they explained that she had been traumatized by the experience of waking up during surgery and she was suffering from post-traumatic stress disorder."

Pathways Level Two Relaxation with basic imagery was implemented as the first Level Two intervention (Halm 2009). In our presence, Vanessa focused on the sensations of relaxation and reported an image of a pleasant scene. Before the next week's appointment Vanessa called to say that she appreciated our help with breathing and healthy eating, but she was not returning to the Pathways program. The relaxation/imagery exercise made her feel "really nervous" and put "scary pictures" in her head. She was asked to come back one more time to give the team feedback and perhaps help other people in the future. She agreed if the purpose was to help other patients and if she would not be asked to do any imagery.

At the next appointment, Vanessa first talked only about helping other patients. She was asked to describe in more detail the frightening images that came into her mind during imagery so that other patients could be counseled if it happened to them. This strategy was both a simple ruse and an honest attempt to anticipate the same phenomenon in future patients. Vanessa talked about trying to relax and see the pleasant scene, but soon the scary pictures came into her head. The images were "heart scary," and then she said: "I remember going crazy during surgery," and "if I tell you, you will send me right to the psych hospital." With reassurance, empathy, and encouragement, Vanessa finally revealed that she awoke during surgery, and heard the sounds of the surgeon cracking her chest. The "heart scary" pictures were the sound of bone cracking, the smell of the operating room and blood, and the terror that she was dying. She said she could never go back to the hospital or to cardiac rehab because it had the same smells. She was terrified that if she went back, she would not be able to get out of the memory and it would overtake her.

The team comforted Vanessa as she cried and they explained that she had been traumatized by the experience of waking up during surgery and she was suffering from post-traumatic stress disorder. It was unfortunate that she had awakened and that the doctor had not revealed the incident to her so that he could debrief her right after the surgery. What had happened was that the attempt to let go, relax, and generate a pleasant image had increased anxiety instead of decreasing it because traumatic images had filled her mind. The Pathways team was supportive of Vanessa, validated her psychological symptoms, and assured her that no psychiatric hospitalization was necessary at that time. If she agreed to return, her sessions could continue across campus from the main hospital. The team discontinued imagery. Instead, trauma-focused therapy, a Level Three intervention was initiated.

Pathways Level Three Vanessa's response to therapy was very positive and her mood stabilized more quickly than had been anticipated. Her trauma had occurred during a life-saving procedure, not perpetrated by a violent individual who wanted to harm her or in a real-world dangerous situation, like a fire or flood. The trauma was reconstructed cognitively as a few seconds long event that did not interfere with the successful outcome of the surgery. The team did not dismiss her memory in any way, but her description was validated; it was labeled as unfortunate and frightening due to lack of information. Vanessa's belief that because she had awakened, the surgery was not successful was countered by the cardiologist who was asked and agreed to read and review the surgical notes with Vanessa. Patient education is necessary before and after serious medical procedures to address patients' unrealistic beliefs or memories directly. Otherwise, these thoughts and perceptions often prevent patients from obtaining the psychiatric help that they need and in addition contribute to patients dropping out from necessary medical follow-up care (Anderson & Emery, 2014; Wu et al., 2013).

"Brief motivational interviewing is effective in clarifying patients' personal decisions to make changes, to adhere to treatment, and to want to move toward health."

Slowly, Vanessa's scary memories lessened in vividness and intensity, while other memories of successful recovery were more frequently present. Her growing physical strength and increased ability to do more were sources of positive mood. Motivational interviewing was then used to garner reasons to change lifestyle. She wanted to return to work and she wanted to be a good influence on her grandkids, so that they would not repeat her or her daughter's experiences with unplanned pregnancy, low paying jobs, and dependence on public assistance. Brief motivational interviewing is effective in clarifying patients' personal decisions to make changes, to adhere to treatment, and to want to move toward health (Lundahl & Burke, 2009; McGrady et al., 2014).

Weekly sessions of psychotherapy continued for 6 months. Relaxation and imagery were re-introduced and implemented and were mastered with much less difficulty. Occasionally, a frightening image came into Vanessa's mind, but she quickly used a cognitive skill to defuse its impact. The use of relaxation in patients post-cardiac surgery has been validated as one way to improve quality of life (Dehdari, Heidarnia, Ramezankhani, Sadeghian, & Ghofranipour, 2009). Then the team asked Vanessa to drive by the hospital while doing mindful breathing to decrease the association between the hospital and the traumatic event. The Pathways team recommended a return to cardiac rehab with some modifications, but Vanessa refused stating, "I promise you that I will walk every day but I can't go back there." The cardiac rehab nurse attended a therapy session with Vanessa's permission. It was finally agreed by everyone that Vanessa's rehab sessions would be scheduled according to the nurse's schedule for the first few weeks and if Vanessa became distressed, she could cut a session short. Usually, after exercise, patients take the monitoring sensors off themselves and leave them in an identified area; however, a different routine was established for Vanessa. The nurse removed the sensors for Vanessa and used that time to dialogue about the previous rehab session, including any aspects that had frightened her or which brought back memories of the surgical trauma. There was regular communication between the nurse and the psychologist to ensure that Vanessa remained in cardiac rehab, which she did complete. Her depression and anxiety scores, measured at the first rehab session and after completion of the program, decreased significantly. Beck Anxiety decreased from 24 (severe) to 8 (minimal) and Beck Depression was reduced from 20 (severe) to 6 (minimal). Sleep was improved and she no longer required the prescribed sleep aid. Most nights, she fell asleep within 30 minutes and only awakened once to use the bathroom.

Conflict between mother and daughter was carefully explored. Vanessa said that she wanted to improve their relationship and did not like the feeling of being used as a convenient, free babysitter. It was agreed that the team would see both mother and daughter for one or two sessions but further therapy would be referred to another provider. Vanessa's daughter, Ariel was a tall, slim beautiful woman who entered the room with eyes downcast and stooped shoulders. The psychologist told both women that they were here to help Vanessa to continue her pathway to health and to return to full functioning in these words: There are many challenges associated with recovery from a major cardiovascular event and Vanessa needs support" (Lawson, 2012). Ariel began by saying that her mother's heart attack was her fault and she would never forgive herself. She had put too much on her mother and that was the result. She said that she was "no good at anything. I barely got out of high school, have had only minimum wage jobs, and do not know how to parent my kids. They listen to my mother but not to me."

Ariel's perception of her mother was that Vanessa was a great parent, had an excellent job, and knew how to take care of a house and family. Vanessa was shocked at the disclosures by Ariel of her low self-esteem and feelings of personal failure. Yet she also spoke of her own beliefs that Ariel did not try hard enough to find meaningful work and disrespected her mother. It became clearer that the session was starting to focus on Ariel instead of Vanessa. Realizing the highly emotional nature of the mother–daughter relationship, the psychologist sought to redirect the goals of the session to Vanessa and her recovery. Ariel validated the intent of the session and offered to be more respectful of Vanessa's time, particularly since her mother was increasing her hours at her job. Nonetheless, joint therapy with another provider was recommended. Vanessa was followed for a year after completion of active treatment. Monthly appointments were used to check on her lifestyle changes, particularly diet and exercise. She continued to practice mindful breathing and relaxation although she discontinued imagery. When she experienced days of lower mood, she recalled the reasons why she wanted to live. She had returned to her job at the church, where she was welcomed back by the pastors and church members. The referral for joint therapy for mother and daughter was not followed, but Vanessa believed that her own improved ability to be assertive had similarly affected her relationship with Ariel. The critical components of the Pathways Model for Vanessa were motivational interviewing (Lundahl & Burke, 2009), the identification of the traumatic memory, its treatment, implementing combinations of skill building and therapy (Dusseldorp, van Genugten, van Buuren, Verheijden, & van Empelen, 2014), and the ability of the Pathways team to cooperate with the rehab and the medical staff personnel at the hospital.

Summary

Two cases of patients with cardiovascular disease were described in this chapter. These patients were quite different. In the case of congestive heart failure, the emergence of symptoms caused a psychological crisis that manifested in anger and depression. The second case exemplified social determinants of health and illness, where the patient has had multiple stressors throughout her life. An unusual occurrence elicited acute stress disorder and PTSD. In both cases, the implementation of

Pathways Model was interrupted: Eduardo had heart valve replacement while Vanessa dropped out of cardiac rehabilitation and later resumed it. Thus, orderly progression through the Pathways levels is not always possible nor is it always necessary. Clients move through the levels at the pace that is agreed upon by the therapist, the medical provider (included as appropriate), and the client.

References

Anderson, D. R., & Emery, C. F. (2014). Irrational health beliefs predict adherence to cardiac rehabilitation: A pilot study. *Health Psychology, 33*(12), 1614–1617.

Bernston, G. G., Norman, G. J., Hawkley, L. C., & Cacioppo, J. (2008). Spirituality and autonomic cardiac control. *Annals of Behavioral Medicine, 35*, 198–208.

Bosworth, H. B., Powers, B. J., & Oddone, E. (2010). Patient self-management support: Novel strategies in hypertension and heart disease. *Cardiology Clinics, 28*(4), 655–663.

Brennan, I. (2011). *Anger antidotes: How not to lose your s#&!* New York, NY: W. W. Norton & Company, Inc.

Dehdari, T., Heidarnia, A., Ramezankhani, A., Sadeghian, S., & Ghofranipour, F. (2009). Effects of progressive muscular relaxation training on quality of life in anxious patients after coronary artery bypass graft surgery. *Indian Journal of Medical Research, 129*(5), 603–608.

Dusseldorp, E., van Genugten, L., van Buuren, S., Verheijden, M. W., & van Empelen, P. (2014). Combinations of techniques that effectively change health behavior: Evidence from meta-CART analysis. *Health Psychology, 33*(12), 1530–1540.

Gallagher, J., & Grimaldi, A. (2012). Psychological management of patients with heart failure. In E. Dornelas (Ed.), *Stress proof the heart: Behavioral interventions for cardiac patients* (pp. 61–91). New York, NY: Springer.

Halm, M. A. (2009). Relaxation: A self-care healing modality reduces harmful effects of anxiety. *American Journal of Critical Care, 18*, 169–172.

Huffman, J. C., Smith, F. A., Blais, M. A., Taylor, M. A., Januzzi, J. L., & Fricchione, G. L. (2008). Pre-existing major depression predicts in-hospital cardiac complications after acute myocardial infarction. *Psychosomatics, 49*(4), 309–316.

Kucharska-Newton, A. M., Williams, J. E., Chang, P. P., Steams, S. C., Sueta, C. A., Blecker, S. B., et al. (2014). Anger proneness, gender, and the risk of heart failure. *Journal of Cardiac Failure, 20*(12), 1020–1026.

Kemper, K., Carmin, C., Mehta, B., & Binkley, P. (2016). Integrative medical care plus mindfulness training for patients with congestive heart failure. *Journal of Evidence-Based Complementary & Alternative Medicine., 21*(4), 282–290. https://doi.org/10.1177/2156587215599470

Kiviruusu, O., Huurre, T., Haukkala, A., & Aro, H. (2013). Changes in psychological resources moderate the effect of socioeconomic status on distress symptoms: A 10-year follow-up among young adults. *Health Psychology, 32*(6), 627–636.

Krietsch, K., Mason, A. E., & Sbarra, D. (2014). Sleep complaints predict increases in resting blood pressure following marital separation. *Health Psychology, 33*(10), 1204–1213.

Lawson, W. (2012). Psychological challenges of coping with coronary artery disease. In E. Dornelas (Ed.), *Stress proof the heart: Behavioral interventions for cardiac patients* (pp. 9–24). New York, NY: Springer.

Li, C., & Shun, S. (2015). Understanding self care coping styles in patients with chronic heart failure: A systematic review. *European Journal of Cardiovascular Nursing, 15*(1), 12–19.

Lundahl, B., & Burke, B. L. (2009). The effectiveness and applicability of motivational interviewing: A practice-friendly review of four meta-analyses. *Journal of Clinical Psychology: In Session, 65*(11), 1232–1245.

Martin, B. J., Hauer, T., Arena, R., Austford, L. D., Galbraith, P. D., Lewin, A. M., et al. (2012). Cardiac rehabilitation attendance and outcomes in coronary artery disease patients. *Circulation, 123*(6), 677–687.

McGrady, A., McGinnis, R., Badenhop, D., Bentle, M., & Rajput, M. (2009). Effects of depression and anxiety on adherence to cardiac rehabilitation. *Journal of Cardiopulmonary Rehabilitation and Prevention, 29*(6), 358–364.

McGrady, A., Burkes, R., Badenhop, D., & McGinnis, R. (2014). Effects of a brief intervention on retention of patients in a cardiac rehabilitation program. *Applied Psychophysiology and Biofeedback, 39*(3-4), 163–170.

Motivala, S. J. (2011). Sleep and inflammation: Psychoneuroimmunology in the context of cardiovascular disease. *Annals of Behavioral Medicine, 42*(2), 141–152. https://doi.org/10.1007/s12160-011-9280-2

Redfern, J., Briffa, T., Ellis, E., & Freedman, S. B. (2008). Patient-centered modular secondary prevention following acute coronary syndrome: A randomized controlled trial. *Journal of Cardiopulmonary Rehabilitation and Prevention, 28*(2), 107–115.

Roepke, S. K., & Grant, I. (2011). Toward a more complete understanding of the effects of personal mastery on cardiometabolic health. *Health Psychology, 30*(5), 615–632. https://doi.org/10.1037/a0023480

Roest, A., Heideveld, A., Martens, E. J., de Jonge, P., & Denollet, J. (2014). Symptom dimensions of anxiety following myocardial infarction: Associations with depressive symptoms and prognosis. *Health Psychology, 33*(12), 1468–1476.

Ruiz, J. M., & Brondolo, E. (2016). Introduction to the special issue disparities in cardiovascular health: Examining the contributions of social and behavioral factors. *Health Psychology, 35*(4), 309–312.

Stewart, J., Janicki, D., & Kamarck, T. (2006). Cardiovascular reactivity to and recovery from psychological challenge as predictors of 3-year change in blood pressure. *Health Psychology, 25*(1), 111–118.

Surtees, P., Wainwright, N., Luben, R., Khaw, K. T., & Day, N. (2006). Mastery, sense of coherence, and mortality: Evidence of independent associations from the EPIC-Norfolk prospective cohort study. *Health Psychology, 25*(1), 102–110.

Wu, J. R., Frazier, S. K., Rayens, M. K., Lennie, T. A., Chung, M. L., & Moser, D. K. (2013). Medication adherence, social support, and event-free survival in patients with heart failure. *Health Psychology, 32*(6), 637–646.

Wulsin, L. (2012). Psychological challenges of coping with coronary artery disease. In E. A. Dornelas (Ed.), *Stress proof the heart: Behavioral interventions for cardiac patients* (pp. 9–24). New York: Springer.

Yu, D. S. F. (2008). Heart failure: The manifestations and impact of negative emotions. In L. Sher (Ed.), *Psychological factors and cardiovascular disorders: The role of psychiatric pathology and maladaptive personality features* (pp. 133–157). New York, NY: Nova Science Publishers.

Chapter 12
A Pathways Approach to Systemic Lupus Erythematosus

Abstract Systemic lupus erythematosus (SLE) is a complex and typically chronic illness, producing a wide variety of symptoms and following an unpredictable course. SLE is an auto-immune condition, commonly affecting the skin, joints, kidneys, the brain, and other organs. This chapter describes the application of a multilevel integrative care plan, following the Pathways Model, to assist a patient with SLE in managing and moderating symptoms, and improving quality of life. The patient, Mary Anne, was a 33-year-old female nurse, with a 14-year history of living with SLE. Her initial response to her diagnosis of lupus was biomedical, with a passive reliance on a wide range of medications, and an increasingly inactive, sedentary lifestyle. Along with lupus she developed obesity, hypertension, migraine, sleep disturbance, depression, and anxiety. Her rheumatologist referred her for behavioral health interventions to help her learn non-pharmacologic forms of pain management and motivate her for illness self-management for her chronic conditions. The interventions were organized according to the three levels of the Pathways Model, developed by McGrady and Moss (Pathways to illness, pathways to health. New York, NY: Springer, 2013), and included: Level One—movement, sleep hygiene, and mindful eating; Level Two—Aquatherapy, an illness self-management support group, and a mindfulness class; and Level Three—heart rate variability (HRV) biofeedback, self-hypnosis training with healing imagery, a nutritional consultation, and a sleep medicine program. This patient mastered excellent skills with self-hypnosis, paced breathing, and HRV biofeedback. She increased physical activity and modified her diet. At the 3-year point, she reported less frequent pain and joint swelling, less nausea and sick feeling, moderate improvement in sleep, and less frequent and less severe Lupus "flares."

Keywords Systemic lupus erythematosus · Lifestyle change · Biofeedback · Hypnosis · Imagery · Nutrition

This chapter is adapted with the permission of the Association for Applied Psychophysiology and Biofeedback from a previous version that appeared as: D. Moss (2016), Pathways interventions and systemic lupus erythematosus: The case of Mary Anne. *Biofeedback, 44*(2), 73-80. doi: 10.5298/1081-5937-44.2.05

Introducing Mary Anne

At the time of her initial contact, Mary Anne was a 33-year-old divorced woman. She described good health and an active involvement in athletics in childhood and adolescence. She began a BSN/nursing program at age 19. After 2 years of college, she began to feel sick and suffer discomfort in her joints; she dropped out of school four times before finally earning her degree. She completed college at 25, passed her licensing boards in nursing and began to work as an intensive care unit (ICU) nurse.

History

Initial Course of Illness

Mary Anne worked rotating shifts in the ICU, but after several months her sleep deteriorated, joint pain and swelling increased, and she frequently felt sick and feverish. Her primary care physician diagnosed depression and prescribed an anti-depressant and then a benzodiazepine. She gained weight on her antidepressant. Her symptoms waxed and waned, and her moods shifted with the course of the illness.

Long diagnostic process   Soon Mary Anne was placed on probation from her job for absenteeism. She encountered medical specialists at work who diagnosed fibro-myalgia, chronic fatigue, and a psychiatric diagnosis of somatoform disorder. She underwent testing for Lyme disease. She suffered similar symptoms, with varying intensity over time, for 7 years before she received a correct diagnosis. A nurse practitioner at the hospital noticed her hair loss and the distinctive skin rash on her face and suggested she see a rheumatologist. The rheumatologist gave her a primary diagnosis of systemic lupus erythematosus, and a secondary diagnosis of antiphospholipid syndrome. Her lab testing showed high anti-nuclear antibody (ANA) levels and elevated antiphospholipid antibody levels.

Systemic lupus erythematosus (SLE) is a complex and typically chronic illness, manifesting in a wide variety of symptoms and an unpredictable course. SLE is an auto-immune condition which affects multiple body systems, most commonly the skin, joints, kidneys, the brain, and other organs. Estimates of prevalence in the US population range from 20 to 150 cases per 100,000 people (Wolters Kluwer, 2017). A recent study reported the prevalence for SLE in two Michigan cities as 72.8 per 100,000 and 128.7 per 100,000 in females (Somers et al., 2014). SLE incidence and prevalence is consistently higher in women and afflicts disproportionate numbers of African-Americans and Asians (Murphy & Isenberg, 2013; Wolters Kluwer, 2017). The most distinctive marker is a butterfly-shaped rash across the cheeks and nose.

Common symptoms of SLE include chest pain when taking a deep breath, fatigue, fever with no other cause, generalized discomfort, feeling sick, hair loss, mouth sores, sensitivity to sunlight, skin rash, swollen lymph nodes, and a variety of other symptoms.

The progression of Mary Anne's illness Mary Anne became increasingly seden-ary, suffering with joint pain and sick feelings. She gained 65 pounds during the time between initial onset and diagnosis, which contributed to her inactivity since the weight gain made movement more difficult and painful. She also developed hypertension and hyperlipidemia. Several of her medications listed adverse effects including weight gain, hypertension, GI distress, depressed mood, headache, and anxiety.

Referral to Behavioral Health

Two years after her lupus diagnosis, Mary Anne was referred for assessment and treatment of depression, anxiety, disturbed sleep, migraine, hypertension, and poor compliance with her medical treatment regimen. Her blood pressure was 165/94 mmHg, even with antihypertensive medication. The rheumatologist requested that a behavioral specialist address non-pharmacologic forms of pain management, which could also motivate her for better self-management of her lupus, near daily migraine headaches, and hypertension.

Medications at intake: Polypharmacy and off-label medications At the time of evaluation, Mary Anne's list of medications was extensive and included several off-label medications (medicines used for a purpose other than their FDA-supported targets). Her medications for lupus included Prednisone (a corticosteroid), Disalcid (a nonsteroidal anti-inflammatory), and Plaquenil (an anti-malarial used as anti-inflammatory). For depression, she was prescribed Celexa (an SSRI), Pamelor (a tricyclic, used especially at bedtime for sleep), Topamax (an anti-seizure medica-tion, used to stabilize mood and sometimes to reduce migraine onset). For head pain, she used Imitrex (a 5 HT agonist, often prescribed for migraine), Methergine (a vasoconstrictor), Ultram (an analgesic), and Migranol (a headache abortive). For anxiety Mary Anne used Klonopin (benzodiazepine) several times a day. For cho-lesterol she used Zocor (a statin), and for hypertension she used Captopril (an ACE inhibitor). For gastrointestinal distress, Prilosec was prescribed, for overactive blad-der she used Ditropan, and for sleep, she was prescribed Lunesta (a hypnotic) and Pamelor.

Each of Mary Anne's medications was appropriate and credible for the symptom it targeted. However, when a patient takes more than 20 medications, the risk of adverse side effects and drug interactions increases. Mary Anne kept regular appointments with her primary care doctor and nine medical specialists, and occa-sionally sought additional prescriptions from physicians at her workplace. Each of the prescribers drew on specialist knowledge to select her medications, yet the over-all effect was that Mary Anne developed a helpless passivity toward her health and health care. She was waiting for her caregivers and prescriptions to reduce her suf-fering, yet her primary care physician now demanded that she begin to take an active role in her health by lifestyle change.

Pathways Assessment

"On the Prochaska scale Mary Anne seemed somewhere between the 'Pre-Contemplation' and 'Contemplation' stages. She expressed anger at the referral to behavioral health, and demanded to know why her request for a stronger analgesic had not been honored."

Initially, Mary Anne was assessed for her "readiness for change" using the Prochaska scale developed by James O. Prochaska (Prochaska, Norcross, & DiClimete, 1994). On the Prochaska scale, Mary Anne seemed somewhere between the "Pre-Contemplation" and "Contemplation" stages. She expressed anger at the referral to behavioral health and demanded to know why her request for a stronger analgesic had not been honored. However, she agreed to participate in behavioral health sessions because her headache specialist refused to continue her migraine and pain medications unless she attended behavioral health appointments three to four times each month, as documented by phone calls by our office to her primary care physician's nurse.

Mary Anne and the Pathway Model

The interventions for Mary Anne were organized into the three levels of the Pathways Model developed by McGrady and Moss (2013). The Pathways Model only proceeds to professional interventions when the patient has already engaged in a number of self-directed lifestyle and behavior changes (Pathways Level One) and engaged in skill-acquisition for improved coping and self-regulation (Level Two). The Pathways Level Three plan consists of interventions delivered by trained health care professionals, including both mainstream and complementary medicine practitioners.

Mary Anne initially exhibited an antagonistic approach of "going through the motions," keeping appointments but sitting sullenly during individual and group appointments. She cooperated only when offered progress notes on activities for her primary care physician and rheumatologist. Given the number and chronicity of Mary Anne's symptoms and her pathogenic lifestyle, a variety of interventions were included in each of her Pathways Level plans. Her progression from Level One to Three was slow, continuing over 5 months. She acknowledged many basic lifestyle behaviors and attitudes undermining her health and wellness. We scheduled weekly health coaching and supportive psychotherapy sessions from the beginning, until she showed solid progress in Level Three.

Lifestyle assessment Mary Anne reported almost no physical exercise. Her nutrition was heavily weighted with fast food and salty snacks, supplemented with occasional micro-waved portions of "lean cuisine"™ and similar products. Her sleep was poor, disrupted by four rotating 10-hours work shifts each week, and daytime use of Red Bull™. She achieved sleep onset only with Pamelor and Lunesta, and then reported nighttime restlessness and nightmares. She qualified for a diagnosis of metabolic syndrome, along with SLE and migraine. She lived alone with a Dachshund and reported few social supports outside of work.

Pathways Intervention Plan

Level One Plan

> "The professional involved in the goal setting utilizes a health-coaching approach, searching with the patient for areas in lifestyle and behavior where the patient him or herself is dissatisfied and wants change."

In the Pathways Model Level One consists of self-directed lifestyle and behavior changes, with the overall goal of restoring more optimal biological rhythms. The choice of Level One activities is collaborative. The professional involved in the goal setting process utilizes a health-coaching approach, searching with the patient for areas in lifestyle and behavior where the patient himself or herself is dissatisfied and wants change. Specific goals then are graduated and realistic: For example, for most patients with chronic illness, minimal increases in movement around the home are realistic and practical, whereas 60 minutes of aerobic exercise is not. No Level One goal is set until the patient expresses belief that he or she is ready to implement it and is determined to follow through with the behavior change.

Level One: Movement Mary Anne acknowledged inactivity was a problem, but perceived herself as unable to make changes in activity due to joint and head pain. We compromised with an initial goal to walk for 5 minutes on the Grand River boardwalk and pier one block from her home and then walk back to her home each day. She also agreed to walk her dog, instead of paying a neighbor boy to walk her. She agreed to keep a log, listing minutes of activity on a daily calendar.

Level One: Sleep hygiene Mary Anne began with a sleep diary, which showed chaotic times of retiring, long sleep onset latencies, frequent awakenings, and multiple non-calming activities in the bedroom. Her diurnal rhythms and behavior were highly disorganized as she ate, watched television, played with her dog, and ran a small cosmetics business from her bed. She made a commitment to improving sleep-relevant behaviors because the poor quality of her sleep was impairing her functionality. Mary Anne agreed to negotiate with her Director to stabilize her work shifts as much as possible. She agreed to limit her Red Bull to one per day, with the long-term goal to eliminate Red Bull and any caffeinated drinks.

Stimulus control We oriented Mary Anne to optimal sleep environments and the impact that stimulation in the bedroom has on sleep. She reluctantly agreed to move her television and her cosmetics business out of the bedroom for 60 days and see if it made any difference. Bootzin (Bootzin, Epstein, & Wood, 1991) pioneered the stimulus control approach to treating sleep disorders and Taylor and Roane (2010) have reviewed the evidence base that supports the effectiveness of stimulus control.

Level One: Mindful eating   Mary Anne discussed weight loss as a possible goal for a Level One activity. We discouraged her from setting specific goals in this area at this time, due to her agitated generalized anger about food, diets, physicians, and pain. Because dysregulated emotions are a major trigger for poor eating patterns, there seemed too much risk of Mary Anne setting herself up for failure.

We instructed her in mindful eating and experimented in the office with mindfully eating a grape. Mary Anne agreed to the goal to practice mindful eating—eating slowly, with attention to savoring each sensory aspect of each food item, each bite, each taste, as well as each color perception of food. On her own, she discovered and benefited from an educational *YouTube* workshop on "mindful eating" by Jan Chozen Bays (2011). Bays (2014) also later published an educational CD on mindful eating and Mary Anne benefited from listening to the CD after its release.

Level One Progress

Progress: Movement   Mary Anne reported being surprised at moments of enjoyment walking on the nearby boardwalk, walking her dog, and being outdoors in nature in daylight. She extended her walks to 15 minutes, which allowed her to reach the Lake Michigan pier and return to her home. She sometimes could smile and laugh when outdoors and with her dog. She initiated an effort to list more of her activities on a calendar.

Progress: Mindful eating   Mary Anne spontaneously started a diary of mindful eating experiences. She reported that she had not intended to cooperate so much with our plan. She discovered pleasure in slowly eating and tasting simple foods at home. She wrote one hilarious narrative on mindfully eating a "double whopper™" with French Fries, and insisted on reading it to her Pathways team and her physician. Based on a comment by a nutritionally minded co-worker, she set a new goal to have more rainbow colors on her plate.

Progress: Sleep   The area of sleep was much more challenging for Mary Anne. Without Red Bull she was less attentive and often drowsy during her shifts at the hospital. She reported staying out of the bed and bedroom until time for sleep, but felt lonelier during the evening hours. Her sleep onset latency slightly improved as she reduced caffeine. She agreed to decrease the dosage of her Lunesta very gradually, in consultation with her physician, and found it made no difference in her sleep onset, concluding that the Lunesta was apparently contributing almost nothing to her ability to initiate sleep. Unfortunately, her director resisted her request to stabilize her nursing shifts and labeled her as "demanding" for this request. She continued to experience delay in sleep onset, and fragmented sleep, with these problems more severe after shift changes. We promised a referral to a cognitive behavioral therapy sleep specialist after Mary Anne completed adequate Level One and Two activities.

Level One Summary

After engaging in Level One activities for 6 weeks, Mary Anne exhibited several significant lifestyle and behavioral changes. Her activity level was consistently higher with daily walks. Her sleep habits were improved and she had nearly eliminated high caffeine drinks, yet her sleep onset was still sometimes delayed and she reported frequent mid-sleep awakening. She expressed enthusiasm for mindful eating and reported a number of more positive food choices. She still showed some mixed motivation about her health, cooperating consistently in her Level One activities, yet asking intermittently how much longer before she could have more opiate analgesics for her pain.

Level Two Plan

"The illness self-management support group supported the central assumption in the Pathways Model, that we can better enlist the coping resources of human beings, when we draw them into an alliance for health emphasizing self-directed lifestyle and behavioral changes."

In the Pathways Model Level Two activities involve the acquisition of self-regulation skills, coping skills, and self-care strategies, often with guidance from educational resources and community-based programs. The choice of Level Two activities is again collaborative and again follows a coaching model. The professional engages the patient in exploring relevant self-regulation skills and self-care strategies, especially those shown in research studies to be efficacious for the patient's symptoms and conditions. The professional also identifies relevant community-based resources, but defers to the patient to narrow the options and select specific resources and goals. The professional remains open to options from the patient that might seem "out of left field," which nevertheless seem relevant and health supportive for this human being with his or her condition.

Level Two: Aquatherapy Mary Anne agreed to attend an Aquatherapy class, designed for people with arthritis and other medical conditions hindering physical exercise. The Aquatherapy class included gentle graded exercise, three times a week, in a therapeutic pool with water temperature in the mid-1990's Fahrenheit. Warm water soothes and relaxes muscles during movement, and the buoyancy of water limits impact on the joints. We recommended gradual and "interval" exercise, that is, increasing the level and time of exertion very slowly and taking frequent rests after fairly short periods.

Level Two: Illness self-management support group Mary Anne agreed to attend a psycho-educational group focused on living with chronic illness. Members of the support group included patients with multiple sclerosis, diabetes, fibromyalgia, and one other woman with systemic lupus erythematosus (SLE). Mary Anne attended the group regularly in exchange for progress reports sent directly to her primary care physician and rheumatologist.

This Level Two intervention was strategically targeted to her rheumatologist's referral recommendation that Mary Anne learn better "self-management" skills. The illness self-management group supported the central assumption in the Pathways Model, that we can better enlist the coping resources of human beings, when we draw them into an alliance for health emphasizing self-directed lifestyle and behavioral changes.

In spite of being a nurse, Mary Anne knew relatively little about SLE and almost nothing about illness self-management. The guidebook used in the group was a free National Institute of Health publication on *Lupus: A Patient Care Guide for Nurses and Other Health Professionals (3rd ed.)* (National Institute of Arthritis and Musculoskeletal and Skin Disease, 2006). The assignments were organized around patient information sheets in the book, such as "Preventing Fatigue Due to Lupus," "Exercise and Lupus," "Preventing a Lupus Flare," "Joint Function and Lupus," and "Skin care and lupus." For the first time, Mary Anne realized that her sporadic use of a tanning bed probably was producing some of her lupus "flares," times of increased symptoms.

Concepts and skills acquisition   In the group, Mary Anne now encountered the idea of becoming a "critical consumer of health care services," and the concept of taking a more "active role in her own health care." She complained that we had not started educating her about illness self-management class on day 1. With the group, she practiced asking questions to health professionals about her illness and symptoms, and about the rationale for each element in her treatment plan. Mary Anne also for the first time learned the side effects of her current medications and compared those possible adverse effects to her current symptoms. She became excited at the ideas of self-care strategies and self-regulation skills, and with the class she selected six self-regulation skills for future mastery.

Level Two: Mindfulness class   Mary Anne enjoyed her Level One mindful eating exercises, and asked for more mindfulness training. We referred her to a mindfulness training class at a local church, supplemented by an audio CD on mindfulness for beginners (Kabat-Zinn, 2006). Mindfulness training involves bringing one's entire attention to one's present experience in this moment, observing events unfold from moment to moment (Kabat-Zinn, 1990). In mindfulness, the individual suspends judgments and evaluations, accepting whatever arises in awareness.

Level Two Progress

Level Two: Aquatherapy   Mary Anne liked the Aquatherapy class. The instructor had been Mary Anne's friend in high school, and they enjoyed stopping for a cup of tea at Starbucks after the class. Mary Anne began to see two of the attendees outside of class. She was surprised that movement in the water evoked only intermittent discomfort. She found by week 3 that she was able to do as much activity in the pool as most of the class members.

Level Two: Illness self-management Mary Anne's background in nursing served her well in building an understanding of her illness. She was frightened to give up any medications, but equally concerned about how many of her medicines frequently produced side effects for which she complained to her physicians. She set the goal of consulting her prescribing physicians about reducing her total medication regimen by one medication every 2 months.

Level Two: Mindfulness Mary Anne described herself as more thoughtful and less edgy. She practiced only basic mindfulness at first, as an experiential practice of observing whatever occurs, with acceptance and without judgment. She later began practicing mindfulness meditation as well, and found this soothing and calming. She became convinced that mindfulness was some kind of magic because when she practiced it at work, her patients and other staff members also seemed calmer and easier to work with.

Level Two Summary

After engaging in both Level One and Level Two activities for 5 months, Mary Anne showed a substantially higher *readiness for change*. She no longer engaged in angry rants with the behavioral health team about wasting time on the Pathways program. Her overall physical activity level had greatly improved with continued Aquatherapy and daily walks. She exhibited enthusiasm for the illness self-management program and was working on combining her nursing knowledge with the concept of assuming a more active role in managing her chronic SLE. She also showed a positive dedication and enthusiasm about mindfulness both as a coping skill and a meditative practice.

Level Three Plan

In the Pathways Model, Level Three involves professional interventions provided by health care and mental health care practitioners. This is the formal professionally delivered treatment phase in the Pathways Model. The selection of the treatments is a collaborative process, based on an evidence-based discussion of the treatment options that have proven valuable for the patient's condition, and the patient's personal preferences.

Level Three: Heart rate variability biofeedback In the human heart, variability correlates positively with health and resilience; the healthy heart is not a metronome. Heart rate variability, the moment to moment change in heart rate is frequently decreased in depression, anxiety, and many medical conditions. Heart rate variability (HRV) biofeedback involves using paced, relaxed breathing to enhance or restore the natural variability of heart rate. HRV biofeedback was chosen for Mary Anne because it has been shown to reduce anxiety and depression and is understood to enhance autonomic nervous system regulation (Moss & Shaffer, 2016).

One example of the health implications of low HRV emerged from research by Kleiger, Miller, Bigger, and Moss (1987), who published a categorization of SDNN into the following ranges:

SDNN 0–50 ms—an unhealthy state
SDNN 51–100 ms—compromised health
SDNN 101 and above—good health

In the Kleiger et al. (1987) research on patients with a past myocardial infarction, the mortality was 5.3 times higher for the patients with an SDNN below 50 ms, compared to those with an SDNN above 100 ms.

At her initial biofeedback assessment, Mary Anne displayed a rapid and irregular breathing baseline, in spite of her months of mindfulness practice. Her baseline respiration rate was 22 breaths per minute. Her heart rate variability was also low, as indicated by her basic HRV statistics. Her baseline SDNN was 43, and her baseline HR Max minus HR Min was 7.[1] Her rapid respiration rate qualified as hyperventilation, and the HRV statistics indicated lower than average heart rate variability, which is common in individuals with chronic illness.

Initially, Mary Anne's biofeedback sessions reduced her mean in-office baseline respiration rate from 22 to 8 breaths per minute. Next, her training helped her to smooth her breathing and to breathe at a fixed rate with a breath pacer on a computer display. Subsequently, the biofeedback sessions assessed Mary Anne's resonance frequency and trained her to breathe at this frequency. The resonance frequency is the breathing rate at which an individual produces the highest heart rate variability. An individual's resonance frequency (RF) is assessed by guiding them to breathe at various breath rates between 4.5 and 8 breaths per minute, and measuring which breath rate produces the highest SDNN, the highest HR Max minus HR Min, and a phase synchronization between the heart rate and respiration waveforms.

We conducted a resonance frequency assessment and established that Mary Anne's RF was seven breaths per minute. She then began in-office HRV training at seven breaths/minute and was given the assignment to breathe at home for 10 minutes one to two times daily with a breath pacer on her smart phone. She logged her practice times by adding HRV and a time to her activity calendar.

Level Three: Hypnosis and healing imagery Mary Anne stated a strong interest in including some form of hypnosis in her Level Three plan. Mary Anne began hypnosis sessions, which focused on slow breathing, relaxation, pain reduction, and

---

[1] SDNN and HR Max minus HR Min are commonly used statistics for heart rate variability. The SDNN is the standard deviation of the normalized interbeat interval, the time between heart beats in milliseconds. The SDNN is frequently cited in medical research as an indicator of heart rate variability and of current health status. The HR Max minus HR Min is the mean difference between the peak (maximum) heart rate and the lowest (minimum) heart rate in a breath cycle, measured in beats per minute (Shaffer & Venner, 2016).

> "Mary Anne began hypnosis sessions, which were focused on slow breathing, relaxation, pain reduction, and soothing her joints."

soothing her joints. She showed high hypnotic ability, which means that she was easily induced into a deep hypnotic trance. She began practicing self-hypnosis at home. She displayed high susceptibility to hypnotic imagery. She practiced visualizing a healing stream of water to cool her joints, soothe pain, and wash away inflammation, and reported feeling a noticeable reduction in pain, burning, and discomfort during and following her self-hypnosis practice sessions.

Level Three: Nutritional consultation Mary Anne was referred to a local physician with training in osteopathic manipulation, acupuncture, and functional medicine. Initially, she received some acupuncture that moderated her joint pain, but the physician's primary focus was to guide her in making better nutritional choices. Mary Anne made standard widely accepted changes in the direction of healthier eating: She reduced alcohol use and decreased her use of prepared foods that contained additives. She increased her intake of leafy greens, spinach, kale, legumes, broccoli, ginger, turmeric, and cinnamon. Later with her physician's guidance she added a probiotic and digestive enzymes and eliminated dairy-based foods.[2] However, she then also added "Mean Green Juice" based on a friend's recommendation (the juice was a recipe from the 2010 documentary film *Fat, Sick, and Nearly Dead* movie) and consumed it every morning. There was no scientific evidence we could identify on the efficacy or safety of this juice intervention, so we watched Mary Anne's condition closely. Mary Anne reported almost immediate benefits with the dietary changes, especially noticeable after she added the juice regimen. She reported a reduction in her skin rashes, a reduction in joint pain and swelling, and a reduction in anxiety.

Level Three: Behavioral sleep medicine clinic Mary Anne continued to make slight progress on improving her sleep habits, but was frustrated. Her new readings from her illness self-management class told her that sleep deprivation often exacerbates SLE symptoms and causes "flares," yet she found herself going to bed and staring at the ceiling for hours and experienced frequent awakening once sleep began. We referred Mary Anne to a Behavioral Sleep Medicine Clinic, which uses a cognitive behavioral approach to sleep. She saw a physician and a psychologist on the sleep team, began to log in regularly to the sleep medicine website, and answered online questions about her behavior and sleep between sessions. The Sleep Medicine Clinic specifically guided her to identify negative or toxic self-statements she was making about herself and her sleep and to confront and modify these self-statements.

---

[2] The selection of a probiotic and dietary supplements in functional medicine is not based on the medical diagnosis. This was not a regimen based on her lupus diagnosis and should not be applied for other lupus patients. Rather in functional medicine the choice of dietary supplements, foods to add, and foods to eliminate is largely based on laboratory testing including blood work and stool sample.

Level Three Progress

Level Three: HRV biofeedback progress After 10 weeks of daily practice of paced breathing at the resonance frequency of seven breaths per minute, Mary Anne showed improved breath control skills and improved heart rate variability. Mary Anne could now breathe at seven breaths/minute in most sessions without using a breath pacer. In biofeedback training sessions, she showed more smooth sinusoidal breath and heart rate line graphs. Her breathing line graph and heart rate line graphs on the computer screen peaked together, and she learned to breathe with the biofeedback display, which enabled her to amplify the heart rate oscillations. Her SDNN in training sessions reached 87 and her HR Max minus HR Min reached 17. Her baselines after 10 weeks of practice were an SDNN of 66 and a HR Max minus HR Min of 11.

The Kleiger et al. (1987) study cited earlier utilized 24-hours Holter monitoring to measure the heart rate variability in a cardiac population, whereas the clinical measurements on Mary Anne's HRV were based on a 5-minutes recording. Although an SDNN measured in a 5-minutes recording is not as reliable as an SDNN taken from a 24-hours measurement, nevertheless, Mary Anne was encouraged by the changes in her SDNN. Mary Anne felt initial success in moving from the unhealthy to the compromised health range and expressed determination to increase her variability further. She could now often self-calm when she was upset and reported less Klonopin use when she was anxious.

Level Three: Hypnosis and guided imagery For Mary Anne, her resonance frequency breathing and self-hypnosis began to merge. She practiced breathing at seven breaths per minute, but also imaged soothing springs and soft morning sunlight on her body as she practiced breathing. On days when her swelling, pain, or sick sensations increased, resonance frequency breathing and imagery often moderated discomfort and lifted mood.

Level Three: Behavioral sleep progress Mary Anne identified a number of self-defeating thought patterns that escalated agitation when sleep onset was delayed. She used a "thought stopping" strategy, snapping a rubber band on her wrist whenever she noticed toxic thought trains beginning. Recognizing and redirecting her thoughts seemed to aid sleep onset; in addition, frequent awakening during the night diminished.

Mary Anne learned to use the awareness of toxic thoughts as a reminder to do her self-hypnosis and self-soothing imagery. She continued to use "stimulus control" to improve her sleep environment. The online sleep diaries and downloaded reports from the sleep clinic objectified her progress and reassured her when she became discouraged. The numbers assured her that she was making progress.

Level Three: Effects of nutritional changes She found that taking her "Mean Green Juice" on mornings when she felt joint swelling was helpful because both pain and swelling were reduced after drinking her juice. After 6 months, she informed her physicians that she was decreasing and then eliminating her Prednisone, Plaquenil, Celexa, and Beta Blocker. Her physicians recommended against stopping these medications, but eventually assisted her to taper the medications very gradually. She continued to suffer fewer symptoms in spite of stopping these medications. Her physicians insisted on regular check-ins and Mary Anne followed their recommendations and kept her appointments with them.

Mary Anne continued her new nutritional regimen, including a probiotic, digestive enzymes, consumed no dairy products, and made much healthier food choices. On her new regimen, the joint swelling and sick feelings occurred only before her menstrual periods. At one point in therapy, after a time of work stress, joint swelling, pain, and skin rashes flared severely. She managed the increased symptoms with her resonance frequency breathing, self-hypnosis, and imagery. After 4 weeks, the symptoms moderated greatly again.

Most Recent Assessment

Mary Anne mastered excellent skills of self-hypnosis, paced breathing, and HRV biofeedback. She continued to sustain more physical activity and a transformed diet. At the 3-year point, she reported less frequent and less severe Lupus "flares." This individual showed substantially more interest in making changes in her own behavior than at intake. Mary Anne's mood was improved, and she was less inclined to intense discouragement. Her sleep onset was faster, she awakened less frequently, and her average hours of sleep per night increased. On the nights that she lay awake for long periods, she was frustrated but she did not resume medical management with Lunesta.

Her Primary care physician and her rheumatologist encouraged Mary Anne to continue her nutritional and lifestyle changes, but both stated that her improvement must be a placebo response. Neither could believe that her lifestyle and nutritional changes could have caused these significant changes in a chronic illness. Nevertheless, Mary Anne's blood work indicated a major, objective improvement in the usual measures accompanying SLE; specifically, her two most recent ANA levels (anti-nuclear antibodies) were in the normal range. Her antiphospholipid antibodies numbers were only moderately elevated.

Summary

Systemic lupus erythematosus is recognized to be a waxing and waning condition, with an unpredictable course. It is not unusual for patients to appear to be in remission one day and report extreme suffering one day later. When a medical condition is this erratic in its course, and one has a case study of one patient, it is not scientifically sound to claim that any specific interventions caused a patient's improvement. Nevertheless, Mary Anne demonstrated dramatic changes in emotional health, activity level, and lifestyle factors associated with higher level wellness. She embraced a determination to become an active agent in her own health. Her suffering was greatly diminished at this time, and she was better able to function in her nursing work, with a reduction in absenteeism and much greater confidence in her ability to perform her professional work effectively.

References

Bays, J. C. (2011). *Mindful eating by Zen master Jan Chozen Bays.* YouTube. Retrieved from https://www.youtube.com/watch?v=tmtNPGZYWOI

Bays, J. C. (2014). *Mindful eating: A guide to rediscovering a healthy and joyful relationship with food* (an audio CD). Boulder, CO: Shambhala Audio.

Bootzin, R. R., Epstein, D., & Wood, J. M. (1991). Stimulus control instructions. In P. J. Hauri (Ed.), *Case studies in insomnia* (pp. 19–28). New York, NY: Plenum.

Kabat-Zinn, J. (1990). *Full catastrophe living: Using the wisdom of your body and mind to face stress, pain and illness.* New York, NY: Delacorte.

Kabat-Zinn, J. (2006). *Mindfulness for beginners: Reclaiming the present moment* (Educational CD). Louisville, CO: Sounds True.

Kleiger, R. E., Miller, J. P., Bigger, J. T., & Moss, A. J. (1987). Decreased heart rate variability and its association with increased mortality after acute myocardial infarction. *American Journal of Cardiology, 59,* 256–262.

McGrady, A., & Moss, D. (2013). *Pathways to illness, pathways to health.* New York, NY: Springer. https://doi.org/10.1007/978-1-4419-1379-1

Moss, D., & Shaffer, F. (Eds.). (2016). *Foundations of heart rate variability.* Wheat Ridge, CO: Association for Applied Psychophysiology and Biofeedback.

Murphy, G., & Isenberg, D. (2013). Effect of gender on clinical presentation in systemic lupus erythematosus. *Rheumatology, 52*(12), 2108–2115. https://doi.org/10.1093/rheumatology/ket160

National Institute of Arthritis and Musculoskeletal and Skin Disease. (2006). *Lupus: A patient care guide for nurses and other health professionals* (3rd ed.). NIH Publication Number 06-4262. Bethesda, MD: National Institutes of Health.

Prochaska, J. O., Norcross, J. C., & DiClemente, C. C. (1994). Changing for good: A revolutionary six-stage program for overcoming bad habits and moving your life positively forward. New York, NY: HarperCollins.

Shaffer, F., & Venner, J. (2016). Heart rate variability anatomy and physiology. In D. Moss & F. Shaffer (Eds.), *Foundations of heart rate variability* (pp. 31–41). Association for Applied Psychophysiology and Biofeedback: Wheat Ridge, CO.

Somers, E. C., Marder, W., Cagnoli, P., Lewis, E. E., DeGuire, P., Gordon, C., et al. (2014). Population-based incidence and prevalence of systemic lupus erythematosus: The Michigan Lupus Epidemiology and Surveillance program. *Arthritis and Rheumatology, 66*(2), 369–378. https://doi.org/10.1002/art.38238

Taylor, D. J., & Roane, B. M. (2010). Treatment of insomnia in adults and children: A practice-friendly review of research. *Journal of Clinical Psychology, 66*(11), 1137–1147. https://doi.org/10.1002/jclp.20733

Wolters Kluwer. (2017). Epidemiology and pathogenesis of systemic lupus erythematosus. *Up to date.* A website of Wolters Kluwer. Retrieved from http://www.uptodate.com/contents/epidemiology-and-pathogenesis-of-systemic-lupus-erythematosus

Chapter 13
A Pathways Approach to Cancer

Alas for those that never sing
And die with all their music in them.

(Oliver Wendell Holmes, *Voiceless*)

Abstract In past decades, cancer was often viewed as a death sentence. Today, the diagnosis of cancer often heralds not sudden death but a transformed mode of living, and a challenge to manage the many adverse effects of treatment, the uncertainty of one's future, and a challenge to quality of life. Cancer survivors frequently report depression and anxiety. Chemotherapy often produces recurring nausea and lingering cognitive deficits. A growing body of research provides evidence that many self-regulation skills, dietary changes, and lifestyle changes can assist cancer survivors to cope with the presence of their diagnosis, manage the adverse effects, and sustain quality of life. This chapter provides a case study of Ellen, illustrating how a Pathways Model can be applied for patients with a cancer diagnosis. Initially, the Pathways Model enabled her to assume self-management of her illness and enhanced coping with the adverse effects of her oncology treatments. When Ellen suffered malignant metastases and required renewed chemotherapy, her efforts to utilize Pathways skills to manage resurgent adverse effects illustrate the adaptation of the Pathways Model for longer term conditions.

Keywords Cancer · Chronic illness · Disease management · Mindfulness · Spirituality

Introducing Ellen

At the time of the initial interview, Ellen was a 46-year-old married woman, with two adult daughters. She reported a positive life adjustment and life satisfaction until mid-life, with an early marriage during her junior year of college, completion of a bachelor's degree, and then a master's degree in education, and a rewarding career as an elementary teacher. She began to suffer moderate depression after her second daughter left home for college. She sensed a loss of joy in her work as a teacher in the same time period. She described her marriage as "committed" with some growing apart. After her daughters' departure from home, she experienced an increasing sense of emptiness in her life. As she grew more anxious, irritable, and sad, her husband retreated into television sports. The onset of cancer aggravated her depression and anxiety, as well as the estrangement at home and at work.

History

Initial Course of Illness

The onset of breast cancer was a shock and, as Ellen experienced it, a wake-up call. She was treated with a lumpectomy and oral medication, and felt relief and a return to normalcy at the apparent success of treatment. The cancer recurred twice further, in the breast and in a lymph node. After her older daughter was also diagnosed with breast cancer, Ellen underwent genetic testing and was diagnosed with the BRCA1 gene mutation. In addition, a pathology report on her second breast tumor showed that the tumor lacked estrogen receptors and progesterone receptors, an indication that hormone therapy regimens would not be effective.

Treatment in oncology After several genetic counseling sessions and further oncology consultations, she underwent bilateral prophylactic mastectomy and inpatient chemotherapy. Ellen's oncologist was supportive of the bilateral mastectomy. She was also scheduled for an annual MRI screening because of her higher risk for metastases/recurrence.

Ellen went into a more sustained remission, but her anxiety and depression deepened and she began to suffer forgetfulness and memory problems.

Referral to behavioral health Ellen's oncologist referred her for psychological treatment for anxiety and clinical depression, and for health coaching to accept a larger role in the self-management of her illness.

> "Leshan concluded that a significant portion of the cancer patients he saw in psychotherapy could benefit from learning how to better "sing their own song.""

During her initial chemotherapy, Ellen read Lawrence Leshan's book, *Cancer as a Turning Point* (Leshan, 1990). Lawrence Leshan is a psychotherapist who worked over three decades with cancer patients. Leshan concluded that a significant portion of the cancer patients he saw in psychotherapy could benefit from learning how to better "sing their own song." In other words, he felt that many individuals with cancer were living lives directed excessively toward fulfilling others' expectations and were not adequately steering their lives in pursuit of their own dreams and values. Ellen reported that several passages in Leshan's text felt uncomfortably close to her own life experiences. She accepted her oncologist's behavioral health referral and asked her behavioral health team (including a health coach and a clinical health psychologist) to help her to better recognize and "sing her own song."

Pathways Assessment

Ellen and the Pathways Model

Ellen's interventions were organized into the three levels of the Pathways Model, developed by McGrady and Moss (2013). The Pathways Model only proceeds to professional interventions when the patient has already engaged in a number of self-directed lifestyle and behavior changes on his/her own or with the guidance of a psychologist, health coach, or counselor (Pathways Level One), and engaged in skill-acquisition for improved coping and self-regulation (Level Two). The Pathways Level Three plan consists of interventions delivered by trained health care professionals, including both mainstream and complementary medicine practitioners.

Ellen described a general dissatisfaction with how she was living, at the time of her initial evaluation. She reported a loss of energy during and following chemotherapy, a decrease in physical activity, a loss of contacts with friends, and a generalized loss of joy. Her therapist described the Pathways Model, and she became excited, stating her readiness for a "life makeover." She described herself as ready to begin making lifestyle changes although she reported some fears that she couldn't control some aspects of her behavior, such as nutrition.

Pathways Lifestyle Assessment

Ellen reported poor sleep, decreased energy, and a reduction in her physical exercise and activity. She also noticed that the poor sleep seemed to aggravate her cognitive deficits. When she occasionally slept through the night, she felt moderately sharper mentally. She frequently took a Tylenol PM at bedtime, but reported delayed onset of sleep and frequent awakening through the night.

Ellen was a cross-country runner in high school and continued to run regularly in her college years. With the birth of her children and increasing responsibilities at work, she stopped running, but continued to take frequent walks and play tennis weekly in good weather. During her chemotherapy and radiation, she felt lethargic and tired and began to sit in her recliner whenever she wasn't at work. She expressed a desire to resume activity in spite of the fatigue and a frequent feeling of heaviness in her limbs. A sensation of heaviness in the limbs is often an indication of lymphedema, due to radiation and/or surgical removal of the lymph nodes. Although exercise is not easy with heavy limbs, exercise can moderate lymphedema.

Ellen had prided herself in preparing healthy meals for her family and herself, throughout the years her daughters were in the home. She used a variety of grains and included an abundance of local vegetables and fruits. She lost her appetite entirely during chemotherapy and began to be repulsed by the smells of many once attractive foods. During and after chemotherapy and radiation, she stopped preparing regular meals and developed a kind of snacking and grazing dietary pattern, with popcorn, cheese curls, and other salty snacks her most consumed foods. She felt no interest in preparing meals and reported feeling no appetite and often repulsion for many healthier foods when her husband prepared a full meal. She gained 25 pounds once the nausea induced by chemotherapy became less frequent. Nutrition was the lifestyle area in which Ellen felt most out of control and incapable of change.

Ellen described a spiritual loss of direction. She grew up in a Catholic home and attended a Catholic College to earn her teaching degree. During her college years, she learned to practice transcendental meditation and became active in a "spiritual conversations" group led by a spiritual director from the "Cenacle," an order of Catholic nuns originating in France. She evolved a kind of open spirituality, embracing her Catholic heritage but also an openness to other traditions. She continued to use meditation and prayer of various kinds through her post-college years and felt very alive spiritually. She wasn't sure when she stopped meditation and prayer, but realized that by the time of her cancer diagnosis she felt spiritually "out of gas." This had not felt like a problem, but with the recurrence of cancer she found herself bitterly questioning why God was punishing a good person. Intellectually, she chided herself and counseled herself that "illness happens to the good and the wicked alike," yet emotionally she felt "cheated" and bitter. She expressed a desire to recover her lost spiritual strength.

Ellen reported a generalized anxiety present most days. She felt most anxious about a recurrence of cancer and any physical sensation that stood out for her seemed to precipitate fears about cancer and other illnesses. When she couldn't remember a conversation or couldn't focus clearly, she feared brain cancer. When she climbed the stairs to her basement laundry room or second floor bedroom, she noticed an increased heart rate and feared both heart disease and cancer in the chest. When she felt tired, she wondered whether a recurrent cancer was sapping her strength. She also felt anxious about leaving her home, anxious about visiting the supermarket, self-conscious about being seen by acquaintances, and anxious about weighing herself. Ellen was still working as a teacher, so she was not housebound, but she dropped most non-essential activities from her life, and rarely left home except for work and urgent grocery needs.

She completed a Beck Anxiety Inventory and scored 41 points, placing her in the severe range for anxiety. She did not qualify for a DSM-V diagnosis of generalized anxiety disorder because her severe anxiety had been present less than 6 months, but her anxiety was seriously disruptive to her functioning (American Psychiatric Association, 2013). A baseline of physiological measures showed a pattern of irregular breathing with a mean breath rate of 18, and an SDNN (an index of heart rate variability and general health and resilience) of 41, showing poor health and low heart rate variability.

Ellen also reported many signs and symptoms of clinical depression, including sadness, discouragement, loss of joy, disappointment in life and in herself, weight gain, frequent tearfulness, social avoidance, and loss of drive or motivation for work or previous recreation. She denied active thoughts of suicide, but acknowledged wondering what she was staying alive for. She recognized the pervasiveness of her depression, yet perceived her anxiety and tensions as more disruptive of her daily life.

Ellen completed a Beck Depression Inventory questionnaire and earned a score of 34 signifying severe depression. She qualified for the DSM-V diagnostic criteria for a major depressive disorder, single episode (296.22) with depressed mood most of each day, loss of interest and pleasure in daily life, daily insomnia, fatigue, and recurrent thoughts of death (American Psychiatric Association, 2013).

Pathways Intervention Plan

Level One Plan

Ellen met three times with her new health coach, discussing areas of her life and behavior in which she desired change, and spent time ranking areas according to how "do-able" or manageable they felt. She decided to initially focus on objectives to address her inactivity, her anxiety, her loss of spiritual directions, and her nutrition.

Level One activity: Walking Ellen set herself an initial goal to walk three to four times each week, doing one circuit around her subdivision, a distance of about three blocks. She was embarrassed to set such a minimal goal, yet even walking to her mail box triggered feelings of heaviness and deadness in her legs and arms. It took enormous effort to continue walking when the heavy sensations became prominent. She set a second goal, for rainy or cold days, of walking for 15 minutes around the corridors of a nearby grade school, which was open in the evenings for community residents to walk.

Level One activity: Mindful breathing Paced, mindful breathing is an effective strategy to reduce the physiological sensations accompanying anxiety. In her initial evaluation, Ellen was observed to breathe irregularly, with alternate rapid breathing and breath holding. Her health coach taught her to breathe more slowly and regularly, at a rate of about six breaths a minute, taking a gentle but long inhalation through her nostrils, pausing briefly, and then initiating an even longer exhalation through pursed lips. She was guided to place her hand on her abdomen to become more aware of her breathing process. She was able to feel the rise and fall of her abdomen with respiration and became both more aware of her breathing patterns, and better able to slow and pace her breathing.

"Ellen set up a small meditation space in a spare bedroom, with a yoga mat for comfort, an inspirational spiritual poster, a statue of the Buddha, and a statue of St. Francis of Assissi, whose attunement with nature touched her."

Ellen set the goal of practicing mindful, diaphragmatic breathing twice daily, using a breath pacer on her smart phone. She chose the Breathe2Relax™ application, which shows a beautiful nature scene as a backdrop and a tube filling as she inhaled and emptying as she exhaled. She set the inhale at 4.0 s and the exhale at 6.0 s initially and found this comfortable. She also learned to focus her awareness mindfully on her breathing, so that her entire awareness became absorbed in the breath process. This mindful absorption also served to distract her from her usual repetitive anxious thoughts.

Level One activity: Meditation Ellen spent approximately 6 years practicing transcendental meditation (TM), in college and in the first few years after college. She associated her past meditation practices with her original sense of spiritual vitality. She chose as her third Level One activity the resumption of TM on a daily basis. Her health coach invited her to establish a special place and time to create a new spiritual home for her meditation practice within her house and daily routines. She chose early morning before her work day for meditation, as a way of beginning her day with a sense of spiritual awakening and serenity. Ellen set up a small meditation space in a spare bedroom, with a yoga mat for comfort, an inspirational spiritual poster, a statue of the Buddha, and a statue of St. Francis of Assissi, whose attunement with nature touched her.

Level One activity: Nutrition Ellen strongly desired to set a goal to modify her current eating patterns, yet felt out of control of her eating. She had a strong fear of failing in this area. Her health coach urged her to set the simplest and smallest possible goal at Level One, in order to recover her confidence and sense of self-efficacy. Ellen decided to set a goal to purchase and prepare some healthy snack foods and to assure that she always had these on hand. She decided not to make any commitments to obligate herself to change her actual food intake. She focused initially on purchasing and cutting up some fresh vegetables and fruit several times a week, keeping them in a sealed container in the refrigerator, and keeping some yoghurt with honey mixed and ready in the refrigerator. She wanted to simply know that if she felt an urge to snack, these foods would be prepared and ready as an option.

Level One Progress

Progress: Walking Ellen initially found that after one half of a circuit around the neighborhood, she felt such extreme fatigue and heaviness in her legs, that she wanted desperately to lie down and sleep on the nearest lawn. She persisted in walking the single circuit 3 days the first week and 5 days in week 2. She began to experience a lessening of the heaviness sensations after her walks. In week 3, she increased her goal to daily walks and added an extra block to the route. She continued to express fatigue, but gained confidence that she was able to move for 15 minutes or more at a time.

Progress: Mindful breathing Ellen began her breathing exercises with enthusiasm and liked following the breath pacer. However, during the first week after setting the breathing goal, doing the breathing exercises triggered light-headedness, which frightened her. Her health coach asked her to demonstrate her breathing in the office and noticed a kind of effortful strain in her breathing, trying to breathe too "deeply." He encouraged her to think of the breath exercises as mindful and gentle breathing, not "deep" breathing. He guided her to breathe more gently, with less effort, and the light-headed sensations ceased. She also reported feeling a moderation of her edginess during the breath sessions and for 1–2 hours afterwards.

Progress: Meditation Ellen was eager to resume her longtime practice of transcendental meditation, which she associated with the vibrant era of college and early marriage. She began to practice daily before work, and the practice felt quite natural and comfortable for her. She also began to experience a convergence between her use of paced breathing and the TM practice of chanting a mantra. Her husband began to tease her about being an aging hippie chanting in the guest room, and this unsettled her. Yet she determined to persist. With the combination of mindful breathing and TM, she experienced that her anxiety and subjective feelings of tension were reduced by about 50%. After 3 weeks, her husband apologized for teasing her and expressed that he could see and feel a significant improvement in her anxiety and mood. He encouraged her to continue her meditation.

Progress: Nutrition Initially, Ellen found herself cutting up fruits and vegetables every 2 days, and each time throwing out the entire supply from the previous chopping session. She continued to graze on popcorn and cheese curls. In her second week, she began to alternate between the popcorn/cheese curls and the fruits and vegetables and ate most of what she chopped. In her fourth week, she threw out her salty snacks and began to prepare a larger volume of fruits and vegetables.

Level One Summary

After 5 weeks Ellen had established a consistent regiment of walking almost daily outdoors and engaging in daily mindful breathing and transcendental meditation. She had also shifted her grazing pattern from junk food to fruits and vegetables and felt physically less stuffed and heavy when mealtimes arrived. She reported a significant reduction in anxiety and subjective edginess and felt more optimistic about moving ahead with additional goals. She said that she was not happy overall, but was experiencing moments of joy during her activities.

Level Two Plan

In the Pathways Model, Level Two activities include lifestyle and behavioral changes supported by educational materials or community-based resources. In weeks 4 and 5 of her health coaching, Ellen began to list possible Level Two activities, and she set the goal of beginning her Level Two activities in week 6.

Level Two activity: Gentle yoga Ellen experienced a sense of success with the walks around the neighborhood and considered a variety of exercise/activity options. She finally set the goal of attending a twice weekly "gentle yoga" class at the community YMCA, designed for persons with arthritis or other medical problems inhibiting more vigorous exercise. The yoga seemed to her a natural complement to her meditation, and she hoped that she could carry out the yoga *asanas* at a gentle level in spite of some lingering limb heaviness and fatigue.

Level Two: Mindfulness training and mindful meditation Ellen had read extensively about the Buddhist tradition and was drawn to Buddhist thinking and practices. She also read Jon Kabat-Zinn's *Full Catastrophe Living* and was fascinated with the idea of mindfulness as a coping strategy (Kabat-Zinn, 2013). Yet she had never attempted mindfulness throughout the period of her cancer and increasing emotional distress. She found her copy of the Kabat-Zinn book and began reading five to ten pages each day. She also identified a mindfulness class available at a local church and decided to attend the class as one of her Level Two activities. Ellen began to practice mindful acceptance toward times of frustration, and in particular began to self-talk patiently and with more acceptance toward herself, when she found herself engaging in self-criticism and self-judgments.

Level Two activity: Pastoral care Ellen had a conversation with the female pastor at the Protestant church where she was attending the mindfulness class. She initially felt hopeful that as a woman, the minister might be able to understand her feelings about breast cancer and her bitterness at God. Ellen realized soon that the minister was proselytizing her to switch denominations and preaching at her about how sinful it was to question God's will. This undermined her trust and comfort with the woman. She expressed frustration that she was gaining more comfort from spiritual practices based in Asian spiritual traditions (transcendental meditation and mindfulness), than in her original Christianity.

Ellen discussed with her coach the options in her community and decided to seek out a spiritual guide at a Catholic-based outreach program operated by Dominican nuns, which was known for a more progressive approach to spirituality. She made an appointment, had an initial positive experience, and decided to participate in an 8-week "spiritual directions" class led by an older Dominican nun who had personally experienced breast cancer.

Level Two activity: Nutrition Ellen felt a sense of accomplishment, having shifted much of her snacking from salty snacks to fresh vegetables. She read Rebekka Katz's book, *The Cancer Fighting Kitchen* (Katz, 2009) and set the initial goal to prepare evening meals three times a week from the Katz book. Katz's approach emphasizes a variety of "cancer-fighting" ingredients such as blueberries, chocolate, honey, and salmon. Katz discusses the "power of yum"; although therapeutic, her menus do not appear medicinal. She promotes recipes high in flavor, yet designed to enhance immune function and diminish the various adverse effects of chemotherapy.

Level Two Progress

Progress: Gentle yoga Ellen attended the gentle yoga class twice weekly and formed a friendship with two other women attending the class. They committed to joining each other two additional times each week for brief yoga practice sessions to extend the impact of the yoga practices. She was the only person in the yoga class with cancer, and she was pleased to see that in spite of her recent inactivity, she was better able to assume the yoga asanas (postural poses) than several other women in the class. She could feel the positive benefit as her flexibility and stamina increased with each week of yoga. The limb heaviness seemed to diminish although it recurred on a sporadic basis, without any apparent trigger.

Progress: Mindfulness training and mindful meditation Ellen began utilizing mindful acceptance as a coping strategy for her fears and worries. She engaged in an inner dialogue counseling herself neither to judge not criticize herself for the fearful thoughts and to simply observe the anxious thoughts unfold in her thought processes. As she progressed in her acceptance exercises, she found the subjective intensity of the fears diminishing. The more acceptance she was able to embrace for the fears, the less anxious she felt at their onset.

She also reached a decision to set aside her transcendental meditation practices, at least for a time, and try out mindfulness meditation. TM is based on the repetition of a mantra, a phrase each practitioner receives from his or her teacher. Instead Ellen began to meditate with a mindfulness-based breath meditation, simply observing the flow and process of her own breathing, accepting whatever aspect presented itself. Later she followed a broader mindfulness approach in her meditation, allowing her thoughts and moments to unfold spontaneously, while observing them passively, noting their impermanence and emphasizing acceptance for whatever emerged in the flow of her experience.

Progress: Pastoral care Ellen described her spiritual directions class as alternately light hearted and "really heavy." Several of the class members were women who rejected all conventional religious beliefs. The class engaged in hilarious moments of recalling strenuous childhood religious beliefs, frightening images of a punishing God, and past guilt, but also engaged the women in discussions of their thoughts and fears about death. Ellen felt a strong trust and attachment growing for both the group leader and several of the women in her group. She was encouraged that she was able to discuss her evolving Buddhist meditation practices and her interest in the Buddhist traditions, without any judgments from others, including the

Catholic nun. After the formal 8-week class ended, the women and their group leader agreed to meet monthly on an indefinite basis, and to schedule a 3-day spiritual retreat weekend soon.

Progress: Nutrition In the first week of cooking from the Katz recipes, Ellen experienced a severe upsurge of revulsion at many of the foods in the recipes. She called her health coach and modified her goal to be one of preparing the Katz menus, so she could achieve some success, whether or not she actually ate the meals. Her repulsions lessened as she handled the ingredients and cooked more frequently. On days when the revulsions blocked enjoying the meals, she reverted to snacking on cut vegetables. In the second month, the repulsions occurred only five times, and in the third month only three times.

Level Two Progress: Summary

Ellen continued her Level Two activities for 12 weeks, before initiating a discussion about starting Level Three. She felt significantly more "functional," since she was engaging in yoga, meditation, and cooking several times a week. She lost seven pounds in the 12 weeks of her Level Two activities and felt more able to move her body. She continued to experience anxiety and depression, but with less intensity and less impact on her ability to carry out her daily activities. Her mindful acceptance and breath exercises helped her manage the onset of anxiety and her mood often lifted with the mindful exercises and after her yoga workouts.

Ellen made a commitment to continue all four Level Two activities although the total time involved in the combination of wellness activities, in combination with her teaching job, was becoming a burden. She decided to attend her yoga class only once weekly, practice once with her new yoga friends weekly, and once alone at home. She looked forward to summer, and offered to do a weeklong "day camp" at her home, for her yoga classmates and the members of her spiritual directions group.

Ellen worked out a plan with her spouse, in which each agreed to prepare a Rebekka Katz meal on two week days and one weekend day. The seventh day was a dining out day, and they experimented with "healthier" restaurants in their community. She now felt more supported by her spouse, who tried out her meditation practice several times, and was now strongly supportive of her new Pathway practices. He now teased her about *two* aging hippies, meditating together in the guest room.

Level Three Plan

Level Three treatments: Acupuncture and acupressure Ellen continued to experience intermittent nausea. She was able to eat and enjoy food more frequently, by this time, but when the nausea was at its worse, it stopped her almost completely from activity and eating. The prevailing feeling of being sick that accompanied the nausea spoiled her sense of joy on many days. Ellen's Pathways health coach suggested and she accepted a referral to a local physician who utilized acupuncture for pain, nausea, and a variety of other symptoms. In a series of research studies, evidence has accumulated that acupuncture can reduce nausea and vomiting produced by chemotherapy and may also have other beneficial effects, including reduction of fatigue and enhanced immune function. Meta-analyses by Towler, Molassiotis, and Brearley (2013) and Wu et al. (2015) reviewed studies on acupuncture and cancer that met current methodological criteria; the Wu et al. study also included Chinese language publications. The evidence base supports including acupuncture as an alternative for patients during and following chemotherapy.

Ellen's acupuncture practitioner recommended a combination of acupuncture and acupressure and suggested that both she and her husband could learn a simple acupressure technique to apply manual pressure to "pressure point P6" or the Neiguan pressure point on the patient's lower arm. He reported that many of his patients with nausea, including first trimester pregnant women, and patients undergoing chemotherapy, were able to moderate their nausea significantly, and sometimes eliminate it.

Level Three treatment: Heart Rate Variability (HRV) biofeedback Ellen now had been practicing mindful breathing for approximately 18 weeks and had found her paced diaphragmatic breathing to be a useful tool for managing anxiety and a useful entry point for meditation. Her health coach encouraged her to participate in heart rate variability biofeedback as her second Level Three therapy, to further build skills for anxiety management, and to assist in restoring autonomic nervous system regulation. Her psychologist also gave her hope that several previous patients with chemotherapy-related nausea had moderated it through heart rate variability training and practice.

Ellen's HRV training began with an in-office practice session to refine her ability to breathe reliably and accurately with a breath pacer. Then in the next session, her biofeedback practitioner assessed her resonance frequency breathing rate. The resonance frequency (RF) is the breath rate at which she exhibits the highest heart rate variability. He guided Ellen through several breathing rates, beginning by breathing for 2 minutes at 7.5 breaths per minute and slowing in half breath steps until she reached 4.5 breaths per minute. At each breath rate, the biofeedback practitioner assessed how closely in synch the line graphs were for breathing and heart rate. At the RF, her inhalation should end just at the moment that her heart rate reaches its maximum level, and the exhalation should end just as the heart rate reaches its minimal level. In addition, at the RF, the patient should produce the largest oscillations in heart rate, the greatest differences from maximal to minimal HR in each breath cycle, and several other statistics for HRV should be at their highest.

Ellen's RF was assessed to be 6.5 breaths per minute. She was guided in the office to breathe at this breath rate and to produce smooth line graphs of respiration and heart rate on the biofeedback display screen. She was also given the homework to set her breath pacer at 6.5 breaths per minute and guide her breathing now to her specific RF. Ellen also purchased the HeartMath®-based Inner Balance system, which measures HRV and displays both an HRV signal and a breath pacer on a smart phone or tablet. She enjoyed practicing her RF breathing and watching her heart rate variability on the Inner Balance.

Level Three treatment: Mindfulness practices Ellen had benefited greatly from her mindfulness class and her experiences of mindfulness meditation. She found that by accepting her anxious thoughts without judgment, she dramatically reduced the sense of struggle and anguish that usually accompanied her anxiety. She had battled her fearful thoughts, trying to squelch or stop the thoughts. She had read about thought stopping as a self-care intervention for anxiety, which is a form of cognitive behavioral therapy. In her case, the effort to stop her thoughts typically failed and led her to self-criticize herself for her miserable lack of cognitive control. Accepting and thoughtfully observing her fearful thoughts, in contrast, seemed to dilute their intensity.

Ellen agreed to attend an 8-week mindfulness-based stress reduction (MBSR) group-based program, which included a follow-up daylong silent retreat. MBSR, developed by Jon Kabat-Zinn, is most closely linked to Buddhist practices of the various mindfulness approaches and includes meditation as an element in the treatment process. Ledesma and Kumano (2009) conducted a meta-analysis of studies applying MBSR for cancer patients and found significant reductions in depression among those studied, and some evidence of improvements in the physical health of the study participants. A later meta-analysis by Cramer et al. (2012) reviewed studies specifically applying MBSR to breast cancer patients and found evidence of reduced anxiety and reduced perceived stress. One of the studies they reviewed showed improved spiritual well-being as well.

Level Three treatment: Narrative psychotherapy Ellen continued to be drawn to Lawrence Leshan's idea of learning to identify and "sing her own song." She explored and read about various forms of psychotherapy for her Level Three Pathways plan. She considered "acceptance and commitment therapy," because it built on her practice of mindfulness. After watching a YouTube video on narrative psychotherapy, Ellen finally asked her health coach and the psychologist who had done her initial assessment to help her find a therapist for narrative psychotherapy,

Narrative medicine and narrative psychotherapy both rest on the recognition that human beings are prone to seek meaning, and that human beings, since primordial times, have often found and defined meaning and identity in story form. Narrative psychotherapists often draw on the myths and stories of the ancient Greeks as well as those from Native Americans and tribal groups worldwide (Mehl-Madrona 2005, 2010). Ellen expressed her hope that narrative psychotherapy would assist her in finding the lost themes in her life story, which she had abandoned or never discovered. She wished to open a new chapter in her life, with more of a sense of embracing a story that felt like her own.

Initial Level Three Progress

Ellen had begun only two of her four Level Three activities—acupuncture and HRV biofeedback— before her Pathways work was interrupted by another medical setback.

Progress: Acupuncture Ellen saw her physician-acupuncturist weekly, for both acupuncture (needling specific points along the meridians of traditional Chinese medicine) and acupressure (applying manual pressure largely to the Neiguan pressure point on her arm). She and her husband practiced applying manual pressure at the Neguan point at home whenever she felt nausea, and she experienced a noticeable decrease in the subjective intensity of her nausea each time. She also reported less onset of nausea after the second session of acupuncture.

Progress: HRV biofeedback Given her extensive practice of paced mindful breathing, Ellen made rapid progress in HRV biofeedback. She quickly produced smooth line graphs, showing large oscillations in heart rate on the biofeedback display. She practiced daily breathing at 6.5 breaths per minute, using the Inner Balance program on her iPhone and was able to breathe at or close to 6.5 breaths per minute without a breath pacer by the end of the third week. She also reported that she was combining her mindful acceptance with the resonance frequency breathing practice. After 2 weeks, she reported minimal sense of strain and effort to produce the desired breath pattern and was able to allow and observe her RF breathing in a mindful fashion.

Metastasis

Three weeks after Ellen commenced her Level Three activities, she returned to her oncologist for her annual MRI and follow-up visit. The MRI showed a small tumor in her left lung. Her oncologist was optimistic about a surgical excision of the tumor and a small wedge of lung tissue around the tumor. However, he was concerned that the cancer had recurred in spite of the double mastectomy and chemotherapy. He recommended a new series of platinum-based chemotherapy sessions in the hospital's outpatient oncology unit.

Ellen was initially heartbroken. She feared that this relapse condemned her to a never-ending sequence of chemotherapy, recurrent nausea and cognitive deficits, new interventions to moderate symptoms, and then another relapse and more chemotherapy. The recurrence of cancer also meant to her that somehow she had failed to enhance her immune function. Ellen was reminded by her health coach that her strain of breast cancer was a virulent one, often prone to relapses, and that the practices in which she was engaging would assist her in living as fully and with the maximal possible wellness, but that any cancer can recur. Her health coach also encouraged her that her Pathways self-care skills should help her now through chemotherapy, as they had in recovering from chemotherapy. Her oncologist also assured her that many of his patients were living for 5 years, 10 years, or more after successful platinum-based chemotherapy.

Ellen underwent surgery to remove the tumor in her lung. Four weeks later, she began a scheduled 10 weeks of outpatient intravenous chemotherapy. Although she was given antiemetic medication prior to each chemotherapy session, Ellen experienced severe nausea with each session of chemotherapy. Her husband applied manual pressure the Neiguan point on her arm, and this reduced her nausea. She also began to practice the Inner Balance application and mindful awareness while seated in a recliner undergoing the chemotherapy. Practicing her resonance frequency breathing helped her further. She explained that even when the nausea persisted, just mindfully watching it occur calmed her and rendered it less upsetting. In addition, she reported diminished anxiety and clearer thinking after the resonance frequency breathing sessions. She experienced recurrent fears of dying, but her RF breathing and mindfulness enabled her to view both the fears and the reality of death with greater acceptance.

Ellen was not able to continue her yoga during chemotherapy, due to weakness. She continued to visit the acupuncturist who continued doing needle-based acupuncture aimed at nausea and fatigue. In addition, the Dominican nun and two members of her spiritual directions class visited her at home during the weeks of chemotherapy, and she found their supportive presence encouraging.

Renewed Level Three Progress

Progress: Mindfulness-Based Stress Reduction Ellen rescheduled her MBSR group for the month following her completion of chemotherapy. She experienced the MBSR as anti-climactic but helpful. Her own mindfulness skills had been so severely tested by her recurrent cancer that she felt her skills were far beyond most of the attendees who were just beginning the mindful path. Yet, she was suffering continued challenges, with very slow regrowth of her hair following chemotherapy, and lingering weakness and fatigue. She reported that the MBSR therapist knew so many different mindfulness exercises and strategies that she learned something new at each session.

"Ellen visualized herself at 80 looking back and telling the story of the second half of her life. She discovered images of herself in a college classroom teaching teachers, and other images of herself teaching cancer patients some of the lessons she was currently learning."

Progress: Narrative psychotherapy Ellen's narrative psychotherapist accepted her objective in her psychotherapy. She engaged Ellen in a variety of imagery exercises and writing activities to sensitize her to themes already present in her life. She read about and chose a Native American totem animal, the swan, for its grace and beauty. Ellen wrote "stories" at least weekly about herself as a young girl, her dreams, and the figures and images who had stirred her own dreams as a child and adolescent. Her therapist used hypnotic age regression to revisit critical moments when Ellen made choices about her education and career. In particular,

Ellen tearfully re-lived her decision to pursue a bachelor's degree in elementary education, after vacillating among nursing, teaching, and social work. She re-experienced a sense of her passion as a college student at the mission of touching young learners' hearts in the classroom. Teaching at least had been "her own song," and not some form of compromise with life. Ellen also used hypnosis to revisit some of the moments of discouragement and disenchantment with teaching in the past 5 years and gained a strong sense that the disappointments had to do with bureaucracy and administration and not her students, who still regularly awakened her enthusiasms.

The therapist also guided her in several hypnotic age progressions. Ellen visualized herself at 80 looking back and telling the story of the second half of her life. She discovered images of herself in a college classroom teaching teachers, and other images of herself teaching cancer patients some of the lessons she was currently learning.

Assessment

Ellen continued her HRV biofeedback training for ten sessions, completed the 8-session MBSR program and the daylong MBSR retreat, continued in regular acupuncture visits for 1 year, and continued in narrative psychotherapy (two times a week) for 10 months. At her last Pathways session, 1 year after the third metastasis, she completed the Beck Depression Inventory and Beck Anxiety Inventory again. Her BDI score was 9 or normal, and her BAI score was 12, or low. A baseline sample of her heart rate variability showed an SDNN, an index of HRV and overall health and resilience, of 94—high in the compromised health range, close to normal. When asked to engage in resonance frequency breathing, she produced a smooth well-organized pattern of breathing and heart rate oscillations.

At last contact, 2 years had passed since Ellen's third metastasis. Nausea and fatigue were present intermittently but mild. She was walking, participating in yoga, and meditating several times a week. Her spiritual conversations group continued to meet monthly, and she expected they might continue indefinitely. She reported that her various self-care skills were strong, but she also emphasized that she needed the skills. She continued to experience anxiety, whenever any physical sensation caught her attention. If she felt confused or could not remember information, she feared brain cancer; if she noticed shortness of breath she feared another tumor in the lungs. She also found herself looking online at statistics about survival rates after three metastases. She had learned to "catch herself" whenever these kinds of fearful ruminations occurred and to engage her RF breathing and her mindful awareness and mindful acceptance.

Ellen's own song Ellen continued in narrative psychotherapy for 10 months. Initially, she was hungry to find any new direction for her life, some new purpose and perhaps a different job and career. As she continued in her narrative psychotherapy, she instead began to find a renewed enthusiasm for her calling as a teacher.

Ellen was a fourth-generation teacher, with men and women in each generation since her great grandfather working in the classroom in elementary school, high school, and University careers.

Ellen felt a new awakening in the year after her psychotherapy ended. She began taking classes toward a doctorate in education, with a focus on elementary education, and added courses on stress management and health education. She also began volunteer activity through the cancer center where she had received her own care. She set up mindfulness classes for women with breast cancer and integrated both breath training and meditation practices. She entertained thoughts of leaving the elementary classroom to teach in a school of education, as well as thoughts of pursuing a full-time career as a health educator. Regardless, she found herself reaffirming her passion for teaching.

Ellen remained painfully aware that she might face a recurrence of her cancer, but remained hopeful to live a full life, as long a life as she could sustain, using her Pathways self-care skills for quality in that life.

References

American Psychiatric Association. (2013). *Diagnostic and statistical manual of mental disorders* (5th ed.). Washington, DC: Author.

Cramer, H. (2012). Mindfulness-based stress reduction for breast cancer: A systematic review and metaanalysis. Current Oncology, 19(5), e343–52. doi: 10.3747/co.19.1016.

Kabat-Zinn, J. (2013). *Full catastrophe living: Using the wisdom of your body and mind to face stress, pain, and illness* (revised edition). New York, NY: Bantam Books.

Katz, R. (2009). *The cancer fighting kitchen: Nourishing, big flavor recipes for cancer treatment and recovery.* New York, NY: Ten Speed Press.

Leshan, L. (1990). *Cancer as a turning point: A handbook for people with cancer, their families, and helping professionals.* New York, NY: Plume.

Ledesma, D., & Kumano, H. (2009). Mindfulness-based stress reduction and cancer: A meta-analysis. Psychooncology, 18(6), 571–9. doi: 10.1002/pon.1400.

McGrady, A., & Moss, D. (2013). *Pathways to illness, pathways to health.* New York, NY: Springer.

Mehl-Madrona, L. (2005). *Coyote wisdom: The power of story in healing.* Rochester, VT: Bear and Company.

Mehl-Madrona, L. (2010). *Healing the mind through the power of story: The power of narrative psychiatry.* Rochester, Vermont: Bear and Company.

Towler, P., Molassiotis, A., & Brearley, S. G. (2013). What is the evidence for the use of acupuncture as an intervention for symptom management in cancer supportive and palliative care: An integrative overview of reviews. *Supportive Care in Cancer, 21*, 2913–2923. https://doi.org/10.1007/s00520-013-1882-8

Wu, X., Chung, V. C., Hui, E. P., Ziea, E. T., Ng, B. F., Ho, R. S., et al. (2015). Effectiveness of acupuncture and related therapies for palliative care of cancer: Overview of systematic reviews. *Science Reports, 5*, 16776. https://doi.org/10.1038/srep16776

Chapter 14
A Pathways Model Approach for Traumatic Brain Injury

Abstract The incidence of traumatic brain injuries (TBI) has increased in recent years, now comprising 2.5 million emergency room visits, hospitalizations, and deaths each year in the United States. TBI is frequently a chronic condition with persisting symptoms and disability. This chapter presents a case study in which self-hypnosis, hypnosis-assisted psychotherapy, and palliative care strategies were provided within a multi-modal integrative treatment program for a 38-year-old woman with TBI secondary to motor vehicle accident. Self-hypnosis was helpful in anxiety reduction and pain management. Hypnosis-assisted psychotherapy was beneficial in desensitizing many post-traumatic memories, and in managing post-concussion pain, including neuropathic pain and post-traumatic migraine headaches. A variety of palliative care techniques and spiritual interventions were applied to enhance sleep, moderate cognitive deficits, and enhance quality of life.

Keywords Traumatic brain injury · Post-traumatic stress disorder · Hypnosis · Palliative care · Spirituality

Neurologically Based Conditions

Neurologically based conditions include seizure disorders, cerebral palsy, multiple sclerosis, Lou Gehrig's disease, Alzheimer's disease, cerebral vascular accidents, traumatic brain injury, and many other conditions. Most of these conditions are chronic and debilitating in nature. The degree and specific nature of incapacity is more closely related to the areas of the brain and central nervous system affected and the severity of the damage, than to the medical diagnoses. As the percentage of persons over 65 years of age increases in the North American and world populations, the global burden of neurologically based conditions will increase sharply. The Family Caregiver Alliance (2011) estimated that 1.2 million Americans are

This chapter is adapted with permission of the Annals of Palliative Care from a previous version that appeared as: D. Moss (2018), I hurt so: Hypnotic interventions and palliative care for traumatic brain injury. Annals of Palliative Medicine, 7(1),151–158.

diagnosed each year with a neurological condition. The World Health Organization (2006) emphasizes that neurologically based conditions, including both communicable diseases and non-communicable diseases and conditions, present a serious burden of death and disability worldwide, with the level of burden varying across the national income categories. For example, the disability-adjusted life years lost from epilepsy varies from 158.3 DALY lives lost per 100,000 people in the lowest income regions to 51.3 in the highest income regions (WHO, 2006, p. 33). Affluence leads to more effective identification of cases, better treatment, and reduced disability.

"With growing recognition of the neuroplasticity of the brain and nervous system, the hope for at least partial recovery of function increases."

In the majority of cases, neurologically based disorders, even those with sudden onset as in motor vehicle accidents, become chronic; they cannot be "cured." With growing recognition of the neuroplasticity of the brain and nervous system, the hope for at least partial recovery of function increases. Rehabilitation and management of neurologically based disorders should begin as soon as possible after the diagnosis of the disorder or condition (WHO, 2006). Palliative care interventions are appropriately used to moderate and manage symptoms, reduce patient distress, and enhance quality of life.

Traumatic Brain Injury

In this chapter, we present a case narrative of a 38-year-old woman with a traumatic brain injury (TBI), based on a motor vehicle accident. The Centers for Disease Control and Prevention has documented a steadily increasing incidence of TBI in the United States, with 2.5 million emergency room visits, hospitalizations, and deaths from TBI in the United States in 2010 (CDC, 2015), and an increase in the incidence of TBI from 2005 to 2014 from 521 to 824 per 100,000 population (CDC, 2016). Motor vehicle accidents contribute heavily to the toll of TBI-related injury and disability. Between 2002 and 2010, there was an annual average of 232,240 emergency room visits with TBI related to motor vehicle accidents and 53,391 hospitalizations for TBI-related motor vehicle accidents.

Clinical hypnosis has proven effective in the management of anxiety and pain symptoms in a variety of populations; hypnosis is also effective in the resolution of traumatic memories and post-trauma symptoms, which frequently accompany TBI. In one recent clinical report, hypnosis was also utilized to facilitate cognitive recovery following brain injury (Vanhaudenhuyse, Laureys, & Faymonville, 2015). This chapter describes the integration of hypnosis and a variety of palliative care strategies into a multi-modal treatment program for a 38-year-old woman with traumatic brain injury secondary to a motor vehicle accident.

Introducing Kay Ellen

At the time of evaluation, Kay Ellen was a 38-year-old married mother of two daughters, previously employed as a bookkeeper. Two years ago, she was involved in an automobile accident while driving to an accounting training program for her job. She had worked only briefly since the accident.

Kay Ellen was driving a small SUV, and another driver ran a stop sign and struck her passenger side door, rolling Kay's SUV onto its roof, and throwing her against her car door. Her air bag inflated, protecting her from the windshield. She suffered a concussion from the impact of her skull with the left-side car door. She recalled a sudden impact and shattering glass, and then lost consciousness. She recovered consciousness while EMTs were working to pry open her door and remove her from the upside-down wreckage. She became aware of sharp pains in her left shoulder, arm, and hip, and an aching in her head.

She was hospitalized for evaluation, and underwent extensive X-rays and CT scans while an inpatient. Her X-rays showed cracked ribs but no fractures. Her CT scans showed swelling of the brain in the left frontal, left temporal, and right temporal areas. The consulting neurologist diagnosed post-concussion syndrome with a coup/contrecoup injury from the collision and rollover, and medicated her with a neuro-modulator, Neurontin (gabapentin).

In the days following the accident, she was mostly concerned with arm and shoulder pain and the emotional trauma of the accident. As her bruising and muscle pain lessened, she suffered increasing head pain, with migraine features including throbbing pain, nausea with the head pain, and sensitivity to light. She also reported a sharp, deep burning pain in her head that never left. At times, she also experienced an intense burning pain in her right leg and right chest.

She also complained of cognitive deficits, with word-finding problems, some stuttering, poor concentration, and a sense of slowed lethargic thought process. The word-finding difficulties, speech problems, and poor concentration occurred daily, but were worse when migraine headaches were present.

Kay Ellen suffered nightmares, often awakening screaming and waiving her arms as she re-lived the car rolling in addition to daytime flashbacks to the accident. She found herself avoiding the intersection where the accident occurred, and at times was reluctant to even drive. She experienced intermittent panic attacks, most often in the car, with rapid heart rate, rapid breathing, and a fear of another driver smashing into her car. Her physician medicated her with an SSRI, Lexapro, for depression and anxiety.

Pathways Assessment

Kay Ellen came to the clinic 2 years after the motor vehicle accident, for depression, anxiety, and pain management. Her mental status exam at the time of her initial evaluation showed that she was well oriented in time, space, and person, but exhibited difficulty with short-term memory, failing to recall three objects, and the inability to recall any sequence of numbers exceeding three digits. She also reported short attention span and a clouding of consciousness. She experienced her thinking as dulled and slowed.

"'I hurt so much,' she said repeat- edly. She often thought that death would be easier than living with the intensity of her pain."

Kay Ellen acknowledged severe depression and reported a sense of loss for her life as it was before the accident. She had briefly returned to work follow- ing the accident, but was unable to focus and manage the detailed bookkeeping required in her job. She also felt less of a mother, because she could no longer comprehend her middle school age chil- dren's homework, nor could she assist them. She had previously volunteered to direct the middle school math club and was especially proud of increasing the participation of middle school girls in the club, but now gave that up as well.

She reported that her worst depressive moods came when her head pain and/or right-sided pain were most intense. "I hurt so," she said repeatedly. She often thought that death would be easier than living with the intensity of her pain.

Psychometric assessment Kay Ellen completed a Beck Depression Inventory (BDI) and a Beck Anxiety Inventory (BAI) (Beck & Beamesderfer, 1974; Fydrich, Dowdall, & Chambless, 1992). On the BDI she scored 35, indicating severe depres- sion, and endorsed items indicating sadness, discouragement, loss of satisfaction in life, self-hate, self-criticism, crying, poor sleep, fatigue, and thoughts of suicide. On the BAS she scored 50, indicating severe anxiety. She endorsed items indicating the inability to relax, fear of the worst happening, terrified feelings, nervousness, and a host of somatic symptoms associated with anxiety disorders and panic episodes. She scored a 19 on the Tellegen Absorption Scale, indicating that she was likely to be a good candidate for therapeutic application of hypnosis and hypnotic sugges- tions (Tellegen & Atkinson, 1974). Finally, she scored a 41 on the Nijmegen Questionnaire; this is an instrument designed in the Netherlands to identify patients whose symptoms are probably caused or aggravated by maladaptive breathing pat- terns (van Dixhoorn & Duivenvoorden, 1985).

Diagnostic assessment Kay Ellen met the criteria for medical diagnoses of post- concussion syndrome with head pain, neuropathic right-sided pain, and intermittent migraine headache. The left-sided brain swelling and bruising coincided with Broca's area in the brain, and probably explained the speech problems. She fit the psychiatric diagnoses of post-traumatic stress disorder and major depression, with anxious distress. She showed significant anxiety, but her anxiety episodes seemed post-traumatic in character; therefore, she did not meet criteria for a separate anxi- ety disorder diagnosis.

Neurophysiology As part of her assessment, Kay Ellen submitted to a quantitative electroencephalogram (QEEG), using the Neuroguide® norms. The QEEG showed an excess of slow wave (Delta and Theta) EEG activity over both hemispheres, specifically in the left frontal, left temporal, right temporal, and occipital areas. The underactive left temporal area included Broca's area (the Brodmann areas 44 and

45, essential for productive speech). There were also smaller areas of elevated high Beta, in the left and right temporal areas and along the mid-line, over the anterior cingulate cortex, a pattern which frequently contributes to heightened anxiety.

Lifestyle assessment Following the accident, Kay Ellen reported unsteadiness in her gait and found that walking aggravated her head pain. She gradually gave up most activity, spending much of the day and night in a reclining chair with the lights turned off and curtains pinned closed to shut out sunlight. She claimed that she had lost appetite as well, and ate sparingly, but had gained 25 pounds since the automobile accident. Kay Ellen's sleep cycle was severely disturbed. Since she kept herself in near total darkness day and night, and watched movies on the television intermittently around the clock, she was often confused as to whether it was day or night. She slept erratically for only brief periods.

Readiness for change Kay Ellen was desperate for any intervention that would relieve pain or moderate her anxiety. However, her depression was so severe that she had little hope that action on her part would cause improvement. She accepted the referral for behaviorally based treatment, but simultaneously she had requested her spouse to investigate deep brain stimulation and neuro-surgery. She agreed to cooperate with the Pathways team's recommendations, yet expressed hopelessness. It remained difficult for her to believe that she could help herself.

Pathways Treatment

Following the Pathways Model (McGrady & Moss, 2013), Kay Ellen's treatment was organized into three levels:

Pathways Level One focuses on self-directed changes in everyday behaviors and lifestyle that are designed to re-establish normal body rhythms.

Pathways Level Two focuses on the individual learning self-regulation skills and utilizing community resources and educational materials to support learning and lifestyle changes.

Pathways Level Three involves professional interventions, the utilization of services provided by a health practitioner, such as hypnosis, energy therapy, psychotherapy, acupuncture, or medication management.

Level One activity: Mindful breathing practice Kay Ellen wanted to focus her treatment initially on her post-traumatic stress symptoms, anxiety, and head pain. Given her high score on the Nijmegen questionnaire, and her pervasive anxiety, her Pathways health coach suggested that she adopt paced mindful breathing as her initial Level One activity. She was aware of rapid and irregular breathing during her anxiety attacks and accepted this suggestion. Her health coach taught her to pace her breathing using a breathing app on her smart phone (Breathe2Relax) and showed her how to monitor her breathing using one hand on her chest and one on her abdomen to increase her awareness of her breathing. She learned to breathe gently, slowly, and fully, at a pace of about six breaths per minute.

Level One activity: Sleep hygiene Kay Ellen agreed to a goal of restoring a diurnal cycle to her sleep and waking. She experimented with opening the curtains in the room where she sat and wore sunglasses to cope with her light sensitivity. She also began lying down in the bedroom between 10 and 11 p.m. and forced herself to get up at 7 a.m. to see her daughters before they left for school. She also consented to sit in the shade on her patio, whenever the outdoor temperature was warm enough, again wearing sunglasses and a hat.

Level One Progress

Kay Ellen experienced the mindful breathing as soothing and calming. She experienced a lessening of her stress and anxiety when she engaged in her breathing practices. However, an intense panic attack occurred while driving, only 5 minutes after engaging in her breath practices, which was very discouraging. When another panic attack happened while driving, she pulled over safely to the side of the road, started the breath pacer on her phone, and slowed her breathing. This time her panic abated and she was able to drive home. She was encouraged by this success.

Restoration of Kay Ellen's sleep cycle was more challenging. She made herself lie down at bedtime, but sleep eluded her. She was encouraged to use some behavioral sleep aids to enhance sleep onset. First, she used a white noise device simulating falling water to create a steady soothing background and shut out environmental noise. Second, she utilized an audio-visual entrainment (AVE) device, a headset, and a set of LED goggles delivering sound and light at a rate gradually ramping down from 8 to 2 Hz[1] to entrain her brain to Delta range sleep rhythms.[2] Tang et al. (Tang, Vitiello, Perlis, Mao, & Riegel, 2014, Tang, Riegel, McCurry, & Vitiello, 2016) have documented the effectiveness of AVE in improving sleep. Sleep diary data in their studies showed faster sleep latency and reduced awakenings.

Using white noise and AVE, Kay Ellen slowly made progress in falling asleep more rapidly—in about 25–35 minutes. She still reported fragmented sleep and daytime sleepiness, but the hours of nighttime sleeping gradually increased. She was also instructed to use the AVE device when she awakened in the night as well, and this gave her additional hours of sleep.

---

[1] The device used was a David Paradise® device, from Mind Alive, Ltd., in Calgary.

[2] Possible adverse effects of audio-visual entrainment were discussed with the patient. Strobe lights can trigger onset of migraine or seizure, usually at faster frequencies. The patient agreed to trials of the AVE device in the office. In her case neither the protocol for sleep onset nor the protocol used later in her treatment for daytime alertness triggered any adverse effects.

Pathways Level Two Pathways Activities

Level Two in the Pathways Model involves the acquisition of coping skills and self-regulation skills and the use of community resources and educational materials for better coping.

Level Two activity: Self-Hypnosis Kay Ellen expressed fascination with hypnosis, and her psychologist suggested she begin with home practice of calming self-hypnosis exercises. In the office, Kay Ellen showed above average hypnotic ability, responding positively to suggestions of arm heaviness and arm levitation. She learned to use eye fixation, slowed breathing, and a descending staircase image to induce trance, and accepted suggestions of a calm scene to calm her emotions and quiet her mind. She also learned a self-hypnosis exercise in dissociation to enter trance and then pictured herself across the room from her body. She learned to disengage herself mentally from the pain, experiencing it as distant.

Level Two activity: Aquatherapy Because Kay Ellen suffered pain much of each day, and the pain seemed to be aggravated by activity, she was resistant to increasing movement. She reluctantly agreed to a trial with Aquatherapy, gentle graded activity in a warm-water therapeutic pool, so she was referred to a program operated by a physical therapy (PT) clinic. The PTs conducted an initial evaluation, found several patterns of muscular bracing and tensing, and assigned her to their gentlest program of in-pool activity, a class composed primarily of men and women with severe rheumatoid arthritis. Kay Ellen found the 94°F pool water soothing, and initially enjoyed lolling in the pool. Gradually, she was encouraged to join in some gentle movements with the class.

Level Two activity. Prayer Kay Ellen's spouse Richard asked her psychologist whether healing prayer could help her mood and hopelessness. He explained that she had been a devout Catholic, who regularly participated in a Bible study group and in a healing prayer circle with women from several area churches that seemed to benefit several women with serious medical and emotional conditions. Since her accident, however, she had lost hope and refused to engage in prayer. When the psychologist spoke with Kay Ellen, she burst into tears, and expressed a wish that the women from the prayer circle would pray over her. Richard made contact with the group facilitator, and a meeting was set up for the circle to pray with Kay Ellen at her home.

Level Two Progress

Kay Ellen reported that she was much calmer and less anxious with the combination of paced mindful breathing and self-hypnosis. On days of extreme tension and anxiety, she was able to achieve a relaxed state, even if for a short time. She found the breathing to be her first response to any anxiety because she was able to slow her breathing even when driving or in public. She still reported flashbacks to the accident, and it took her longer to calm at those times, but her breath practices at least reduced the intensity of the anxiety. When she took the time to sit quietly and do her self-hypnosis exercises, the process calmed her deeply.

She reported after 4 weeks of self-hypnosis that she was suffering less with her deep burning pain in the head and the right-sided leg and chest pain. When she mentally disconnected from her body in her self-induced trance, she experienced the pain as distant and weaker. Kay Ellen reported that her migraine headaches continued, but were now less frequent (down from four times weekly to one to two times weekly).

Kay Ellen gradually increased her movement in the Aquatherapy classes. She reported that she felt less "twisted" in her body, and the physical therapist supervising her participation reported less muscular bracing.

Kay Ellen's prayer circle visited her four times in the month after her husband relayed her request. Each time they began by "praying over her"—praying for healing. Two of the group members felt spiritually moved and prayed in tongues over her. Then they invited her to pray with them for herself and others. She felt cared for and supported in these sessions, and the prayer sessions lifted her mood. On one occasion, she suffered a severe migraine headache with onset an hour before the prayer session, but she decided not to cancel the group. She experienced a spontaneous lessening of the migraine pain during the prayer. She was afraid to feel hopeful, yet experienced a further lessening of the intensity and frequency of the headaches in the coming weeks. The prayer visits also led to telephone contact with three of the group members, who had felt shut out by Kay Ellen's not returning their phone calls, in the months after the accident.

Kay Ellen was encouraged that she was at least "moving in the right direction." She reported her depression was more moderate; her days dominated by discomfort and distress were fewer.

Pathways Level Three Treatments

Level Three in the Pathways Model consists of professional treatment interventions. In Kay Ellen's case, the treatment interventions were *palliative*, aiming to reduce both the symptoms and her distress secondary to the traumatic brain injury.

Level Three treatment: Clinical hypnosis Kay Ellen had responded positively to self-hypnosis, with both calming and reduction in pain intensity. She eagerly consented to a series of psychotherapy sessions focused on hypnosis both for pain and traumatic memories of the accident. Her psychologist began doing a hypnosis induction at the beginning of each session. Kay Ellen entered hypnosis easily and responded positively to suggestions to deepen her hypnotic state.

Hypnosis for traumatic memories Kay Ellen's psychologist initially focused the hypnotically assisted psychotherapy on revisiting the accident scene. The purpose was to help her to face each phase of the accident, the moment when the other car was racing toward her passenger door, the impact which she so frequently re-lived in nightmares, and the minutes in which she hung from the seat belt upside down in

"Kay Ellen's psychologist initially focused the hypnotically assisted psychotherapy on revisiting the accident scene, and assisting her to face each phase of the accident, the moment when the other car was racing toward her passenger door ....".

her overturned car. He invited Kay Ellen to see herself from a distance, then to approach more closely, and then to see the accident in slow motion. Whenever she grew agitated, he invited her to withdraw to her safe place and recover an inward calm and strength.

Next, he guided Kay Ellen into the future, in an age progression, to join herself on a balmy tropical beach where she is celebrating progress in her healing. Kay Ellen saw herself walking steadily into the warm salty water, and then lying on the beach soaking up the sun. She spoke quietly through this age progression, inviting her sunning future self to describe some of her struggles and some of her progress.

Hypnosis for pain management Next, Kay Ellen's psychologist guided her through a series of hypnotic exercises to transform her sensory experience of her pain, changing its shape, its color, moving it from right side to left, from deep in her head to her foot, and shrinking the pain to a small capsule in her toenail. Finally, he used a "glove anesthesia" script to create tingling numbness throughout Kay Ellen's left hand, then suggested that wherever and whenever she touched herself with this numb glove-like hand, and said the word "tingle," that body area touched would also become numb and tingly (Crasilneck & Hall, 1985, pp. 76–77; Yapko, 2012, pp. 505–506).

Level Three treatment: Neurofeedback Given her baseline QEEG readings, and the pattern of cognitive deficits, Kay Ellen appeared to be a good candidate for neurofeedback (EEG biofeedback) to modify cortical activation patterns, with the intent to moderate both cognitive deficits and centrally mediated pain. A growing number of researchers have documented the efficacy of neurofeedback for addressing pain and cognitive deficits in traumatic brain injury (Ayers, 1999; Thomas & Smith, 2015; Thornton & Carmody, 2008). Unfortunately, the case manager managing her auto insurance benefits absolutely refused any payments for neurofeedback. Kay Ellen was eligible for worker's compensation benefits for services not covered by auto insurance, but the worker's compensation office also refused to pay for this necessary intervention. An attempt was made to negotiate a reduced fee for neurofeedback but the family's resources had been severely strained, and they declined to pay even a token amount for any services not covered by insurance.

Instead, Kay Ellen's therapist suggested using audio-visual entrainment to modify daytime cortical rhythms. Kay Ellen had utilized AVE at home for sleep onset, with substantial benefit. AVE is also often effective in inducing faster attention-enhancing cortical patterns in inattentive persons, but unlike neurofeedback the effect is generally time limited, so the AVE device must continue to be used daily for any effects.

Level Three treatment: Audio-visual entrainment (AVE) Kay Ellen continued to experience cognitive deficits including a lack of mental sharpness and a kind of cognitive fog. Kay Ellen's psychotherapist taught her to select a daytime AVE protocol with a much higher target rate, about 15 Hz, to entrain her brain to a dominant Beta rhythm. In the office, this AVE protocol produced a moderately more awake and alert state, with noticeably sharper thinking. Kay Ellen decided to use the AVE each morning and early afternoon to enhance her daytime alertness and attentiveness.

Level Three treatment: Spiritual counseling Kay Ellen's sessions with her prayer circle rekindled her desire for a spiritual recovery. She was ashamed at how she had cut herself off from her church and prayer and become so cynical about any spiritual help. She wanted to speak with a priest or minister, but not her own pastor, who she saw as a parrot mouthing empty formulas. One of the women in her prayer circle introduced her to a Franciscan monk, who was a spiritual guide at a retreat center 30 minutes from Kay Ellen's home. She began to meet with him whenever she was able to arrange a ride to the retreat center.

Level Three Progress

Kay Ellen almost always responded positively to hypnotic induction. She found the hypnotic sessions consistently soothing and calming. Her response to the various hypnotic scripts and suggestions varied greatly. She found herself less frequently troubled by flashbacks and nightmares, as the hypnotic regressions to the accident served to de-sensitize her reactions to the accident scene. She also felt bolstered by the hypnotic visit to her vacationing future self and set herself the goal to plan a tropical vacation with her husband within a year. She returned from that hypnotic age progression hearing her own words from the future saying to herself: "breathe, pray, and use trance."

Kay Ellen found little initial effect in the hypnotic suggestions to change the sensory aspect of her pain. Even when she visualized the pain shrunken down to a tiny space within her toenail that tiny space hurt so intensely she wanted to cut off her toe. The glove anesthesia surprised her however. She could tangibly feel her left hand becoming numb and tingly, and losing its fleshy substance, feeling like gauzy, cottony fluff. Then when she touched her aching right leg, the numbing, cottony glove-like sensations began to spread through her leg. Kay Ellen decided to use this strategy and numb her leg and chest before her Aquatherapy class, which enabled her to increase her activity further in the class.

However, Kay Ellen plunged into anger and discouragement at her insurance companies' refusal to pay for neurofeedback treatment. So she was assured that at least some of the potential benefit of neurofeedback could probably be accomplished by audio-visual entrainment. Kay Ellen experienced a moderate clearing of her thought processes and enhanced alertness initially with AVE. With daily repetition of the AVE sessions, she reported occasional days when she felt more like "herself" mentally. She did not feel ready to take on heavy accounting tasks or head the math club, yet she found herself better able to plan some of the meals for her family, and prepare a shopping list.

Kay Ellen found her spiritual counseling sessions helpful in coping with her changed life. She decided to use the Franciscan brother as a spiritual director for the next phase of her recovery. He taught her to pray in new ways, with simple meditations, and biblical imagery exercises. In one of her visualizations, she imagined the biblical figure Job, who had suffered the loss of his health, family, and wealth, holding her hand and encouraging her (Job, New International Version, 2015). She felt a strange validation in this visualization that someone whose name had become synonymous with suffering could acknowledge her suffering. In another visualization, she pictured herself as the woman described in the books of Mark (5:26–33, New International Version) and Luke (8:47, New International Version), who touched Christ's cloak, and felt healing power go into her.

Kay Ellen felt positive effects both in mood and in concentration with the meditation and imagery. Her spiritual guide also recommended books about meditation and spiritual practices, and she found herself able to concentrate on reading more than at any time since the accident.

Discussion: Life with a Damaged Brain

Kay Ellen continued to suffer pain, anxiety, and cognitive deficits. She experienced a variety of palliative effects from her self-regulation activities and her new spiritual practices, yet her brain was still damaged. She was not able to resume her work as a bookkeeper, nor to ride a bicycle with her daughters. However, she now was awake most days, shared breakfast with the daughters, and resumed much of the meal preparation for her family. She and her husband set up a vacation fund and began to plan for a trip to the beach sometime in the coming year.

She continued to utilize breathing practices, self-hypnosis, and a variety of visual images for calming and pain relief daily. She drove her car more freely now, with less anxiety, and regularly passed through the intersection where her accident had occurred. She "strobed herself" to sleep with slow frequency Delta range AVE and "strobed" herself into greater alertness with low Beta range fast frequency AVE. When the battery failed in her AVE device, and it took her 2 days to replace it, she realized the difference this device was making: She was less mentally clear during the day and found sleep onset more difficult at night, until she replaced the battery.

Kay Ellen continued in her Aquatherapy class, now paying for her sessions, as part of her own ongoing health maintenance program. Spiritually, she felt more awake and alive again. She began to search for a pathway of community service for herself, visiting a rehabilitation center and encouraging some of the women with TBI in their recovery process.

She continued to suffer occasional episodes of depression and bitterness at the loss of her former life. But she found that she could manage the intensity of depression now both with her self-regulation skills (breathing, hypnosis, and spiritual practices) and contact with her prayer circle (the group offered her "prn prayer sessions," on 24-hours' notice). In most cases, the prayer circles nudged her mood at least partially out of the darkness.

Kay Ellen was offered the option to schedule hypnosis sessions and sessions to refresh her breathing skills as needed. Her spiritual guide continued to provide intermittent guidance about every 4 months. Initially, she felt some shame and embarrassment at the idea of ongoing psychological and pastoral support, until her therapist reminded her that traumatic brain injury is a chronic condition like heart disease and diabetes all of which require monitoring, support, and intermittent interventions.

References

Ayers, M. E. (1999). Assessing and treating open head trauma, coma, and stroke using real-time digital EEG neurofeedback. In J. R. Evans & A. Abarbanel (Eds.), *Introduction to quantitative EEG and neurofeedback* (pp. 203–222). New York: Academic Press.

Beck, A. T., & Beamesderfer, A. (1974). Assessment of depression: The depression inventory. *Modern Problems of Pharmacopsychiatry, 7,* 151–169.

Centers for Disease Control and Prevention. (2015). *Report to congress on traumatic brain injury in the United States: Epidemiology and rehabilitation.* Atlanta, GA: National Center for Injury Prevention and Control; Division of Unintentional Injury Prevention. Retrieved from https://www.cdc.gov/traumaticbraininjury/pdf/tbi_report_to_congress_epi_and_rehab-a.pdf

Centers for Disease Control and Prevention. (2016). *Rates of TBI-related emergency department visits, hospitalizations, and deaths — United States, 2001–2010.* Atlanta, GA: CDC. Retrieved from http://www.cdc.gov/traumaticbraininjury/data/rates.html

Crasilneck, H. B., & Hall, J. A. (1985). *Clinical hypnosis: Principles and applications* (2nd ed.). Orlando, FL: Grune & Stratton.

Family Caregiver Alliance (2011). Incidence and prevalence of the major causes of brain impairment. Website of the Family Caregiver Alliance. Retrieved from https://www.caregiver.org/incidence-and-prevalence-major-causes-brain-impairment

Fydrich, T., Dowdall, D., & Chambless, D. L. (1992). Reliability and validity of the Beck anxiety inventory. *Journal of Anxiety Disorders, 6*(10), 55–61.

McGrady, A., & Moss, D. (2013). Pathways to illness, pathways to health. New York, NY: Springer.

Tang, H.-Y., Vitiello, M. V., Perlis, M., Mao, J. J., & Riegel, B. (2014). A pilot study of audio visual stimulation as a self-care treatment for insomnia in adults with insomnia and chronic pain. *Applied Psychophysiology and Biofeedback, 39*(3–4), 219–225.

Tang, H.-Y., Riegel, B., McCurry, S., & Vitiello, M. (2016). Open-loop audio-visual stimulation (AVS): A useful tool for management of insomnia. *Applied Psychophysiology and Biofeedback, 41*(1), 39–46.

Tellegen, A., & Atkinson, G. (1974). Openness to absorbing and self-altering experiences (absorption), a trait related to hypnotic susceptibility. *Journal of Abnormal Psychology, 83*(3), 268–277.

Thomas, J. L., & Smith, M. (2015). Neurofeedback for traumatic brain injury: Current trends. *Biofeedback, 43*(1), 31–37.

Thornton, K. E., & Carmody, D. P. (2008). Efficacy of traumatic brain injury rehabilitation: Interventions of QEEG-guided biofeedback, computers, strategies, and medications. *Applied Psychophysiology and Biofeedback, 33,* 101–124.

van Dixhoorn, J., & Duivenvoorden, H. J. (1985). Efficacy of Nijmegen questionnaire in recognition of the hyperventilation syndrome. *Journal of Psychosomatic Research, 29,* 199–206.

Vanhaudenhuyse, A., Laureys, S., & Faymonville, M.-E. (2015). The use of hypnosis in severe brain injury rehabilitation: A case report. *Acta Neurologica Belgica, 115*(4), 771–772. https://doi.org/10.1007/s13760-015-0459-3

WHO. (2006). *Neurological disorders: Public health challenges.* Publication of the World Health Organization (NLM classification: WL 140). Retrieved from http://www.who.int/mental_health/neurology/neurological_disorders_report_web.pdf

Yapko, M. D. (2012). *Trancework: An introduction to the practice of clinical hypnosis* (4th ed.). New York, NY: Routledge.

Chapter 15
Pathways Interventions for Chronic, Relapsing Substance Abuse Disorders

Abstract The authors regard substance abuse and addictive behavior as a chronic recurrent illness, with psychological, behavioral, and medical components. They call for multi-modal intermittent treatment throughout the life span, addressing the emotional, social, and biological dimensions of the disorder. A case study of a life-long alcohol and drug-dependent male illustrates the often chronic relapsing course of the illness. The patient, Colin, was a gifted trial attorney, who struggled with alcohol, marijuana, and cocaine use for decades. The chapter provides an example of a Pathways Model treatment program, integrating lifestyle changes, complementary therapies, spiritual intervention, and professional treatment for addiction to assist this individual in managing his condition, and recovering his life.

Keywords Substance abuse · Addiction · Recovery · Relapse · Second phase recovery · Intervention

Introduction: Substance Abuse as a Chronic, Recurrent Illness

For many, substance abuse and addictive behavior are chronic recurrent conditions, marked by a progression in severity, eventual disasters in career and relationships, contrite, and heartfelt declarations of intent to make a new beginning, and then relapse. Previously, we have argued that substance abuse should be recognized as a chronic disease and not simply a moral or behavioral problem (McGrady & Moss, 2013, pp. 99–101). Substance abuse is an excellent model for understanding all chronic diseases because it is both behavioral and medical, psychological and biological. Treatment that ignores this complex etiology and the multiple mechanisms reinforcing addiction will fail.

There are several features of substance abuse that qualify it as a chronic illness. Substance abuse disorders, especially alcohol, marijuana, and cigarette dependency, have a higher heritability rate than essential hypertension and Type 1 diabetes and heritability rates comparable to Type 2 diabetes and asthma (McLellan, Lewis, O'Brien, & Kieber, 2000). The evidence for alcohol dependence is strongest. It is

© Springer International Publishing AG, part of Springer Nature 2018　　　251
A. McGrady, D. Moss, *Integrative Pathways*,
https://doi.org/10.1007/978-3-319-89313-6_15

polygenic; that is, multiple genes contribute to an individual's vulnerability to addiction. Alcohol dependence shares a poly-genetic profile with other disorders, including attention-deficit disorder, bipolar disorder, and other disorders (Cross Disorder Group, 2013). Substance abuse has a measurable pathophysiology, including dysregulation of the autonomic nervous system and endocrine system. Substance abuse follows a relapsing and remitting course similar to other chronic conditions. We do not expect one episode of treatment to cure asthma or diabetes, nor should we expect one intervention to cure substance abuse. Rather, chronic conditions call for careful evaluations sometimes from several providers, more intense initial treatment, ongoing management, and scheduled follow-up, with an emphasis on a comprehensive recovery plan, ongoing support, and monitoring for early signs of relapse.

History

Initial Course of Illness

Colin was the first-born son of Irish parents. His father, Colin, Sr., was a physician and a chronic alcoholic, with repeated arrests for driving under the influence; he was a charismatic personality when sober or mildly intoxicated and an abusive monster when drunk. Colin described his mother as a "saint" and an enabler. She was the mother of six children, and a stay-at-home housewife, who guided all six children through college and into professional careers. She remained a loyal supporter of the husband through arrests, temporary loss of his medical license, and episodes of spousal abuse. After his final arrest at 46, Colin Sr. was admitted to the hospital for detoxification, but died of a heart attack mid-way through the process. The story among his friends was that "alcohol never hurt an Irishman, but take away his whiskey and you kill him."

Colin, Jr., began drinking alcohol and using marijuana in high school and was apprehended for driving under the influence for the first time during his sophomore year of college. His father's attorney used his contacts to have the charges dismissed. Additional arrests for driving under the influence were dismissed during law school and during his first year of law practice.

Colin, Jr., excelled in high school, college, and law school. He served on the Law Review and graduated second in his class. He joined a prestigious legal firm upon graduation as a criminal trial lawyer and rapidly developed a reputation for thorough preparation and successful courtroom arguments.

Colin continued to drink daily and used marijuana almost daily through the early years of his legal practice. His professional contacts with criminals facilitated his access to drugs and he began intermittent cocaine use during his fourth year with the law firm. He managed to contain the effects of his drug and alcohol use, with no apparent impact on his work. Like his father, he was magnetic and the life of the party when sober and when mildly intoxicated or high on marijuana. When drunk on alcohol or high on cocaine, however, he was explosive, verbally abusive, and violent.

At age 32, Colin married Mindy, one of the paralegals in his law firm; he promised both Mindy and himself that he would curtail his use of drugs and limit his consumption of alcohol. Mindy had seen him several times at his worst; on two occasions, his abusive moods resulted in fistfights with strangers and once he and Mindy were escorted by security out of an elegant restaurant due to his verbal tirades at the wait staff. Mindy gave birth to their first son in their second year of marriage, and a daughter followed 18 months later. Colin drank less and used no cocaine for the first two years of the marriage, but gradually began to stay out late several nights a week. He returned to his favorite bars and began to use cocaine again.

At age 35, at 3 a.m. on a Sunday morning, Colin was driving while high on cocaine, after a party in a crack house run by one of his criminal law clients. He sideswiped another car, rolled his Mercedes, and was arrested with cocaine in his possession. The partners in Colin's firm were shocked and appalled at the arrest and the publicity. Colin was a persuasive man, and initially convinced the law partners that this incident was an aberration, and that he did not have a serious substance problem. As the stories emerged about his presence at a crack house party with a current client facing meth and cocaine sales charges, the partners became irate. The senior partner in the firm was able to bargain the charges down to driving under the influence, and Colin received a 90-day suspension of his driver's license and a fine. The managing partners suspended him from practice with the firm for 120 days and mandated that he enter a treatment facility. They also gave him notice that any further incident would result in dismissal, and the partners would pursue suspension or disbarment with the state bar association.

Colin completed 3 weeks in a residential treatment facility, cooperating as a model patient. He was released with no clear after-care plan, and soon resumed both alcohol and marijuana use. His wife moved home to her parents with the two children during the period of his residential treatment and threatened divorce. He wooed her with flowers and promises and she agreed to reconcile if he committed to cease all drug use.

Colin followed a similar trajectory over the next two decades, leaving his law firm after one cocaine arrest and receiving two suspensions of his law license for repeated arrests. His practice thrived in spite of the intermittent scandals because he was one of the most successful trial lawyers in the region. But the typical progression in severity of an addiction was evident over the decades. His wife divorced him when he was 45, and he saw his children less over time. He married and divorced two additional times, and both of these spouses were alcoholics and drug users. His social circle narrowed to include only other drug users and common criminals. At age 50, following an auto accident that occurred while he was high on cocaine, he was disbarred, and this time he served 90 days in jail. He worked as a paralegal for two friends in their practice for 5 years, and finally won re-instatement by documenting 2 years of attendance at Alcoholics Anonymous and Narcotics Anonymous and weekly participation in addictions counseling. He also submitted to random urine checks for 1 year following his re-instatement at the bar.

At age 61 he was arrested again, for driving while intoxicated and high and causing an accident in which another driver was injured. His blood alcohol level was 1.6.

The drunk driving law in the State of Michigan, where Colin was arrested, makes it illegal to drive with a blood alcohol of 0.8 or above. He had marijuana in his possession when arrested.

Pathways Model

Referral

Colin's attorney referred him for poly-substance abuse treatment, after his sixth conviction for drunk driving, following a hospitalization for detoxification, a 3-week inpatient treatment at Hazelden in Minnesota, and 120 days of jail time. He was released from jail with a mandate for regular probation, random urine testing, participation in professional substance abuse treatment, and regular AA and NA attendance, to be logged and documented to his probation officer. Colin was a gifted trial attorney, 61 years old, who had struggled with alcohol, marijuana, and cocaine use for decades. Now he faced probable permanent disbarment, loss of income, and restrictions on contact with known drug users.

Colin presented himself at his initial evaluation as a "new man," sober, clean, and determined to begin his life anew. He expressed gratitude for his arrest because it had forced him to confront his problems. His past treatment records were reviewed and included descriptions of similar loud vocal repentance following each previous arrest.

Pathways Assessment

Family history Colin checked with several older relatives and was able to document serious alcohol problems dating back six generations. The male line in his paternal family had two or more recognized alcoholics in each generation for six successive generations, and in the past three decades four of Colin's first cousins either committed suicide or were arrested for alcohol problems.

Lifestyle assessment Colin's lifestyle raised multiple red flags. He was unable to name any friend with whom he had current ongoing contact, who was not also a drug user. Three of the individuals he listed as his closest friends had histories of cocaine use and jail time and two of them had arrest records for petty crimes to pay for drug use. Colin had not seen his siblings or children in 8 months.

A home visit by a probation officer showed 12 bottles of hard liquor in his kitchen cabinets and no food in the refrigerator or cabinets. Colin denied current alcohol use, but protested vehemently against pouring out the bottles and wasting expensive liquor.

In high school, Colin had been a varsity track and tennis player; during his college years, he remained physically active and participated in debate, chorus, and the literary magazine. Now, however, he had no regular recreation, no regular exercise, and could name no church, civic, or community contacts.

Psychodiagnostic assessment Colin's substance use, behavior, social deterioration, and emotional symptoms supported multiple diagnoses in the DSM-V nomenclature (American Psychiatric Association, 2013). On the substance abuse/addiction side, at the time of his most recent arrest, Colin met the diagnostic criteria for *303.90 Alcohol use disorder, severe, 304.30 Cannabis use disorder, severe,* and *304.20 Stimulant (cocaine) use disorder, severe.* His use of alcohol and marijuana was daily through his adult life, except for brief periods after arrests, and during periods of urine testing. His use of cocaine was more intermittent, but he acknowledged using cocaine whenever he had access. The use of all three substances persisted in the face of job loss, legal consequences, loss of relationships, loss of reputation, and financial hardship. He showed patterns of increased volume of alcohol and marijuana consumption over time. In recent years, he consumed a fifth of whiskey a day and an ounce of marijuana every other day. Much of his day now revolved around obtaining alcohol and drugs, seeking opportunities for use, and using in risky situations (for example, he had begun to smoke marijuana and snort cocaine in his car in daylight while parked on public streets). He also showed a progressive pattern of increased craving for both alcohol and cocaine, after a few hours without use and severe symptoms of withdrawal during detoxification.

During the interviews, Colin acknowledged a significant number of symptoms of *303.81 post-traumatic stress disorder.* Colin was tense and fidgeted constantly in his initial evaluation. He acknowledged a sense of edgy nervousness and restlessness since his most recent detoxification. He suffered severe sleep problems and utilized alcohol to induce sleep onset. He reported terrible nightmares of his father beating his mother and Colin, and the images of his father in the nightmares blurred into images of Colin himself. He suffered daytime flashbacks of his father's rages, which sometimes triggered his explosive outbursts at others. He reported anxiety and occasional flashbacks triggered by contact with family; as a result, he avoided the funerals of both parents and stayed away from most family gatherings. Early on he always excused himself with family by stating that he was ill, but the family eventually stopped contacting him.

Readiness for change Colin acknowledged the overall progression of his substance abuse over the decades of his life, and his regular relapses in spite of declared good intentions. He rated himself at a nine, "already making changes," on the Readiness for Change ruler (DeSalle & Agley, 2015). Yet, he could not identify one change beyond what was being controlled and monitored by the court and probation; therefore, the treatment team was in consensus in rating Colin as a 2 on the Readiness for Change ruler, in the Low Readiness range.

Colin's Pathways counselor used *motivational interviewing* at this stage to identify and utilize Colin's own intrinsic motives (Miller & Rollnick, 2013; Rollnick, Miller, & Butler, 2008). Colin admitted that his first thoughts about treatment had to do with "building a good case" and "presenting well" to the court, but also expressed his determination not to live the remainder of his life like his father. He concluded that we had his attention, and he would cooperate. The treatment team reminded him of the need for significant behavioral changes beyond the requirements of the court.

Pathways Interventions

Acceleration of Treatment Timeline

Because of the severity of Colin's addictive behaviors, the lack of positive recovery supports in his current life, and the court orders for intensive treatment, the treatment team reached an agreement with Colin to modify the usual Pathways approach and develop a Pathways treatment plan providing Levels One, Two, and Three simultaneously and overlapping with one another. His Pathways counselor continued to utilize motivational interviewing during weekly sessions, as a tool to facilitate his engagement and commitment in the treatment. The team had serious doubts whether he could sustain any self-directed activity without regular contact with the counselor. In addition, Colin was once again suspended from practicing law, leaving him with only 10 hours a week of paralegal work. Colin was barely surviving on the income from his paralegal work and the remnants of his inheritance, but was available for a variety of recovery and lifestyle change activities.

Level One Pathways Activities

Level One Pathways activities involve self-directed behavioral changes and lifestyle modifications.

Level One Pathways activity: Walking   The initial assessment showed a complete void of structured physical activity and exercise in Colin's life. His most strenuous endeavor involved walking about 150 ft from his parking place to his first-floor office. Colin suggested walking as his initial self-directed activity. He enjoyed walking on a nature path less than one block from his home and found it calming. He committed to walking four times a week, initially for 15 minutes, with gradual increases in time.

Level One Pathways activity: Mindful breathing   Colin's second Level One activity was mindful breathing. Slow even diaphragmatic respiration is an effective and easily mastered relaxation tool. Colin reported that anxiety was a trigger in many of his relapses. When he felt like he would explode with tension, he often had used alcohol to calm himself.

Colin had trouble initially slowing and pacing his breathing. His baseline breathing was rapid, irregular, and punctuated by breath holding and sighs. He was eventually able to increase his awareness and control over his breathing by lying on his back on the floor, with a large book balanced on his stomach, and using counting (1, 2, 3, 4 in, 1 hold, 1, 2, 3, 4 out, 1 hold), to pace his breaths which caused the book to rise and fall with his abdomen. Then he used a breath pacer on a computer monitor in the office, and a pacer on his smart phone at home, to pace his breathing at six breaths a minute.

Level One Pathways activity: Family contact As described in the assessment section, Colin had almost no contact with his family and minimal social supports. With encouragement to set a goal in this area, Colin concluded it would be easiest for him to begin with resuming contact with the two siblings next in line after him, a sister Colleen and a brother Liam. The three had been close growing up, and both had remained encouraging whenever he made contact. Liam had a similar early history with alcohol and marijuana use and drunk driving arrests, but had stopped all substance use by age 30.

Level One Progress

Progress: Walking Colin found himself making excuses for not walking. A home visit by his probation officer shook him up because Colin had mentioned several goals to him, and the officer quizzed him on his walking and family contact. He began to walk again, and discovered that the walks through a meadow and a forest quieted his usually racing thoughts, and evoked a kind of comfortable reverie. Periodically though, that reverie state seemed to trigger painful memories and emotions. His Pathways counselor encouraged him to mindfully accept whatever memories and emotions emerged, as a pathway to identifying and healing traumatic experiences.

Human beings often suppress painful emotions related to past painful experiences and utilize a tensing and bracing of the musculature to implement the suppression of emotions. Mind-body practices such as relaxation exercises or relaxed walking often lead to a loosening of the bracing process and release of emotions (Moss, 2005, 2008). The released material can be useful for self-understanding and long-term resolution of trauma. Colin's breakthrough trauma experiences also led the Pathways team to add an additional Level One assignment: *emotional journaling*. Colin was encouraged to keep a journal by his easy chair at home and to engage in 15–20 minutes of journaling after his walks, writing about his emotions, any painful memories, or any other upsurges in awareness.

Progress: Mindful breathing Colin continued to experience difficulty breathing in a relaxed and mindful fashion on his own, but with the breath pacer on his iPhone he was able to establish a fairly smooth pattern of relaxed breathing. Within 2 weeks he was staying with the pacer quite well at six breaths per minute. Once the breathing became more automatic for him, he began to find that it relaxed him. He was encouraged to slow and pace his breathing whenever he found himself tense or restless, until the tensions moderated. Slow breathing sometimes triggered painful memories, similar to what happened during his walks. He was again instructed to mindfully accept whatever memories and emotions entered his awareness and to journal about the experiences following his breathing exercises.

Progress: Family contact Colin's brother and sister were cautious at first, but delighted to see him when he made contact with them. They began to have lunch together once a week. His brother encouraged Colin to stick with his overall recovery plan and not to sabotage progress as he had before. Colin mentioned that he was still experiencing nightmares of their father's rages, and some breakthrough memories while walking and doing his breathing exercises. His sister reported similar nightmares and painful memories. She called it the *family curse*, because their father had suffered similar nightmares, and often drank to subdue strong daytime emotions.

Summary of Level One Pathways Progress

"He found both the walks and the breathing exercises calming, although he continued to experience episodic upsurges of painful memories and emotions."

During the initial month of Level One activities, Colin increased his commitment to a program of lifestyle and behavioral changes, especially after the surprise home visit by his probation officer. The counselors encouraged him. They *cognitively re-framed* his actions by explaining that even extrinsically coerced wellness behaviors can have positive transformative effects. As he entered his second month of treatment with the Pathways team, he walked and carried out his mindful breathing almost daily. He found both the walks and the breathing exercises calming although he continued to experience episodic upsurges of painful memories and emotions. He continued to journal about the increased awareness of past trauma. He also appreciated the increased contact with his siblings Colleen and Liam. Their disclosure of similar emotions reassured him that his own recovery was possible.

Level Two Activities

Level Two Pathways activities involve acquiring self-regulation skills and drawing on community resources and educational materials, including support groups, educational CDs, DVDs, websites, and smart phone "apps."

Level Two activity: Alcoholics Anonymous (AA) and Narcotics Anonymous (NA) Colin was court ordered to attend AA and NA weekly, and to carry a log book to be signed by another attendee, to verify his attendance at each meeting. The treatment team discussed with Colin the traditional 12-step recovery goal of making 90 meetings in his first 90 days. He committed to attending "90 in 90," which he had never done before. He also committed to asking his most effective past sponsor to work with him again since most individuals in recovery go through their 12-step program more effectively when they choose a sponsor to hold them accountable. The team also discussed Colin's "bullshit factor." He was a trial attorney used to creating positive impressions and knew exactly what 12-step groups wanted to hear from an addict in recovery. He decided to drive twice a week to a community 40 minutes away, which had particularly confrontational NA meetings. He had attended there before with a sponsor and found that the attendees there were able to recognize when he was just talking, and when he was more seriously engaging himself in the meetings.

Level Two activity: Mindfulness training Colin was introduced to mindfulness as a strategy to cope with the painful memories and emotions that emerged during his walks and breathing exercises. He was encouraged to simply observe the unfolding of the feelings and memories, and accept whatever emerged, as ongoing tools for self-awareness. When traumatic memories intruded into the present, he found that mindfulness was effective in restoring a calmer state. For years, he had tried to combat any painful memories with thought suppression, driving them from his mind or drinking to neutralize them. For a Level Two activity, he began practicing mindfulness guided by a CD program developed by Jon Kabat-Zinn (2006).

Level Two activity: Heart rate variability (HRV) biofeedback self-training Colin found that his breathing exercises were better for reducing his tensions than other strategies he had previously used. Heart rate variability (HRV) biofeedback training is a natural extension of breathing practices. Heart rate variability is lower than normal in alcohol-dependent populations, and HRV biofeedback has been found in one recent study to reduce anxiety, reduce cravings, and normalize HRV and vasomotor functions in alcoholics (Penzlin, Siepmann, Illigens, Weidner, & Siepmann, 2015).

In order to pursue HRV training on his own at home, Colin purchased the InnerBalance™ Trainer from the HeartMath Institute. The InnerBalance™ sensor plugged into his iPhone and operated with a downloaded InnerBalance™ app on the phone. The app tracked variations in his heart rate (HR), displayed the moment to moment variations in HR, and rated his increased *coherence*[1] in heart rhythms as he used his breathing to create smooth organized oscillations in HR. The software also tracked his practice sessions, and his progress in increasing coherence over the weeks of practice.

---

[1] Coherence is a HeartMath concept indicating a global state of optimal functioning; physiological systems, emotional life, and interpersonal relationships can show coherence. On the InnerBalance device, physiological coherence is measured as a peak of heart rate variability in the low frequency range, accompanying a breathing rate close to six breaths a minute. McCraty (2016) has hypothesized that emotional coherence and physiological coherence coincide, and encourages trainees to cultivate positive emotional states as well as smooth relaxed breathing.

Level Two activity: Pastoral counseling Colin's NA sponsor suggested he pursue pastoral counseling as part of his recovery. Colin described himself as a "lapsed Catholic," someone who believed in a personal God he could talk to in prayer, but who had not been active in his faith since college. His sister's parish priest, a recovering alcoholic himself, had a reputation for being helpful to many addicts in providing spiritual guidance supportive of their recovery. Colin met him after an AA meeting and agreed to speak with him regularly.

Progress in Level Two Activities

Progress: AA and NA Colin averaged six to eight 12-step meetings each week during the first 90 days after he began his 12-step work. He attended one to two meetings with his sponsor weekly, and the sponsor dropped in on Colin at home intermittently. Colin began "step-work," pursuit of the recovery process organized in the Twelve Steps and Twelve Traditions published by Alcoholics Anonymous (AA, 2004). Colin struggled with the process of acknowledging his own powerlessness over alcohol (and drugs) and surrendering his recovery to a higher power. His sponsor kept at him through these first three steps in the 12-step process, and Colin's pastoral counseling, going on simultaneously, also helped. After he made a "good enough" initial progress through steps one to three, he committed to revisit them again in the future and proceeded to step four, making a moral inventory of his own wrongs and character defects that contributed to his difficulties. He discussed a great deal of this "personal housekeeping" process with his sponsor and his siblings, who had encountered in themselves many of the negative qualities Colin found in himself.

> "When one becomes newly aware of negative aspects of oneself and other human beings, the guideline of mindfulness is to adopt compassionate acceptance. This coming together of a searching self-discovery process, with the guidelines of mindfulness proved beneficial for Colin."

Progress: Mindfulness Colin's attention to learning mindfulness coincided with his initial AA/NA step-work. The key guideline in mindfulness is to pay attention to everything that enters one's awareness, in a particular way, without judging, without self-criticism, and with acceptance (Kabat-Zinn, 1990, 1994). When one becomes newly aware of negative aspects of oneself and other human beings, the guideline of mindfulness is to adopt compassionate acceptance. This coming together of a searching self-discovery process, with the guidelines of mindfulness, proved beneficial for Colin. In the past, when Colin tried to take AA-based step-work seriously, he subsequently experienced serious self-hatred at the negative qualities he discovered in himself. This self-loathing turned into rages at himself, life, God, and his father, and triggered renewed alcohol and drug abuse.

This time, the mindfulness emphasis on compassionate acceptance seemed to temper his self-hatred. He accepted responsibility and felt deep regret for the person he had become in his addiction, but judged himself less. He committed to continued practice of mindfulness and began reading Kabat-Zinn's books as well (Kabat-Zinn, 1990, 1994).

Progress: HRV training Colin found the InnerBalance appealing because it was a short step from his breathing with an iPhone pacer to practicing breathing *and* HRV. He found increasingly that when he was agitated or had stray thoughts of drug use, he could use his breathing/HRV practices to self-calm. He reported that his cravings for alcohol and drugs were still present at times, but less intense. His Pathways team encouraged him to use the InnerBalance twice daily, and whenever negative emotions or painful memories emerged.

Progress: Pastoral counseling Colin's anger and bitterness against his father colored his religious beliefs and spiritual experiences. He remembered the words of the Lord's prayer, "Our *Father*, who art in heaven ...," but when he repeated those words he remembered his father slamming his mother against the refrigerator at home. The priest shared a similar story from his own childhood and confided that he had changed the words of the Lord's prayer to "Our Mother, who art in heaven," because he was convinced that the deeper intent of the prayer was to portray a personal and loving spiritual being, in the best words human beings had to draw on. For the priest's life, like Colin's life, the *Father* word and *Fathe*r image were tarnished, perhaps beyond salvage in one lifetime.

Colin's sessions with the priest helped him with his 12-step work as well. Reminding him that some of his black and white religious beliefs were childish, grade-school level versions of something beyond human understanding helped Colin with the concept of surrendering to a higher power.

Summary of Level Two Activities

Colin achieved his goal of "90 in 90," attending 93 AA and NA meetings in the first 90 days after his discharge from jail. He committed to continuing to attend AA and NA meetings at least four to five times weekly and continued to engage in step-work with his sponsor's guidance. He suffered one relapse when he encountered one of his previous law clients in a car parked on the street outside an NA meeting one night and began to drink from a bottle of Jameson's Irish whiskey the man offered him. A woman from the NA meeting rapped on the car window and called out to Colin to come with her. Colin felt outside himself, watching himself sit in the car sipping whiskey, with his addict client pulling him down and the woman from NA pulling him up. He felt himself snap like a rubber band breaking and got out of the car. His NA friend helped him call his sponsor and went with him to a nearby restaurant to drink coffee and meet with the sponsor. His sponsor emphasized what

Colin knew: The world of the addict is full of opportunities to relapse, and the addict is only one drink or one cocaine "line" away from relapse.

Colin continued to use mindfulness, breathing, and his iPhone-based HRV exercises daily, and whenever he experienced painful memories and emotions. He struggled with prayer and the AA emphasis to surrender to a higher power, but used his mindfulness and his mindful breathing to slow himself down, observe, and learn from these difficulties.

Level Three Activities

In the Pathways Model, Level Three consists of professional services, including psychotherapy, CAM therapies, and medical care. Level One and Two practices frequently seem to prepare the individual to make better use of professional services and also sustain the positive effects of professional interventions long term.

Level Three intervention: Addiction counseling Hazelden referred Colin to an experienced addiction recovery specialist in his community. This counselor was a certified chemical dependency counselor, with a reputation for guiding addicts into sobriety and drug-free living. She communicated her intention to Colin and the Pathways team of focusing on relapse prevention, adherence to a 12-step-oriented recovery plan, and recognition of warning signs for possible relapse. She encouraged the Pathways team to focus on lifestyle change supportive of recovery and on "second-stage" addiction issues. First-stage-oriented treatment focuses on getting sober and drug free, establishing a recovery plan, and avoiding relapse. Second-stage treatment focuses on the many psychological, behavioral, and social changes needed to actually live and enjoy life sober (Learsen, 1985; Mooney, Eisenberg, & Eisenberg, 1992, p. 506). Addicts, especially those like Colin who begin substance use early, bypass much of the basic life learning—the learning of social skills, coping skills, and adaptive behavioral patterns—necessary for daily life.

Level Three intervention: Acupuncture Auricular acupuncture, which involves inserting acupuncture needles into specific sites in the ears, is widely used to support addiction recovery (Margolin, 2003). Auricular acupressure uses the same acupuncture points, located by the meridian system, and applies physical pressure on the point, usually manually. Electrical acupoint stimulation applies electrical stimulation to the same acupuncture points. Auricular acupuncture, acupressure, and electrical acupoint stimulation are often used in detoxification to reduce the symptoms and distress in the withdrawal period (Lin, Chan, & Chen, 2012; Meade et al., 2010). They are also utilized during the extended recovery period to reduce cravings, induce a relaxed state conducive to continued recovery, and reduce relapse. The World Health Organization designated acupuncture in 2003 as an appropriate intervention to reduce relapse (Zhang, 2003). Subsequent research has been mixed, yet some research reports and many clinical reports suggest reduced cravings for alcohol (Lee, Kim, Jung, Jung, & Kim, 2015), as well as reduced cravings and reduced relapse rates in opioid addiction.

> "The Peniston protocol is a form of intense psychodynamic therapy assisted by neurofeedback to sustain a brain state conducive to emotional abreaction and trauma resolution."

Colin underwent an initial evaluation with a physician trained in acupuncture and agreed to attend two auricular acupuncture sessions each week, for a period of 12 weeks.

Level Three intervention: Neurofeedback The Pathways team proposed neurofeedback training as Colin's third Level Three intervention. One of the typical neurophysiological features in alcoholics and drug-addicted individuals is an excess in faster wave (Beta range) cortical activation patterns and a deficiency in slower wave (Alpha, Theta, and Delta range) cortical activity (Pollock et al., 1983). Porjesz and Begleiter (2004) reviewed several studies on electrophysiological patterns in the brains of alcoholics. They concluded that an imbalance between excitation and inhibition in the brains of alcoholics contributes to the predisposition to alcoholism (Begleiter & Porjesz, 1999). Subjectively, many alcoholics and drug users report that they cannot relax without substance use, which corresponds to a deficit in slow wave activity.

Eugene Peniston developed a neurofeedback training protocol for alcoholics, based on earlier research at the Menninger Clinic (Peniston & Kulkosky, 1989). The protocol combines a number of biofeedback and neurofeedback-assisted interventions. Autogenic training and thermal biofeedback (hand warming training guided by biofeedback instrumentation) is intended to produce deep autonomic nervous system relaxation; imagery techniques are used to visually rehearse successful abstinence and better coping without alcohol. Neurofeedback training is used to increase Alpha- and Theta-range cortical activity producing a deeply relaxed mental state, and abreaction of painful emotional experiences, while in the Alpha-Theta state. The Peniston protocol is a form of intense psychodynamic therapy assisted by neurofeedback to sustain a brain state conducive to emotional abreaction and trauma resolution.

Peniston conducted clinical trials of this neurofeedback intervention in a Veterans Administration Hospital, with veterans with severe alcohol dependence and PTSD; the intervention produced significant reductions in relapse rates. Scott and Kaiser later added another pre-training intervention to the original Peniston protocol, for stimulus abusing addicts, training them to mentally focus prior to beginning the Alpha-Theta training (Scott & Kaiser, 1998; Scott, Kaiser, Othmer, & Sideroff, 2005). Sokhadze and Trudeau (2016) recently reviewed nearly three decades of studies that applied neurofeedback for substance abuse and rated this intervention as "probably efficacious."

Progress in Level Three Interventions

Progress: Addictions counseling   Colin's addictions counselor was encouraged by his persistence in both 12-step meeting attendance and "step-work." The counseling focused on relapse prevention, especially reviewing cravings, vulnerabilities, negative emotions, and past patterns of relapse. The counselor encouraged Colin in the full range of coping strategies he was learning—mindfulness, mindful breathing, HRV exercises, and renewed spiritual awareness. Apart from the week he sipped the Jameson's whiskey, Colin felt less vulnerable to relapse. In the past, he often felt doomed to fail and made bets with himself on which day of the week his relapse would come on. He joked about preferring to relapse on days associated with his father, such as his birthday and his father's patron saint's day. Now he carried his sponsor's phone number in his cell and dialed him intermittently to test his supports. He expressed extreme gratitude both to the NA group member who disrupted his relapse and his sponsor who met him that evening and spent several hours talking him through the incident.

Progress: Acupuncture   Colin kept his appointments for acupuncture and initially felt that nothing was happening. Then he attended acupuncture appointments on several days when he was anxious, and once after a night of terrifying and brutal nightmares. He experienced tensions leaving his body even as the physician inserted and rotated the needles. This lessening of tension continued during the time he sat with needles inserted and persisted through the day afterwards. Colin had experienced renewed cravings for alcohol for several days after the encounter described above with Jameson's Irish whiskey and acknowledged feeling frightened of the intensity of the cravings. However, after an acupuncture session, those cravings diminished greatly, and he felt renewed control.

Progress: Neurofeedback   Because of his cocaine use, Colin's neurotherapist initially applied an attention deficit-type training to produce more low range Beta activity in frontal sites of the cortex to improve his ability to focus in sessions. An initial QEEG (a digital brain map comparing Colin's EEG patterns at 19 cortical sites to databases of other adults with known mental and medical conditions) on Colin showed unusually high cortical activity in the 20–38 Hz range in frontal and central areas of the cortex, along the mid-line. This pattern is typically associated with heightened anxiety, rumination, and traumatic experiences, and one study (Bauer, 2001) found that elevations in the high Beta range correlate strongly with relapse. Consequently, the initial stage in his neurofeedback therapy also included down-training his "high Beta" activity. Colin reported feeling both calmer and more focused after this initial training increasing low Beta and reducing high Beta.

Then Colin began the Peniston protocol, learning to produce and remain in a strong Alpha-Theta state, conducive to imagery, visualization, and emotion discharges. His neurotherapist guided Colin in the Alpha-Theta state to explore painful memories related to his nightmares. During the neurofeedback sessions, he re-experienced many episodes of domestic violence in his childhood home and began to see more clearly his mental confusion between his father's emotions and actions and his own. He began to differentially label his father as "rage-man" and himself as Alpha-man because he was encountering his rage-filled father, while he himself was cultivating a high Alpha relaxed and receptive state. Colin used his emotional journaling after neurofeedback to record his experiences in his Alpha-Theta states. He described painful memories and flashes of emotional pain, but felt some relief at recording the pain on paper.

The Peniston protocol also includes imagery-mediated mental rehearsals of interacting socially without alcohol or drugs. Initially, Colin could not feel himself engaged in the social settings; as his Alpha-Theta sessions continued the subjective emotional reality of the visualizations increased.

Colin was encouraged that a follow-up QEEG after 1 year of neurofeedback showed only mildly activated cortical activity in the high Beta range. With this change, he hoped his prognosis was more hopeful. Colin also felt emotionally unburdened at this new experience in neurofeedback of himself and his father as not the same. He had hated his father for his abuse and emotional cruelty and hated himself for seeming to become his father. It was a dramatic shift when Colin lessened his experience of rage, which had haunted him for much of his life.

Summary of Level Three Progress

Colin continued his Level One and Two practices while he participated in Level Three treatment processes. He regularly practiced mindful breathing and mindful awareness of moments of trauma and negative emotion. He continued intermittent contact with the pastoral counselor and arranged to drive him to the confrontational NA meetings, which the priest also found refreshing. Colin called his addictions counselor the "handout queen," because he never left her office without a fresh handout depicting something like the symptoms of relapse, the cycle of addiction, or coping strategies. Yet he bought a binder and organized the handouts so he could find any handout when he wanted to refresh his memory. Colin concluded that the acupuncture was alleviating anxiety and lessening cravings, so he continued intermittent sessions after the initially scheduled 12 weeks.

Colin's neurotherapy was the most intense element in his Pathways treatment. He continued to experience upsurges of pain, anger, and grief as he revisited his childhood and the early years of his first marriage. He continued journaling after his neurotherapy sessions and periodically re-read his journals to assure himself of progress.

Summary: The Future

The prognosis for relapse in poly-substance addiction is high, and Colin's QEEG showed one of the markers predicting high risk for relapse, but following specific neurofeedback training to modify central and frontal high Beta activity, the relapse marker was no longer evident.

After an initial period of going through the motions, Colin participated with significant enthusiasm and motivation in a multi-modality recovery program with elements of traditional substance abuse treatment as well as complementary therapies. Two years following his release from jail, his only relapse was the 20-minute encounter with Irish whiskey. His contact with his siblings continued, and their encouragement helped him through a number of challenges. With his sister's help he made contact with his son and daughter, and the daughter has seen him twice.

Colin continues to engage in most of the activities and strategies making up his Pathways treatment. He is working as an attorney again, on a probationary "action plan" with the state bar association. Colin is guardedly hopeful. His addiction counselor, his NA/AA sponsor, and his Pathways counselor share that guarded optimism but remind him that addictions are a chronic condition, with a relapsing and remitting pattern. He is welcome to begin his entire Pathways program again at any time to prevent relapse or to abort a relapse.

References

Alcoholics Anonymous. (2004). *Twelve steps and twelve traditions*. New York, NY: Alcoholic Anonymous World Services.

American Psychiatric Association. (2013). *Diagnostic and statistical manual of mental disorder* (5th ed.). Washington, DC: Author.

Bauer, L. O. (2001). Predicting relapse to alcohol and drug abuse via quantitative electroencephalography. *Neuropharmacology, 23*, 332–340. https://doi.org/10.1016/S0893-133X(01)00236-

Begleiter, H., & Porjesz, B. (1999). What is inherited in the predisposition toward alcoholism? A proposed model. Alcoholism: Clinical and Experimental Research, 23, 1125–1135.

Cross Disorder Group of the Psychiatric Genomics Consortium. (2013). Identification of risk loci with shared effects on five major psychiatric disorders: A genome-wide analysis. *Lancet 381*(9875), 1371–1379. https://doi.org/10.1016/S0140-6736(12)62129-1

DeSalle, M., & Agley, J. (2015, September 24). SBIRT: Identifying and managing risky substance abuse. *Counseling Today.* a publication of the American Counseling Association. Retrieved from http://ct.counseling.org/2015/09/sbirt-identifying-and-managing-risky-substance-use/

Kabat-Zinn, J. (1990). *Full catastrophe living: Using the wisdom of your body and mind to face stress, pain and illness*. New York, NY: Delacorte.

Kabat-Zinn, J. (1994). *Wherever you go, there you are: Mindfulness meditation in everyday life* New York, NY: Hyperion.

Kabat-Zinn, J. (2006). *Mindfulness for beginners: Reclaiming the present moment*. (Educational CD). Louisville, CO: Sounds True.

Learsen, E. (1985). *Stage two recovery: Living beyond addiction*. New York, NY: HarperCollins.

Lee, J. D., Kim, S. G., Jung, T. G., Jung, W. Y., & Kim, S. Y. (2015). Effect of Zhubin (KI9 acupuncture in reducing alcohol craving in patients with alcohol dependence: A randomized placebo-controlled trial. *Chinese Journal of Integrative Medicine, 21*(4), 307–311. https://doi. org/10.1007/s11655-014-1851-1

Lin, J. -G., Chan, Y. -Y., & Chen, Y. -H. (2012). Acupuncture for the treatment of opiate addiction. *Evidence-based Complementary and Alternative Medicine*, 739045.doi: https://doi. org/10.1155/2012/739045

Margolin, A. (2003). Acupuncture for substance abuse. *Current Psychiatry Reports, 5*(5), 333–339.

McCraty, R. (2016). From depletion to renewal: Positive emotions and heart rhythm coherence feedback. In D. Moss & F. Shaffer (Eds.), *Foundations of heart rate variability* (pp. 82–84). Wheat Ridge, CO: Association for Applied Psychophysiology and Biofeedback.

McGrady, A., & Moss, D. (2013). *Pathways to illness, pathways to health*. New York, NY: Springer. https://doi.org/10.1007/978-1-4419-1379-1

McLellan, A. T., Lewis, D. C., O'Brien, C. P., & Kieber, H. D. (2000). Drug dependency: A chronic medical illness. *Journal of the American Medical Association, 284*(13), 1689–1695.

Meade, C. S., Lukas, S. E., McDonald, L. J., Fitzmaurice, G. M., Eldrige, J. A., Merrill, N., et al. (2010). A randomized trial of transcutaneous electrical stimulation as adjunctive treatment for opioid detoxification. *Journal of Substance Abuse Treatment, 28*(1), 12–21. https://doi.org/10.1016/j.jsat.2009.05.010

Miller, W. R., & Rollnick, S. (2013). *Motivational interviewing: Helping people change* (3rd ed.). New York, NY: Guilford.

Mooney, A. J., Eisenberg, A., & Eisenberg, H. (1992). *The recovery book*. New York, NY: Workman Publishing.

Moss, D. (2005). Psychophysiological psychotherapy: The use of biofeedback, biological monitoring, and stress management principles in psychotherapy. *Psychophysiology Today: The Magazine for Mind-Body Medicine, 2*(1), 14–18.

Moss, D. (2008). Zur psychosomatischen Psychotherapie (Toward a psychosomatic psychotherapy). *Biofeedback in der Praxis, Band II. Erwachsene.* (Biofeedback in practice: vol. 2. Adults). Vienna/New York: Springer Medizin.

Peniston, E. G., & Kulkosky, P. J. (1989). Alpha-theta brainwave training and beta endorphin levels in alcoholics. *Alcoholism: Clinical and Experimental Results, 13*(2), 271–279.

Penzlin, A. I., Siepmann, T., Illigens, B. M.-W., Weidner, K., & Siepmann, M. (2015). Heart rate variability biofeedback in patients with alcohol dependence: A randomized controlled study. *Neuropsychiatric Disease and Treatment, 11*, 2619–2627.

Pollock, V. E., Volavka, J., Goodwin, D. W., Mednick, S. A., Gabrielli, W. F., Knop, J., et al. (1983). The EEG after alcohol in men at risk for alcoholism. *Archives of General Psychiatry, 40*, 857–864.

Porjesz, B., & Begleiter, H. (2003). Alcoholism and human electrophysiology. Alcohol Research and Health, 27(2),153–60.

Rollnick, S., Miller, W. R., & Butler, C. C. (2008). *Motivational interviewing in health care*. New York: Guilford Press.

Sokhadze, E. M., & Trudeau, D. (2016). Alcohol substance use disorders. In G. Tan, F. Shaffer, R. Lyle, & I. Teo (Eds.), *Evidence-based treatment in biofeedback and neurofeedback* (3rd ed., pp. 22–26). Wheat Ridge, CO: Association for Applied Psychophysiology and Biofeedback.

Scott, W. C., & Kaiser, S. (1998). Augmenting chemical dependency treatment with neurofeedback training. *Journal of Neurotherapy, 3*(1), 66.

Scott, W. C., Kaiser, D., Othmer, S., & Sideroff, S. S. (2005). Effects of an EEG biofeedback protocol on a mixed substance abusing population. *The American Journal of Drug and Alcohol Abuse, 31*(3), 455–469.

Zhang, X. (2003). *Acupuncture: Review and analysis of reports on controlled clinical trials*. Geneva, Switzerland: World Health Organization.

Chapter 16
Special Applications of the Pathways Model

Abstract This chapter summarizes unique applications of the Pathways concepts. Several examples are provided, including applications of the Pathways Model in support groups, in intensive outpatient services, and in patients with lifestyle issues and patients with vague, diffuse symptoms, among others. When a group intervention is the most practical, then the Pathways principles are adapted to provide the best care. Some patients with complex psychiatric and medical comorbid chronic illnesses need more than weekly sessions, so an intensive outpatient program using the Pathways Model is detailed. Patients with medically unexplained symptoms often search for ways to cope with their daily suffering, but also the negative reactions of medical professionals to them. This chapter will also attempt to project the Pathways Model into the future, particularly to anticipate what advances people with chronic illness can expect. The use of technology, self-help programs, and better understanding of the biological basis of illness hold great promise for those who struggle every day with pain or depression. Finally, the chapter described the application of the Pathways Model for those who are biologically and psychologically healthy—"not sick"—but who desire to be fully well, mentally, emotionally, and spiritually, with suggestions for implementation.

Keywords Pathways Model · Biopsychosocial model · Group format · Intensive outpatient · Optimal performance

The Biopsychosocial Model and the Pathways Model

> "Major depression is a *mind-body-spirit* illness, characterized by emotional symptoms in addition to physical manifestations such as poor sleep, loss of appetite, and fatigue …".

This book has emphasized that chronic illnesses are complex biopsychosocial entities and therefore require a multimodal approach to care. Major depression is a *mind-body-spirit* illness, characterized by emotional symptoms in addition to physical manifestations such as poor sleep, loss of appetite, and fatigue

© Springer International Publishing AG, part of Springer Nature 2018

A. McGrady, D. Moss, *Integrative Pathways*,

https://doi.org/10.1007/978-3-319-89313-6_16

(Capuron et al., 2008). Type 2 diabetes is a *mind-body-spirit* illness, affecting the endocrine system primarily, but also disturbing mood and motivation. Most physicians agree that strictly one-dimensional medical care is not enough for these patients, nor is it cost-effective. Patients may seek out multiple specialty providers, who often do not communicate with each other, fragmenting care and increasing expenditures.

Sometimes the illness has emerged slowly after decades of personal neglect and unhealthy choices. Or, the initial insults, such as emotional or physical abuse, occurred in infancy and childhood, resulting in changes in the brain, but the patient only presents for care of migraine at 40 years of age (Tietjen, 2016). Many practices other than psychiatry are asking questions about the history of abuse, but sadly, the emotional consequences of informing the patient about the relationship between childhood traumatic events and their current pain or disability are not sufficiently recognized by some members of the medical profession. When patients are told by their physician (or come upon the information during their own website searches), they may become tearful or feel doomed to continue to suffer from earlier events where they were victims not perpetrators. Abuse during adulthood certainly has its serious effects, such as fear, anxiety, and depression, but it does not have the impact of childhood abuse where the child was helpless and was realistically unable to escape. Eliciting the information about childhood traumatic events in a cardiology, surgical, or pulmonary medicine practice can bring back memories and strong emotions that further complicate the treatment of the presenting problem.

An astute college professor patient of a local psychiatrist understood the *mind-body-spirit* connection. During a medical management session, she said to her psychiatrist: "What else can you offer me besides medicine? I am so lethargic, feel so sad; I am alone; I often feel physically ill, but I have had tests and nothing shows up. How does a pill fix these problems?" Twenty-year-old Leon, a college freshman, came to the realization that his stress load had been extreme during the early years of his life. He had had asthma since age 6 and noticed that during times when he was under family or school stress, his breathing was more labored.

Pathways Applications in a Group Setting

Leon was given the opportunity to attend a private college on a full scholarship because of his abilities in math and science. But he felt estranged from his classmates. They talked about where they came from and he felt that he had nothing in common with them. Leon worried about interacting with his roommates, and whether the differences among them would make them enemies. He was suspicious of others and began to think about leaving school.

A counselor at the school talked to Leon and his freshmen class about a personal growth program based on principles of positive psychology and the Pathways Model. The idea of structured education and skill development was appealing to Leon and he signed up for it. The first session consisted of an introduction and description of the model. In addition, the counselor requested that the participants complete the Social Readjustment Scale, which measures life events during the past year (Hobson et al., 1998). There were five freshmen in his group and they met once a week. The three girls and two boys were tentative and hesitant, speaking little, so the counselor did most of the talking, introducing the idea of support among the participants and explaining the goals of the program. One of the girls said that "support group" sounded like "we can't stand on our own two feet—can we call ourselves something else?" The counselor responded: "sure—you get to name it." By the end of the second session, the group was called "*Amazing Paths.*"

Pathways Level One mainly emphasized slow mindful breathing which Leon found calming. He was able to practice the breathing outside of the group sessions and reported back to the group that he liked being able to control his breath. He was surprised that he could do the breathing exercise despite his asthma. Level Two began with specific skill building including progressive relaxation and basic cognitive skills. Leon reported that he realized that his muscles were tense most of the time, so the concept of creating more tension in order to relax was difficult for him to grasp. Other group participants chimed in that he was creating too much tension and should tense his muscles in small increments. Leon followed this suggestion and over several weeks came to recognize that his sensations of tension had lessened and he was more relaxed. In contrast, he displayed minimal push back to the cognitive restructuring portion of the program because, as he stated: "I have had to counter criticism and negativity my whole life." "My mom tried to be positive about my future, but the main message from the rest of the family was that my goals of a college education were unrealistic." Nevertheless, there were still cognitive challenges. Leon worked on countering his suspicious thoughts about his roommate and his fear of never fitting in.

The counselor provided feedback on the life events instrument that the group members completed early in the program. She told them that all group members had scored above 400, indicating higher than average risk for physical and emotional illness. However, the group process was designed to teach specific skills to decrease the impact of previous life events. Leon and the others accepted this explanation.

Over the weeks, the group interacted more easily. Leon revealed that he was the third child of a single mother. The family received government assistance but it was difficult for his mother to keep up with what the kids needed. There was no abuse, only minimal neglect by a busy mom, but there were frequent environmental stressors. His neighborhood was dirty and the only place to play outside was a sandlot. Often, when the younger Leon went out to play, he would return seriously out of breath, asking his mother for a breathing treatment. The family moved four times during his school years, resulting in a loss of class time, so at age 20, he was older than his classmates. Leon was performing at a high level in his classes. His calculus teacher remarked that Leon was very well prepared for college math, so he asked him to help another student. Leon knew the person, "Jackson the 3rd," from a math camp that both had attended, and recalled that Jackson's father was a very successful and wealthy engineer. Jackson believed that sons of fathers such as his have "good genes" and would automatically succeed in school. Leon was too embarrassed to say anything about his father, who had left the family and never returned. Now Leon's feelings were mixed; he was proud to be able to help Jackson, but also admitted to a certain feeling of "who is top dog now?"

Pathways Level Three consisted of thermal biofeedback and heart rate variability biofeedback (HRV) using simple devices. Members of the group first tried to outdo each other in a healthy, fun competition. Then, they got serious and came into the moment to control their breathing and gain a sense of both control and peacefulness. The skill practice occurred at the beginning of each session because the counselor believed that positive energy was generated by group relaxation which made it easier for the group to engage in conversation. After one of the HRV sessions, Leon opened up to the group. He said that he had experienced more in his 20 years than most people live through in 40 years. He had already buried two guys from the old neighborhood, one from a drug overdose and another who was murdered in a gang fight. The other group members had similar stories and one of the guys said: "Our group name says it all. We are going beyond others' expectations and our past history to travel Amazing Paths."

At the end of the freshmen year, Leon felt that he had benefited greatly and wanted to have access to the counselor and to keep in contact with the other participants. He had not had an asthma attack in several months, but maintained a supply of his asthma medication. The group was encouraged to continue on its own and the Center provided a space for them. The counselor also offered psychotherapy, but Leon felt that the group interaction would suffice. He appreciated the offer and agreed to make contact if needed. Drop in services were also available at the center. Leon utilized those services once or twice during the next year to discuss his sorrow at news of the death of another boyhood friend who overdosed and died.

> "The example of Leon highlights not only the use of the Pathways Model in a group setting, but the presentation of Levels One, Two, and Three spread out over an entire academic year for individuals who had no current diagnosed psychiatric problems."

The example of Leon highlights not only the use of the Pathways Model in a group setting, but also the presentation of Levels One, Two, and Three spread out over an entire academic year for individuals who had no current diagnosed psychiatric problems. When the life events total is very high, it means that the person has used a lot of energy to cope with change and may not be able to move through the Pathways levels as quickly as someone who has more energy reserves.

It is important for the group leader to frame the results of the life events scale in a positive way, so as not to engender fear in those who score relatively high. Slow introduction of the Pathways concepts and spending ample time in each level is critical for those individuals who have possibly used many coping resources during the past year. The college student group also discussed other issues during the course of the year, problems related to interacting with professors and keeping on track for studying. All were also working part-time jobs, so time management was an important part of the goals for the group.

Pathways applications in Intensive Outpatient Programs A different type of group work can be used as an adjunct to individual therapy in the Pathways Model. Patients with multiple chronic illnesses often need intervention and a network of support to be available more frequently than weekly. Waiting weeks for an evaluation and additional weeks for treatment to begin, then sessions spaced 1 or 2 weeks apart will not serve those with several comorbid conditions. In contrast, intensive outpatient programs (IOP) consist of sessions held for at least 2 hours per day, for a minimum of 3 days per week. The group process is mobilized and the Pathways Model can be included for the benefit of participants who often suffer disruptions in daily rhythms and a lack of stress management skills, as well as medical and emotional problems. The IOP can also include physical activity for those who have clearance from their medical provider.

Shadonna, aged 52, carried multiple medical and psychiatric diagnoses. She had fibromyalgia, migraine headaches, insomnia, and major depressive disorder with occasional psychotic features and generalized anxiety disorder. She had a history of alcohol overuse, but had been sober for 10 years. One year ago, she began to smoke marijuana because she said it eased her pain from the fibromyalgia, which was sometimes severe and nearly incapacitated her. Her use of marijuana became excessive, impacting her functionality. She was employed part time as a medical assistant in a busy internal medicine practice, but her mood and most importantly her substance use had affected her work. Her employer told her that she was on leave until she could once again be the conscientious worker that she had been previously. Shadonna was devastated by this because her work gave her meaning in life. She spent her time outside of work watching television, posting to *Facebook,* and playing online games. She had been divorced for many years and her adult son had little time for her. She was currently in an abusive relationship, but believed that she couldn't get out of it because she feared being alone.

"Shadonna expressed her belief that the suggestions were too drastic and told the group that she couldn't change her eating habits, move more, and try to sleep better all at once."

Shadonna made the commitment to the IOP plan, which was 2 hours, 3 days a week for 6 weeks, and signed a contract to attend a minimum of 90% of the sessions. A comprehensive medical, psychiatric, and lifestyle evaluation was completed by all participants. All of the normal biological rhythms were disrupted in Shadonna's life as well as in most of the other group members. Therefore, the Pathways Level One components: breathe, feed, sleep, soothe, and move were introduced and explained. Shadonna expressed her opinion that the suggestions were too drastic and told the group that she couldn't change her eating habits, move more, and try to sleep better all at once. The group leader, an experienced social worker, responded that no one expected immediate change. He reminded the group that they had goals to improve function and the changes were necessary to meet those goals. They could proceed at their own pace within the 6-week framework and then continue in individual psychotherapy.

Shadonna wanted to tackle her sleep schedule first because she believed that she had developed unhealthy sleep habits since she went on leave from work. In order to improve sleep, caffeine had to be decreased from six cups a day to about three with no caffeine after 6 p.m. Sleep restriction therapy, an evidenced-based intervention (Morgenthaler et al., 2006), was initiated to limit all activities in bed except for sleep and intimacy. She followed the recommendations of sleep restriction and added mindful breathing to her pre-bedtime ritual. The length of time necessary to fall asleep was reduced to 30 minutes and sleep became more restful so her fatigue on most mornings gradually lessened. The primary Level Two intervention was *cognitive renewal*. Many of Shadonna's thought patterns were catastrophic in theme. She had developed the habit of negative thinking for many years, and it was almost as if her physical illnesses were proof that her negative beliefs were correct. Building awareness of the negative thoughts and documenting them in a journal along with her mood state at the time showed Shadonna the relationship between the two entities: cognitions and mood.

The Level Three interventions consisted of psychodynamic therapy, cognitive behavioral therapy (CBT), and biofeedback-assisted relaxation. Shadonna was a victim of serious childhood abuse; she had been molested for 3 years by a neighborhood adult. Now she was in an abusive relationship. She stated: "How could this happen? I suffered so much as a child and now I am still suffering with my boyfriend. Maybe I deserve it and I am what he says I am—a loser. Nobody else will want to be with me, so I stay with him. I think about dying and finally getting relief from this horrible life. I used to use alcohol to numb the pain and it worked for a while, until I lost a job that I loved because I showed up to work drunk. Then I was sober for 10 years, but my pain worsened so I found pot, which helped my body and emotional pain. But too much of it led to my current work problems."

Although some of the group had dropped out by the 6th session (12 hours), the remaining members had developed trust in each other and were able to process their past histories and the effects of their early experiences on current functioning. Some of the sessions became very emotional for Shadonna as she described the abuse she suffered as a child, but the support offered by the clinician and other group members was real and helped her to feel calmer and more at peace. The CBT followed her earlier exposure to cognitive renewal in Level Two. The group therapist explained *thought countering*, and the group practiced together, resulting in a growing awareness for Shadonna that she did not have to be at the mercy of her negative thoughts and their effects on her mood, her body, and her behavior. Maybe she did not have to be so hard on herself.

The type of biofeedback used with Shadonna varied between thermal biofeedback and HRV. Shadonna became very adept at warming her hands using simple relaxation tools and imagery of pleasant, warm, calming locales. She had a lovely voice, almost musical, so the provider asked her to lead the group in relaxation for one of the practice experiences. This simple event, her first experience as a leader (of anything, ever, as she put it), had an important consequence for Shadonna. She saw herself in a different light, and started to believe that she could consider escaping from the abusive relationship as well as getting back to work.

The examples of Leon and Shadonna highlight several important concepts related to the Pathways Model. First the application of the Pathways Model in a group setting shows that the model can be flexible, can be utilized with a group of late teens on a college campus, or can be implemented with patients with serious and highly complex medical and psychiatric disorders. It was noteworthy that the college counselor was challenged in the first session by criticism of the word "support," but the IOP participants welcomed the idea of mutual support from group members. The college counselor allowed the group to pick their own name, giving them a sense of control over the group process. The model was introduced slowly and requirements for home practice were minimal at first. These five college freshmen had gone through many changes in their lives and had experienced many stressors, all of which could potentially derail them from making the necessary adjustments to college life.

The IOP group presented different challenges. Most of the literature on intensive intervention reports on substance abusing clients, some who have just completed detoxification and others who are mandated by the legal system (Center for Substance Abuse Treatment, 2006; Drake, Mueser, Brunette, & McHugo, 2004). Other applications are to patients with co-occurring psychiatric and substance overuse problems (Bottlender & Soyka, 2005). In the above example, the Pathways Model is applied in an IOP format for patients with medical and psychiatric disorders. Common to all IOP programs is the requirement for attendance, goal setting, and participation. Patients may be passive outwardly and seem to accept suggestions, but resist intervention in other ways, by being late to group or by questioning homework assignments. They may want to assert themselves openly by confronting each other or the provider, refusing to do "homework," stating that the interventions do not work or they don't need to be re-taught how to breathe.

In Shadonna's group, control was offered to participants in several ways to decrease the resistance to Pathways recommendations. For example, they were given the opportunity to choose which of the Level One interventions would be the starting point. Motivational interviewing can be used to develop personal motivation for change, by eliciting change talk and proceeding to discuss the pros and cons of change (Hettema, Steele, & Miller, 2005). The more control the patient perceives in decision-making, the easier the perceived demands for change are transformed into choices for change (Duhigg, 2016). Shadonna's acceptance of the offer to lead her group in relaxation and imagery was a critical point in her recovery. After the IOP, she participated in weekly therapy for another 6 months and in monthly follow-up for 2 years. During that time, medical management of her fibromyalgia continued, but increased movement, better sleep, and daily relaxation provided the most benefit in decreasing pain. Psychopharmcological intervention for the depression was maintained, with no acute episodes of severe depression at last contact.

The Pathways Model for Patients with Lifestyle Issues

Richard was a 50-year-old Caucasian male who presented to the Pathways team "horror struck" as he described himself. He was a strategic analyst for a large health care organization. He had been a daily smoker, drank on weekends, sometimes to excess and lived a sedentary life. His body mass index was over 30 indicating obesity. He had many responsibilities at work, including presentations to groups of physicians (which he disliked doing), writing software, and formulating prediction models (which he loved). The hours were long and sometimes Richard got home at 8 p.m. and ate a hasty dinner. He got to bed at midnight and woke with difficulty at 6 a.m. A year ago, Richard was encouraged to attend a retreat for men at his church which he did reluctantly, because he believed that he was fundamentally not a religious person. To his surprise, the weekend was a very powerful experience. Richard felt as if he was waking up from a long sleep. He recommitted to his Catholic faith and more broadly a spiritual renewal.

A segment of the retreat was concerned with taking care of the body given to us by God, so Richard decided to cut back on smoking and drinking, which he succeeded in doing, finally quitting smoking and significantly reducing his drinking. He joined a Bible study group and practiced religious meditation daily. One year after the retreat Richard began to increase his activity by biking or walking briskly. Although he experienced discomfort in his chest during both of these activities, he disregarded these symptoms and told himself he was just out of shape. Fortunately he scheduled a long overdue physical with an internal medicine physician. The results were horrifying to Richard. He had pre-diabetes, high blood pressure, and an unhealthy lipid profile; besides, a stress test suggested that he might have blockage in his arteries. His breathing was also compromised and he had early signs of possible emphysema. The results of the cardiac catheterization did not indicate the need for stent placement at that time, but Richard was to be monitored every 6 months. Compounding his "horror," he was referred to the Pathways team, "the final blow" as he put it, because he scored high on a screener for anxiety and obsessive thoughts.

At the evaluation by the Pathways team, Richard expressed anger, confusion, and deep regret. He realized that years of personal neglect, destructive eating behaviors, choosing a sedentary lifestyle, and high job stress were major contributors to his current situation. Naively, he had believed that rediscovering his faith and daily prayer would give him buffers against physical illness and emotional turmoil. He certainly had felt more peaceful and more centered, and his life had more meaning after the retreat. In addition, he had changed two unhealthy behaviors, smoking and drinking. Nonetheless, damage to the body cannot always be reversed.

The construction worker, Tony, age 58, smoked, ate fatty foods, and disregarded his chest pain when it occurred. He eventually had a heart attack and was referred to cardiac rehabilitation. During rehab, he frequently stated: "I have to go back to work." When the rehab staff told patients that those who complete the program will have improved tremendously, he listened and assumed that he would be able to work at the same physical level as before. At the 10-week point (2 weeks, 6 hours remaining), Tony wanted to try to work for a couple of days on a relatively minor painting project. One weekend he contracted to paint a garage. Unfortunately, the job took him twice the time as before his heart attack and he was exhausted at the end. The devastation created by this experience was hard for the staff to watch. Tony had come to every rehab session and he had done everything he was asked to do outside of rehab. At the rehab group, he expressed his sorrow over the past and his worry about supporting his family and finding other work that he could do. Construction and manual labor were all that he knew.

Application of the Pathways Model with patients such as Richard and Tony poses major challenges. Both men were desperate but for different reasons. Richard had an occupation that required mental work, but his crisis was an emotional and religious one. Tony was angry and anxious about his inability to return to physical work. Both men were experiencing a crisis of meaning in their lives. The Pathways team must be prepared to work with patients who are grieving the loss of physical ability or deeply regretting past decisions. The desperation invades the office and the provider smells the fear emanating from the patient. If this patient consents to be evaluated by a mental health provider, the first challenge will be supporting the patient enough to keep him or her in treatment. Level One interventions may seem too simple, too slow to these patients who want resolution quickly. Admittedly, the provider can get caught up in the fear and negative energy and considers rushing into Levels Two and Three. Furthermore, some of the medical Level Three interventions such as psychopharmacology are already in place. In addition, some patients may have already had surgery, stent placement, pacemakers, or ports for better access to the vascular system.

The Pathways team and the primary therapist recognize and validate current treatment from other health care providers. They summarize the Pathways levels for the patient and explain that their medical management is Level Three, but it is necessary to begin psychological repair at Level One. Both Richard and Tony had been compromised by unhealthy lifestyles for years so bypassing the Level One modules would be seriously ill advised. The Level Two interventions, pause, relaxation, and cognitive restructuring, were beneficial in decreasing anxious over-reactions. The concept of *pause* was very new to both Richard and Tony. When Richard was at work, he responded to email immediately because a software problem demanded a fix right away. Tony was used to being the group leader at his job; difficult construction issues were brought to him and he would respond quickly. Learning and practicing *pausing* before reacting was challenging, but both slowly accepted the suggestions and found that the moment of pause actually helped them think through a response before answering; they became aware of lower physiological reactions and clearer thinking.

However, Tony persisted in his questions about returning to construction work. He asked the team—is this program going to get me back to work? To head off the possibility of his dropping out, Tony met with a social worker in the practice who explored the options with him. He applied for social security disability, was turned down the first time, and reapplied with a positive result for partial disability. A glimmer of hope then emerged from an unexpected source. Tony was also referred to a vocational rehabilitation counselor. That appointment was difficult for Tony to keep because it was an admission that he could no longer do the work that he loved, at least on a full-time basis. When the counselor met with Tony, she told him that job coaches were needed in the construction industry. Young healthy men and women began their jobs as painters and laborers after serving their apprenticeship, but were tentative and needed guidance on the job. So, Tony was offered a part-time position as a job coach. He accepted the offer, grudgingly but also gratefully. He could stay involved with construction, teach young people beginning their careers, and maybe mentor them with suggestions about lifestyle. In time, he might be able to actually do some of the work himself, if it did not demand excessive physical effort. Of course, not every "Tony" will have this opportunity; but the Pathways team must be prepared to bring in ancillary services, such as case managers, social workers, and rehabilitation counselors to help the patient improve function and restore meaning in their lives when they believe that they have lost everything.

> "The constant barrage of stress hormones affects the hippocampus (learning to react), amygdale (fear), and prefrontal cortex (executive function). The entire system "learns" to see neutral stimuli as negative, to perceive negative stimuli as catastrophic, and to leave no time for recovery."

Patients such as Richard and Tony become motivated to make lifestyle changes at some point in their lives. The impetus for change can occur because of a crisis, a diagnosis, encouragement from a family member, or through an activity such as a church retreat. By the time that the decision is made to improve eating habits, increase activity, and manage stress, the years of unhealthy living have taken a toll on the *body-mind-spirit*. Multiple physical and emotional stressors over time have often depleted adaptation energy, built up allostatic load, and caused damage to the heart, lungs, and other organs. Overload for months and years, with a background of heredity and environment, set the stage for pathophysiology and emotional illness (McEwen, 2004). The constant barrage of stress hormones affects the hippocampus (learning to react), amygdale (fear), and prefrontal cortex (executive function). The entire system "learns" to see neutral stimuli as negative, to perceive negative stimuli as catastrophic, and to leave no time for recovery. In our experience, patients grasp the concept of allostatic load (Beauchaine, Neuhaus, Zalewski, Crowell, & Potapova, 2011) as described above and are then more willing to begin treatment with Level One intervention.

The Challenge of Medically Unexplained Physical Symptoms

Patients with medically unexplained physical symptoms (MUPS) experience deteriorating health and impaired function with no name for symptoms and vague reassurances from medical doctors that the unnamed condition may resolve. Alternatively, patients may be told to seek a referral to a psychiatrist implying that the symptoms are "in the head" or not real. It is difficult to deal with uncertainty and ambiguity about one's own body. Patients experience physical malaise, the feeling that something is wrong within the body, but only receive vague reassurance that answers will be found. Grief over loss of the ability to work a full day, or to care for children in the way that the patient is used to creates emotional stress. Having no answers to questions from friends and families, such as "what do you have/is there a name for it?" compounds the patients' frustration with the medical system and eventually isolates patients from their friends.

Based on the DSM-5 (APA, 2013), these patients may be diagnosed with somatic symptom disorder, characterized by excessive concern about physical symptoms or over-reactions to bodily sensations that are not confirmed by testing. Patients often carry a diagnosis of major depression or generalized anxiety disorder, but it is not clear whether the frustration, sadness, or worry about the physical condition has exacerbated an emotional disruption that was already present or if emotional problems have intensified physical symptoms. However, in most cases, patient acceptance of a psychiatric diagnosis without confirmation of a medical condition adds to their frustration instead of decreasing uncertainty and fear. At the point of entry into Pathways-based treatment, it does not matter which came first since the physical and emotional symptoms are intertwined.

The Pathways approach can assist patients with ambiguous symptoms to re-establish normal rhythms, to acquire skills, and to work through uncertainty. First, they must learn to tolerate the state of *not knowing* instead of continuing to seek medical management and medication. Patients work to re-establish some balance in the new reality, while medical science catches up with what the patient feels to be true, that they are ill (Fennell, 2003). Support and validation of what they are experiencing is critical. In Level One, emphasis is placed on restoring normal basic physiological functioning, obtaining enough rest, movement as tolerated, soothing the self, and laying the foundation for meditation which will be taught in Level Two. Being in the moment is difficult for patients with MUPS because they fear experiencing symptoms more vividly. The Pathways team emphasizes that not every moment is saturated with pain or sad mood. They instruct patients to be in the moment nonjudgmentally. "Enjoy the moments where you are not in distress physically or mentally. Disconnect and uncouple from stress and discomfort, even for a few seconds at first, then gradually increasing the time to minutes several times a day" (Victorson et al., 2015).

The concept of ambiguous grief is a relatively new one that has been more commonly applied to those individuals who have lost a loved one in an accident that has no explanation, sudden break ups of relationships, or instances of an absent father who goes out for gasoline and never comes back (Worden, 2009). However, this concept can be effective in treating patients with MUPS. Their reactions, their frustration about their symptoms is not abnormal in itself, but in fact a type of grieving; the ambiguity comes from an unknown etiology, suffering with no diagnosis, and vagueness in predicted outcome. The Pathways Model will teach the interventions as one would to individuals overcome with grief. Journaling will be added to Pathways Level Two so that the individual can become more aware of their thoughts and feelings, observe their grief coming through on a written page, and begin to see patterns in their emotional reactions (Pennebaker & Smyth, 2016). Supportive therapy will be one of the critical components of Level Three in addition to gaining control of one or more physiological functions through biofeedback.

The Pathways Model in Patients with Sudden Onset of Illness

Rolf, a 22-year-old soccer player, haltingly relayed his story:

> I was told since 6th grade that I was going to play soccer. In high school, I was the star goalie and we won our league. There was interest in me from eight colleges. I left school after my sophomore year in college and have been playing in a professional league for 18 months. Two weeks ago, I sustained a serious injury to my knee which required surgery. The surgery was successful, but my future ability to play is uncertain. The rehab is very difficult and I am in pain. My agent, the club's trainer, referred me here because my anxiety is affecting my recovery.

During the initial evaluation of Rolf, it became clear why he was referred so soon after his surgery. Rolf's devastation at the injury had rendered him virtually incapacitated and non-functional. He became emotional during the first part of the history and continued to cry during the entire session. He stated:

> I am worth nothing. My life doesn't mean anything. I may have to face the situation that I can't play professionally any more. Who is Rolf now? I don't want to live if I can't play again. I did not finish college and while I was there, I barely made the grades necessary to maintain eligibility. There is no other future for me other than soccer. I have never cried this much in my entire life. But I truly believe that my life is over, and I don't care if big strong Rolf is crying in front of strangers.

The first step for Rolf in the Pathways Model was to gradually move away from the fixed mindset—that his natural talent was his only asset and using his talent in soccer was his only reason to live (Dweck, 2006). Yes, the natural ability was there and yes the injury ruined a career, but it cannot destroy the person unless the person allows himself to be destroyed. While always aware of the potential for self-harm, providing support in every session, the provider stayed with the Pathways Model, building the growth mindset, gently encouraging personal control. For example, the therapist focused on slow breathing and paced her breath with Rolf's, slowly decreasing rapid, anxious breathing to calm, peaceful breathing. Building skills in Level Two laid the foundation for regaining stability. Again, the provider relaxed with Rolf so that he felt her positive, calming energy. Both psychodynamic and cognitive behavioral therapy, and HRV biofeedback were the mainstays of Level Three. In the growth mindset, adversity is acknowledged, then used as a vehicle for expansion of the self, broadening of interests, creation of opportunities in a new way that the patient originally believed to be impossible (Edwards, 2008).

Initially, Rolf met with the therapist twice a week until the acute crisis had lessened, then weekly for 4 months. Assessment of suicidal thoughts occurred at every session and a plan for dealing with them when they occurred was formulated and often reviewed. Rolf healed physically to about 85% and gradually was able to accept that he cannot play as a professional again. He would have some pain and limitation of function for a long time, but more importantly, finding meaning in another occupation was a major challenge. At the 6 month point of therapy, Rolf returned to school where to his surprise he did well and found computer courses interesting. He decided to major in statistics and pursue a career in sports analytics.

Therapy continued for another year, but the crisis reaction did not recur. Fortunately, the 2 years of professional playing had allowed Rolf to save a significant amount of money so financing his education was not a problem. Rolf attributed his mental recovery to the Pathways Model, stating at the last session: "I hope I am never as terrified and frantic as I was after the injury. Thank you for bringing me out of that abyss and helping me find meaning in my life again."

The Patient with Overwhelming Fear

Another example of the fixed mindset is the patient who is consumed by fear and cannot think of change without experiencing anxiety or near panic. A true panic attack would be an unusual or extreme reaction to change, but the impact of fear and fearful thoughts in persons with chronic illness must always be considered. It is recommended to take a fear history during the initial evaluation. Many patients who present with a chronic anxiety disorder were shy and fearful as children. They inherited a tendency to be fearful from parents, then, the environment factored in, particularly if their childhood was stressful. When parents are authoritarian in their discipline or abusive, the child learns to fear punishment or even the disapproving look or sneer. Some adults with anxiety disorders report that as children, they had to anticipate two or three steps beyond the moment to avoid being smacked or punched by their parent. The sound of Dad's car going into the garage or his footsteps led to the 10-year-old questioning how Dad would act when he comes into the home. "Do I run to my room and hide or can I stay out in the family room and finish watching my TV show?" These patients are rarely in the moment, continuing to try to anticipate the future based on past experience.

A 25-year-old woman, married for 2 years, described how fear controlled her life. She heard her husband's car coming into the garage and his footsteps and went into vigilance mode, just like she did when she was a child. Her husband had never hit or threatened her but of course they had disagreements. When she was tired or they had argued, she mobilized physically, emotionally, and mentally as if preparing for disaster. When her boss did not praise her work, she believed that she would be fired. When she saw a police officer entering the shop where she stopped for lunch, she assumed that he was suspicious of her.

Stimuli or situations experienced as threatening activate the survival portion of the brain and the autonomic nervous system. The next time the same stressor is presented, the *mind-body-spirit* responds with a survival response again because it is primed for that stimulus. Instead, if the stress is conceptualized as a challenge, the second experience with that stressor will activate the challenge parts of the brain, with positive energy instead of negative energy. These patients will benefit most from the Level Two intervention, mindfulness, with basic skills taught in Level Two and mindfulness mediation with acceptance and commitment therapy used in Level Three.

The Pathways Model in the Returning Patient

Laurie, a 50-year-old married woman with three children and a demanding job as an accountant, told the team:

> Unfortunately, I didn't realize what was happening. Our family has had so much going during the past three months, and besides that, my boss gave me a huge project for my company. I had no time for exercise, our food choices became unhealthy because they had to be quick, and I fell asleep at night exhausted and without doing the relaxation exercises that you taught me. My blood pressure is up and I can't sleep because I am so anxious. My mood is getting worse and I feel stuck. But, she smiled ruefully, I got the best evaluation ever from my boss. My doctor wants to increase my antihypertensive and medicate my mood but I came back to you instead. 'Do I have to start the Pathways plan from the beginning?'

Patients returning to Pathways after months or years of stability should be evaluated similarly to a new client, with one major difference. The team first assesses what has led to the return of symptoms, such as an addition to the family, illness in a close friend, marital stress, or changes at the workplace. The team should obtain old records and evaluate what has been helpful in the first treatment, then assess what the patient has continued to utilize and what has been neglected. A brief review of Level One intervention can be offered if the biological and emotional normal rhythms have been compromised again. Skills in Level Two are refreshed if they were taught previously or added to the skill set if they were not used the first time. Similarly, the patient in a new stage of life with different challenges may require additional Level Three interventions compared to the one or two utilized in the past. For example, the 30-year-old Laurie had a history of conflict with birth parents and did well with psychodynamic therapy; she resolved her anger at her mother for ignoring and neglecting her. She forgave her father for never praising her for excellent grades or being a sports star. Laurie returned at 50. Both parents were now deceased but she had developed a pattern of negative thinking about her own performance at work and the success of her marriage. She had developed several unhealthy lifestyle habits. At this time, she was a more appropriate candidate for cognitive behavioral therapy.

The length of treatment for returning patients is variable, depending on the severity of the relapse or the new illness, the patient's motivation, and the commitment to returning to health. The primary therapist told Laurie that he was glad that she returned, that the assessment and review of her previous work with Pathways would help in setting goals and designing the intervention. She would not have to redo anything unless it would be helpful for the current condition. Her blood pressure and mood would be monitored by staff and she would also measure blood pressure and log mood herself. If there was a dangerous rise in blood pressure, her physician would be contacted.

The Pathways Model in Patients Requiring Repeated Hospitalizations

Some patients with chronic illness suffer with acute exacerbations and require repeated hospitalizations for short-term worsening of the illness. These patients attempt to live in two different worlds, the world of the sick, which comprises the hospital, nurses and doctors, and the world of the well. The onset of illness shifts the person into the world of the sick, and they often feel like they are in a foreign country where they don't know the language, the social ways, or the expectations (Edwards, 2008). Because the person is so ill that they required hospitalization, they make the transition, becoming passive and accepting of care.

"Surprisingly, the re-entry into the normal world after a hospital stay is more difficult than assuming the role of the sick ...".

Surprisingly, the re-entry into the normal world after a hospital stay is typically more difficult than assuming the role of the sick (Edwards, 2014). Kristy, a 22-year-old graduate student with uncontrolled Type 1 diabetes, stated:

I feel like I am an alien when I return to school; I have enough support from tutors through the Students with Disability Center and my friends take my absences and returns without much comment. This is on me. I feel like the pace is way too fast. I have missed the latest gossip. Part of me resents the healthy; the other part believes that being with the healthy is in itself therapeutic.

The provider spoke as follows: "Sometimes Kristy is part of the kingdom of the sick and then attempts to transition to the normal life of the kingdom of the well and it is very difficult emotionally as well as physically" (Edwards, 2014).

The Pathways team welcomed Kristy into treatment and first provided support for her transition. The Level One strategies are particularly important to patients after hospitalization since their sleep and eating schedules have been disrupted and their movement restricted. Kristy needed to center herself in the world of the well, relying on her internal healing energy to resume normal activities. A useful approach to re-grounding is to use a values wheel to determine how much energy is devoted to the domains of life, for example: family, work, faith, and adding illness as a domain (https://www.mindtools.com/pages/article/newHTE_93.htm).

Frequently, when the primary provider goes over the wheel with clients, such as Kristy, it is obvious that she is devoting almost all her energy to illness and other aspects of her life are neglected. Pathways Level Two cognitive renewal addresses the allocation of energy and how decisions are made to attend to illness or to work, home life, and friends. The client is reminded that the illness is one spoke of the wheel, not every spoke or the entire wheel. Kristy's life had been controlled by diabetes since age 7. At one point, she was measuring her blood glucose eight times a day and still worrying about the values. As she worried more and became more anxious, the blood glucose levels were elevated, causing more anxiety and worry.

Kristy's hospitalizations for ketoacidosis furthered her anxiety and sense of hopelessness about the future.

The provider must find a way to create success for Kristy to move her into the kingdom of hope. Skill building with relaxation and imagery in Level Two builds self-confidence, which is manifested in less anxiety and some mental calming. During Level Two, the primary pathways provider brought in a diabetes educator to co-facilitate the skills sessions. The experienced educator who herself had had diabetes since age 3 was an excellent addition to the team, very knowledgeable, empathetic, and committed to helping Kristy achieve glycemic control. Pathways Level Three consisted mostly of cognitive behavioral therapy and biofeedback. One year later, Kristy had had only one additional hospital stay; she transitioned much more easily to the world of the well because she had come to see diabetes as part of her but not all of her. Her values wheel showed a much more balanced life. She would have Type 1 diabetes the rest of her life since at this time, there is no cure, but the emotional toll of the illness was sharply reduced and Kristy was able to thrive in the kingdom of the well.

Pathways to Wellness in Chronic Illness

Wellness, a state characterized by good quality of life, solid relationships, and emotional and spiritual health, is more than just not being sick. Patients experience themselves as well when their diabetes is controlled with lifestyle and medication, when blood pressure does not increase dramatically after stressful stimuli or when the patient with bipolar disorder maintains stable mood without cycling. The person does not identify themselves as ill, nor does it dominate their every moment; their values wheel supports what they believe to be important in life. They are not focused on merely surviving or being safe, but seek to function at Maslow's highest level, self-actualization (Taormina & Gao, 2013). Motivational interviewing is applied in a new way in chronic illness. Instead of identifying problems and reasons to change, it is used to find areas of potential growth so that time can be allocated to meaningful activities.

Patients with chronic illness often feel that the illness has robbed them of their health, but also of their ability to contribute to society. Activities that they engaged in before they became sick are no longer on the priority list. Slowly the person disengages from more and more of the normal work and becomes isolated in pain and sickness. The topic of wellness for these patients is often not even considered by patients or their doctors. Patients are absorbed in regretting the past and their loss of health or a fear of the future, instead of living in real time (Strosahl & Robinson, 2015).

Fortunately, achieving a higher level of wellness is possible for those with chronic illness and building resiliency is one of the tools appropriate for this challenge. The resiliency literature more commonly focuses on performance in sport, dealing with extreme stressors, or reducing burnout in medical practitioners (Epstein & Krasner, 2013). Resiliency has three components: insight (awareness of strengths, weaknesses, and risk factors for burnout), self-care (relaxation, healthy lifestyle), and values (meaningfulness). The Pathways Model allows for an integration of resiliency research into the three levels of intervention. Resiliency is defined as moving through the adversity of setbacks of a chronic illness. This can take many forms: having another surgery when it is necessary; returning to psychotherapy because of a new emotional challenge; taking a leave from a job to spend more time in self-care; realizing that rest is not sufficient; accepting that that activity needs to increase more slowly; and confronting situations that are draining energy. Pathways uses positive psychology, i.e., the patients' personality traits and strengths to mobilize psychological forces to aid the patient in building resiliency (Hassett & Finan, 2016). The adverse circumstances are acknowledged and then used as vehicles for personal growth. The patients' movement through adversity in their illness has meaning; it builds emotional, cognitive, and spiritual strength (Kaufman & Gregoire, 2015; Shostak & Whitehouse, 1999). The primary provider discusses aspirational health: what the patient desires and seeks in terms of health. The patient learns to manage physical, mental, and emotional energy; selected activities are undertaken at the 100% energy level.

Full engagement is described as invigorated, confident, challenged, joyful, and connected. However, energy use must be balanced with energy renewal. Rest and relaxation are as much a part of successful performance in an activity as the engagement itself (Greitens, 2015; Loehr & Schwartz, 2003). Recovery must include: (1) physical recovery after strenuous physical activity or workouts, (2) emotional recovery after a draining day with young children or caregiving for an elderly parent, (3) cognitive recovery after writing a term paper or learning a complex subject; (4) spiritual recovery after a faith crisis, and (5) social recovery, for example, times of solitude after heavy social obligations. A chronic illness may test all of these domains and therefore the patient in Pathways is advised to rest in each of these dimensions. The concept of physical rest is quite easily understandable, but the recommendation to rest the emotions, the mind, and the spirit requires education, practice, and feedback from the primary provider. The domains of engagement are also known to overlap. An interesting example has been described of relaxation after a high intensity workout. The body is very fatigued after physical activity, but the mind is energized by the stimulation. A period of physical rest and relaxation can bring about a creative burst, a mental leap into a new area of thinking. Disruption of routine or change in a familiar pattern (looking at a problem with fresh eyes) can also benefit creativity (Benson, 2015; Benson & Proctor, 2010; Kaufman & Gregoire, 2015). In summary, chronic illnesses cannot be excised, eradicated, blocked, or genetically re-engineered, but the patient can live a good, meaningful self-actualized life.

Pathways to Wellness in Individuals Without Illness

Janice came to the Pathways team with neither a medical nor a psychiatric diagnosis, so she was not sick, but she certainly was not well. She was the 45-year-old mother of a drug-addicted son, Jeff, from her first marriage. She was currently married to a man whom she knew loved her very much; he was the father of her two teen-aged children. Janice's worry about Jeff was threatening to destroy her second marriage. Janice believed that her son would die as a result of his addiction. She had been supportive, shown tough love, and driven Jeff to appointments when he lost his driver's license. She recalled a recent obituary from the local newspaper, written by a mother mourning her 25-year-old daughter. Janice commented:

> I know I did everything that I could for him, but nothing could overcome the addiction. I am blessed with good health but I am wracked with worry. I am starting to take less good care of myself. My husband is losing patience and I don't blame him. Jeff has stolen from us, so we don't want him in the house or around our teens. But all I can think about is when I am going to get the phone call that my son is dead.

Janice had no psychiatric diagnosis at the time of entry into Pathways, but definitely needed help in coping with the severe stress of dealing with her drug-addicted son. The Pathways Level One interventions—breathe and feed—helped her regain her internal focus.

> I have been so tense that I forgot how to breathe, and forget about eating; I cook for the family but the food sticks in my throat.

Mindful breathing was introduced and practiced with the psychologist, but Janice had great difficulty in concentrating on her breath. Finding an app on her phone was helpful to Janice in maintaining her focus. She very slowly began to feel some control over her breath. She was instructed to breathe slowly and not rush while she was making dinner for the family, then to shift her focus to the food. Eating mindfully was also difficult, but Janice was committed to the program. She found that mindful eating was actually easier for breakfast, when she ate alone and her "worry machine was not yet in top gear."

Level Two emphasized mindfulness and exercise. Being in the moment during physical activity was very helpful in resting the mind and working the body nearly to exhaustion, so that sleep was easier at night. Level Three emphasized mindfulness meditation, particularly the nonjudgmental nature of attending to the moment. This skill slowed Janice's racing thoughts and her tendency to rethink her decisions regarding her son (Levitin, 2014). Psychodynamic therapy was also used in Level Three to address her conflicts about making tough choices with her son and the constant emotional drain of waiting for the phone call.

Six months after the beginning of therapy, Janice received the phone call that she dreaded and expected. Her son had overdosed and was barely alive; she was instructed to come to the hospital immediately. Jeff died 2 days later without regaining consciousness. For the next 2 months, Janice mourned acutely; she was entitled to 1 week bereavement leave from her job and took additional weeks without pay. She spent most of her days practicing mindfulness, walking along the beach by their home, reading favorite books, and praying. She came to therapy twice a week and consulted her church pastor. Gradually, she came to terms with her grief. She finally said:

> I did everything that I could for Jeff. It is not my fault that he got into drugs and that he died from them. If I let this ruin my health or my marriage, it does not bring Jeff back; it continues the tragedy.

This example is not what typically comes to mind when we think about wellness in the Pathways Model. But the Pathways team must be prepared to work with clients such as Janice, who are not ill in the traditional sense but are torn apart by awful things happening to their loved ones. Janice needed both healing strategies and permission to resume living.

The Future

Telemedicine Many patients with chronic pain find travel to the clinic for weekly or bimonthly sessions to be very difficult. If these patients also reside a distance from the clinic or transportation is tenuous, fidelity to appointments is even more problematic. Individuals suffering from severe social anxiety disorder may not be able to leave their homes to come in for appointments. Traveling and then sitting in a crowded waiting room is impossible in the severest periods of illness so many give up and discontinue treatment when they need it the most. Patients can be "fired" by their providers because of missed appointments. Pain management through tele-health solves some of these problems in providing care, assuming that the intervention can be adapted to the electronic medium (Bender, Radhakrishnan, Diorio, Englesakis, & Jadad, 2011; Lorig, Ritter, Luarent, & Plant, 2006; McGeary, McGeary, & Gatchel, 2012). Online modules, with worksheets that the patient completes and deposits in a "drop box," are constructed similarly to online academic classes. The provider, just like the professor, still interacts with the patients in real time, using *FaceTime, GotoMeeting, Zoom, Skype,* or similar technology.

In recent years, controlled trials of telemedicine and telepsychiatry have been reported in the clinical literature. Relevant to the Pathways Model are the applications of internet-based interventions to chronic pain, sleep disorders, and mood disturbances. It is well known that sleep problems accompany many physical and psychiatric disorders and are one component of several psychiatric diagnoses (APA, 2013). In addition, short sleep, disrupted nights with multiple awakenings and sometimes nightmares, increases severity of the same disorders. Ho et al. (2014) performed a meta-analysis of self-help programs with internet components for patients with disrupted sleep. Patients responded well and achieved significant improvements in sleep efficiency, a shorter time to get to sleep, and fewer awakenings.

Psychiatrists, psychologists, counselors, and others in the mental health field rely heavily on direct observation of the patient in their evaluation by interview and the mental status exam. Appearance, tone of voice, posture, and behavior are important components of the evaluation. It will be critical in the expansion of telepsychiatry that these observations be possible. Seeing the patient's face on the computer screen is not sufficient. Instead, the provider must see the patient walking into the room, sitting down at the computer, and interacting throughout the session. Beyond the initial evaluation, the experienced mental health provider needs to be able to capture subtle changes over time in the patient's mood. This means that accurate voice transmission and viewing the whole patient is critical throughout the therapeutic process.

When patients are being followed for a disorder that tends to recur, the provider still must see the whole patient and hear the patient clearly in order to prevent relapse.

Ruehlman, Karoly, and Enders (2011) tested the effects of an online totally self-directed program in 162 individuals with chronic pain and compared their results with 143 in a wait list control group. The program comprised modules devoted to learning about pain, changing negative thinking, increasing physical activity, acquiring relaxation skills, and interacting more positively with others. Patients in both groups underwent a comprehensive assessment prior to and after the intervention (or control periods). Those in the intervention group sustained significant improvements in four pain factors: severity, interference, pain induced fear, and perceived disability. Depression and anxiety were also decreased at the completion of the program. Although these results are very encouraging, the authors acknowledge that not every patient with chronic pain will be a good candidate for this type of intervention. Some may not be at a sufficient reading level, may not be able to understand instructions, or may be too ill emotionally to motivate enough to complete the learning modules.

For psychophysiology interventions, a monitoring device is necessary but there are ways to achieve this during telemedicine appointments. Patients can access a small biofeedback device to measure breathing rate, heart rate, HRV, and finger temperature. Data can be relayed to the provider via internet connections and reviewed by the provider. Similarly to the description for psychotherapy, seeing the patient practicing slow breathing, relaxing, or visualizing is important for the provider to reinforce desired responses. Phone apps can be used to capture data and transmit the information via the internet to the clinic. Kristjánsdóttir et al. (2013) tested the use of a Smartphone-based intervention in women with chronic pain. These patients were released from an inpatient chronic pain rehabilitation program and entered the 4-week Smartphone-based trial. The results were promising for the intervention group who sustained improvements in function and symptoms and also reduced catastrophic thinking.

Progress in understanding the mechanisms of *mind-body-spirit* **illnesses** Significant progress in understanding the concept of *mind-body-spirit* illnesses is anticipated, through advances in genetics, neuroscience, psychophysiology, and psychiatry (Ferris, Williams, & Shen, 2007; Kramer & Erickson, 2007). As genetic markers are identified for medical and mental illnesses, the overlap between these domains will be more striking. Shared risk among depression, anxiety, and panic disorder occurs with post-traumatic stress disorder, paving the way for understanding the probability of a victim of trauma developing PTSD (Pittman et al., 2012). Better prediction models will allow providers to refine treatment plans so that patients do not have to endure so many trials of medications to find the best outcome, or in some cases physicians will be able to forego medicines entirely when psychotherapy has a better chance to help the patient (Harley, Luty, Carter, Mulder, & Joyce, 2010). Further, neuroscience research will define the biochemical basis of the non-pharmacological interventions, which will provide greater credibility on the part of practitioners and patients (Buric, Farias, Jong, Mee, & Brazil, 2017; Levitin, 2014; Tang & Leve, 2016).

New concepts of stress Concepts of stress have evolved over years and decades, to the present time and will continue to evolve in the future. Walter B. Cannon defined the very basic flight, fight, and freeze responses to be the only ways that animals responded to stress. Hans Selye focused on a nonspecific physical neural and endocrine response to stress. Claude Bernard studied homeostasis—the constancy of the internal environment. More recently, Bruce McEwen defined allostasis, the constantly changing environment and allostatic load, the buildup of physiological toll and repeated attempts at coping, which may at times overwhelm the system. A newer view is that stress provides the challenges that make life exciting and help the individual grow. It is well known that boredom or unchanging routine can be as stressful as a heavy workload or constant risk. The former leads to cognitive sluggishness and eventual loss of interest and physical fatigue. Risk takers are those who seek out challenges, sometimes to the extreme and to their own detriment. McGonigal (2015) puts a different perspective on stress. It is good for us if we can get good at it. The author recommends looking forward, anticipating the next day's potential stressors, and labeling them challenges and excitement. The individual is encouraged to create a good day, being proactive through anticipatory coping (Webb, 2016). Patients with chronic illness frequently anticipate the next day with dread, fearing pain, or dysfunction. Instead of fear and dread, the patient is encouraged to consider multiple options for the day so that success is prescribed, no matter what the pain or disability level.

The Pathways Model is not in conflict with any of these emerging trends; coping with stress is the foundation, then building resiliency, then going beyond and embracing life experiences, and at the highest levels pursuing self-actualization and transcendence. The Pathways *mind-body-spirit* approach culminates in assisting human beings with chronic illness, even those with terminal illness, to achieve their highest possible physical, emotional, and spiritual well-being.

Conclusion

In summary, this chapter provides examples to showcase the flexibility of the Pathways Model. The examples include intensive outpatient therapy, group sessions, patients who are frequently hospitalized, and patients who return after years of recovery to re-engage with the team. People come to the Pathways team with many different types of physical and emotional illness; others have no diagnoses, but are clearly in distress. In the future, the model can be modified to accommodate technology and treatment of patients via internet connections. A clearer and deeper understanding of the biology of mental illness and the emotional components of physical illness will only enhance the model. In addition, psychophysiological interventions will have a significantly greater impact on disorders that are currently believed to be primarily physical in nature. Prevention of illness in patients with histories of trauma will be more successful as the risk factors are identified and patients educated and treated efficiently. Better approaches to counseling patients about heritable disorders will be developed to arm patients with facts without creating anxiety and fear. Prevention can also be achieved by building avenues for individuals to maintain a healthy lifestyle. This is expected to be a slow process as it requires changes in families and neighborhoods and a dedication of society to improved health.

References

American Psychiatric Association. (2013). *Diagnostic and statistical manual of mental disorders* (5th ed.). Arlington, VA: American Psychiatric Publishing.

Bender, J. L., Radhakrishnan, A., Diorio, C., Englesakis, M., & Jadad, A. R. (2011). Pain. Can pain be managed through the internet? A systematic review of randomized controlled trials. *Pain, 152*(8), 1740–1750.

Benson, H., & Proctor, W. (2010). *Relaxation revolution: The science and genetics of mind body healing*. New York, NY: Simon and Schuster.

Benson, H. (2015). *Mind-body effect: How to counteract the harmful effects of stress*. New York, NY: Simon and Schuster.

Beauchaine, T., Neuhaus, E., Zalewski, M., Crowell, S., & Potapova, N. (2011). The effects of allostatic load on neural systems subserving motivation, mood regulation, and social affiliation. *Development and Psychopathology, 23*, 975–999. https://doi.org/10.1017/S0954579411000459

Buric, I., Farias, M., Jong, J., Mee, C., & Brazil, A. I. (2017). What is the molecular signature of mind-body interventions? A systematic review of gene expression changes induced by meditation and related practices. *Frontiers in Immunology, 8*, 670. https://doi.org/10.3389/fimmu.2017.00670

Capuron, L., Su, S., Miller, A., Bremner, D., Goldberg, J., Vogt, G., et al. (2008). Depressive symptoms and metabolic syndrome: Is inflammation the underlying link? Biological Psychiatry, 64(10), 896–900. doi:https://doi.org/10.1016/j.biopsych.2008.05.019.

Center for Substance Abuse Treatment (2006). *Substance abuse: Clinical issues in intensive outpatient treatment*. Treatment Improvement Protocol (TIP) Series 47. DHHS Publication No. (SMA) 06–4182. Rockville, MD: Substance Abuse and Mental Health Services Administration.

Duhigg, C. (2016). *Smarter faster better*. New York: Random House.

Drake, R. E., Mueser, K. T., Brunette, M. F., & McHugo, G. J. (2004). A review of treatments for people with severe mental illnesses and co-occurring substance use disorders. *Psychiatric Rehabilitation Journal, 27*(4), 360–374.

Dweck, C. S. (2006). *Mindset: The new psychology of success*. New York, NY: Random House.

Edwards, L. (2008). *Life disrupted*. New York, NY: Walker and Company.

Edwards, L. (2014). *In the kingdom of the sick: A social history of chronic illness in America*. New York, NY: Bloomsbury.

Bottlender, M., & Soyka, M. (2005). Efficacy of an intensive outpatient rehabilitation program in alcoholism: Predictors of outcome six months after treatment. *European Addiction Research, 11*(3), 132–137. https://doi.org/10.1159/000085548

Epstein, R. M., & Krasner, M. S. (2013). Physician resilience: What it means, why it matters, and how to promote it. *Academic Medicine, 88*(3), 301–303. https://doi.org/10.1097/ACM.0b013e318280cff0

Fennell, P. A. (2003). *Managing chronic illness*. Hoboken, NJ: Wiley.

Ferris, L. T., Williams, J. S., & Shen, C. L. (2007). The effect of acute exercise on serum brain-derived neuotophic factor levels and cognitive function. *Medicine and Science in Sports and Exercise, 39*(4), 728–734.

Greitens, E. (2015). *Resilience: Hard-won wisdom for living a better life.* Boston, MA: Houghton Mifflin Harcourt.

Harley, J., Luty, S., Carter, J., Mulder, R., & Joyce, P. (2010). Elevated C-reactive protein in depression: A predictor of good long-term outcome with antidepressants and poor outcome with psychotherapy. *Journal of Psychopharmacology, 24*(4), 625–626. https://doi.org/10.1177/0269881109102770

Hassett, A. L., & Finan, P. H. (2016). The role of resilience in the clinical management of chronic pain. *Current Pain and Headache Reports, 20*(39), 1–9.

Hettema, J., Steele, J., & Miller, W. R. (2005). Motivational interviewing. *Annual Review of Clinical Psychology, 1,* 91–111.

Ho, F., Chung, K., Yeung, W., Ng, T., Kwan, K., Yung, K., et al. (2014). Self- help cognitive-behavioral therapy for insomnia: A meta-analysis of randomized controlled trials. Sleep Medicine Reviews, 19, 17–28.

Hobson, C. J., Kamen, J., Szostek, J., Nethercut, C. M., Tiedman, J. W., & Wojnarowicz, S. (1998). Stressful life events: A revision and update of the Social Readjustment Rating Scale. *International Journal of Stress Management, 5*(1), 1–23. https://doi.org/10.1023/A:1022978019315

Kaufman, S. B., & Gregoire, C. (2015). *Wired to create.* New York, NY: Penguin Publishing Group.

Kramer, A. F., & Erickson, K. I. (2007). Capitalizing on cortical plasticity: Influence of physical activity on cognition and brain function. *Trends in Cognitive Science, 11*(8), 342–348.

Kristjánsdóttir, Ó. B, Fors, E. A, Eide, E., Finset, A., Stensrud, T.L., van Dulmen, S., et al. (2013). A smartphone-based intervention with diaries and therapist-feedback to reduce catastrophizing and increase functioning in women with chronic widespread pain: Randomized controlled trial. Journal of Medical Internet Research, 15(1), e5. doi: https://doi.org/10.2196/jmir.2249.

Levitin, D. J. (2014). *The organized mind: Thinking straight in the age of information overload.* New York, NY: Penguin Random House.

Loehr, J., & Schwartz, T. (2003). *The power of full engagement.* New York, NY: The Free Press.

Lorig, K., Ritter, P., Luarent, D., & Plant, K. (2006). Internet-based chronic disease self-management: A randomized trial. *Medical Care, 44*(11), 964–971.

McEwen, B. (2004). Protection and damage from acute and chronic stress: Allostasis and allostatic overload and relevance to the pathophysiology of psychiatric disorders. *Annals of the New York Academy of Sciences, 1032,* 1–7.

McGeary, D., McGeary, C., & Gatchel, R. (2012). A comprehensive review of telehealth for pain management: Where we are and the way ahead. *Pain Practice, 12*(7), 570–577.

McGonigal, K. (2015). *The upside of stress.* New York, NY: Avery.

Mind Tools (n.d.) *The wheel of life: Finding balance in your life.* Retrieved from https://www.mindtools.com/pages/article/newHTE_93.htm

Morgenthaler, T., Kramer, M., Alessi, C., Friedman, L., Boehlecke, B., Brown, T., et al. (2006). Practice parameters for psychological and behavioral treatment of insomnia: An update. An American Academy of Sleep Medicine Report. *Sleep, 29*(11), 1415–1419.

Pennebaker, J., & Smyth, J. (2016). *Opening up by writing it down: How expressive writing improves health and eases emotional pain.* New York, NY: Guilford Press.

Pittman, R., Rasmusson, A., Koenen, K., Shin, L., Orr, S., Gilbertson, M., et al. (2012). Biological studies of post-traumatic stress disorder. *Nature Reviews. Neuroscience, 13*(11), 769–787.

Ruehlman, L. S., Karoly, P., & Enders, C. (2011). A randomized controlled evaluation of an online chronic pain self-management program. *Pain, 153*(2), 319–330.

Strosahl, K. D., & Robinson, P. J. (2015). *In this moment. Five steps to transcending stress using mindfulness and neuroscience.* Oakland, CA: New Harbinger.

Shostak, D., & Whitehouse, P. (1999). Diseases of meaning, manifestations of health, and metaphor. *The Journal of Alternative and Complementary Medicine, 5*(6), 495–502.

Tang, Y., & Leve, L. (2016). A translational neuroscience perspective on mindfulness meditation as a prevention strategy. *Translational Behavioral Medicine, 6*(1), 63–72.

Taormina, R. J., & Gao, J. H. (2013). Maslow and the motivational hierarchy: Measuring satisfaction of the needs. *The American Journal of Psychology, 126*(2), 155–177.

Tietjen, G. (2016). Childhood maltreatment and headache disorders. *Current Pain and Headache Reports, 20*(4), 26. https://doi.org/10.1007/s11916-016-0554-z

Victorson, D., Kentor, M., Maletich, C., Lawton, R., Kaufman, V. H., Borrero, M., et al. (2015). Mindfulness meditation to promote wellness and manage chronic disease: A systematic review and meta-analysis of mindfulness-based randomized controlled trial. *American Journal of Lifestyle Medicine, 9*(3), 185–211.

Webb, C. (2016). *How to have a good day. Harness the power of behavioral science to transform your waking life*. New York: Crown Business.

Worden, W. J. (2009). *Grief counseling and grief therapy: A handbook for the mental health practitioner* (4th ed.). New York, NY: Springer.

Index

© Springer International Publishing AG, part of Springer Nature 2018
A. McGrady, D. Moss, *Integrative Pathways*,
https://doi.org/10.1007/978-3-319-89313-6

CPSIA information can be obtained
at www.ICGtesting.com
Printed in the USA
LVHW021721230521
688265LV00002B/148